THE
THYROID30
COOKBOOK

Quarto.com

First Published in 2026 by Fair Winds Press, an imprint of The Quarto Group,
100 Cummings Center, Suite 265-D, Beverly, MA 01915, USA.
T (978) 282-9590 F (978) 283-2742

Thyroid30® is a registered trademark of MAHAR CREATIVE, LLC. All rights reserved.

EEA Representation, WTS Tax d.o.o.,
Žanova ulica 3, 4000 Kranj, Slovenia.
www.wts-tax.si

Fair Winds Press titles are also available at discount for retail, wholesale, promotional, and bulk purchase. For details, contact the Special Sales Manager by email at specialsales@quarto.com or by mail at The Quarto Group, Attn: Special Sales Manager, 100 Cummings Center, Suite 265-D, Beverly, MA 01915, USA.

30 29 28 27 26   1 2 3 4 5

ISBN: 978-0-7603-9814-2

Digital edition published in 2026
eISBN: 978-0-7603-9815-9

Library of Congress Cataloging-in-Publication Data available

Design and Page Layout: Samantha J. Bednarek, samanthabednarek.com
Photography: Mahar Creative, LLC, except Stella Throop on pages 6, 10, 19, 20, 30, 35, 45, 49, 62, 70, 74, and 82

Printed in Guangdong, China TT102025

The information in this book is for educational purposes only. It is not intended to replace the advice of a physician or medical practitioner. Please see your health care provider before beginning any new health program.

THE
THYROID30
COOKBOOK

Three 30-Day Meal Plans and 100 Delicious Recipes to Restore Your Energy and Help You Thrive

GINNY MAHAR
FMCHC, CREATOR OF HYPOTHYROID CHEF

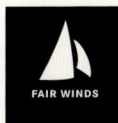

FAIR WINDS

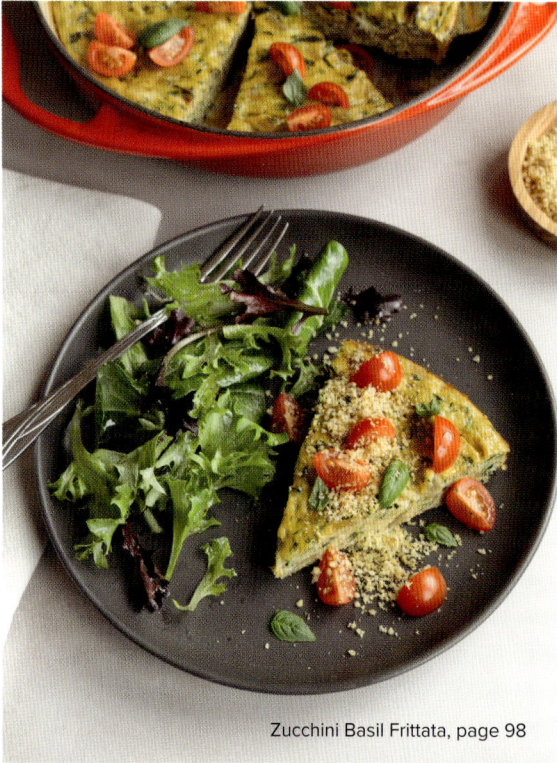
Zucchini Basil Frittata, page 98

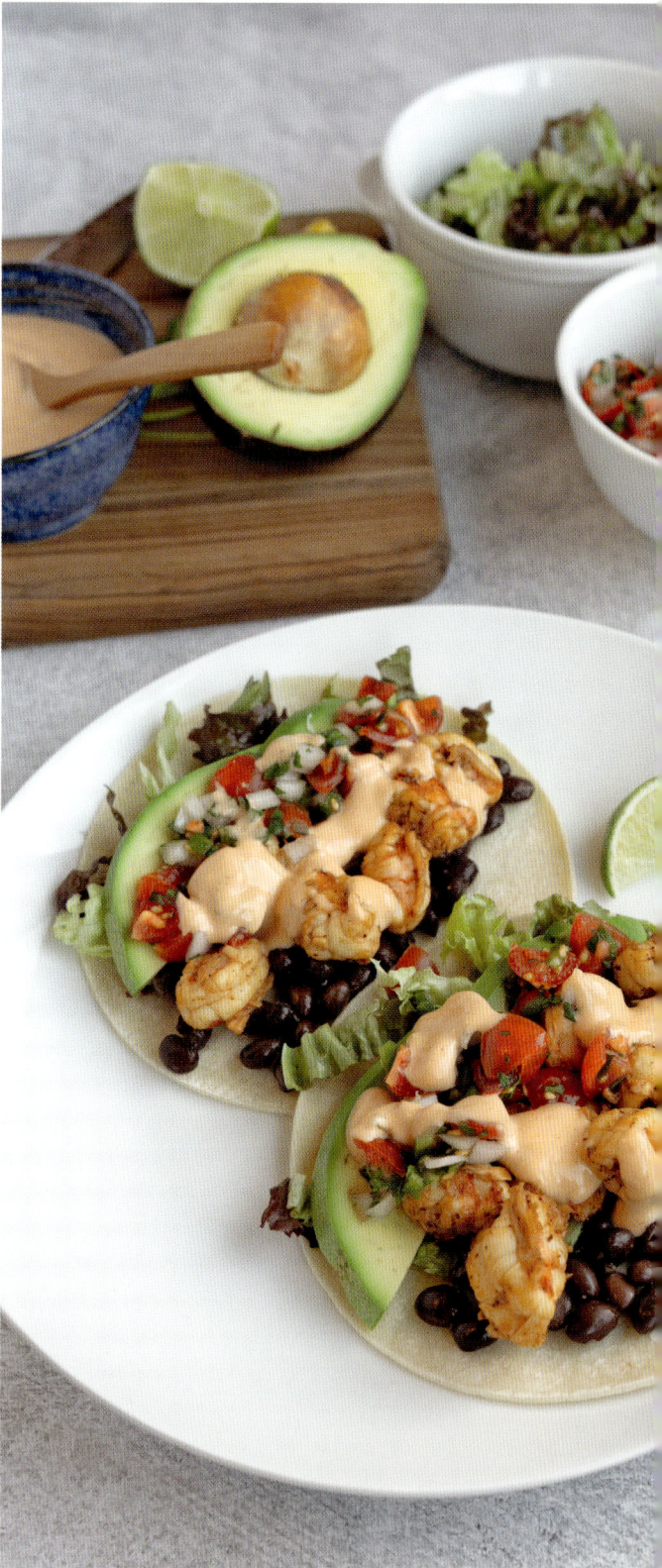

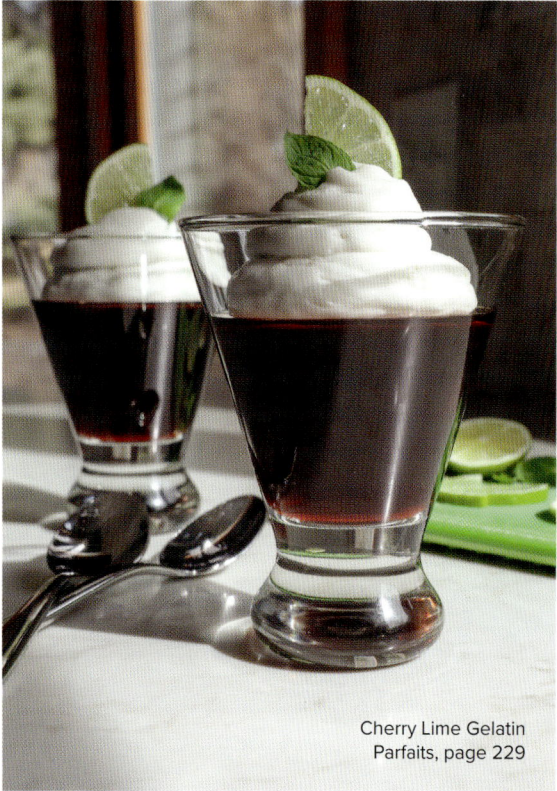
Cherry Lime Gelatin
Parfaits, page 229

CONTENTS

Chile Lime Shrimp
(or Fish) Tacos, page 182

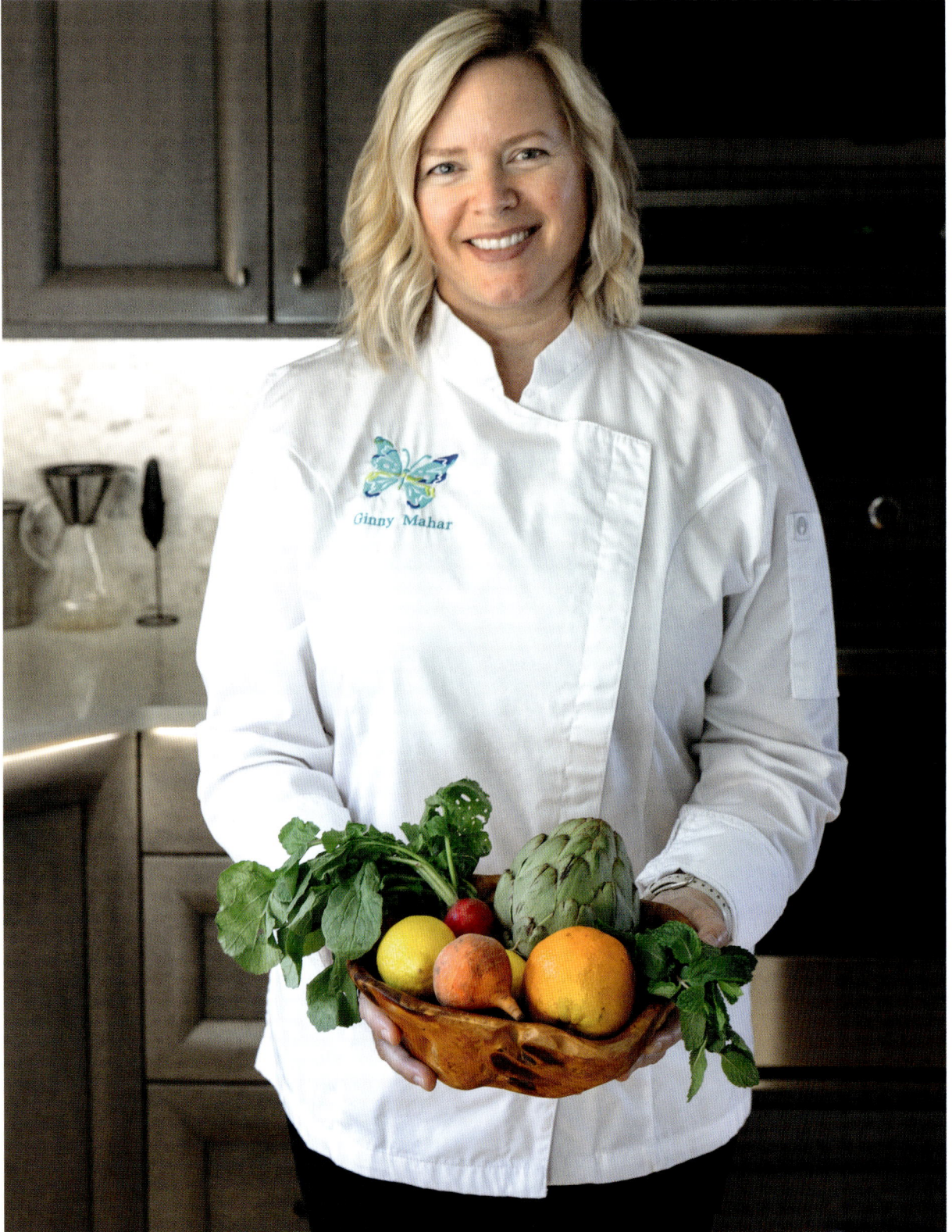

INTRODUCTION
Getting My Life Back, One Bite at a Time

IF YOU'RE HOLDING THIS BOOK IN YOUR HANDS— excited, curious, maybe a little wary—I want you to know that you're not alone. I've been there, and there's so much hope on the other side.

Thyroid-friendly eating didn't just change my health: It changed my life. It helped me reverse debilitating symptoms, cut my antibodies in half, and reclaim energy and clarity I thought I'd lost for good. It also shifted the course of my career and led me to become the thyroid health advocate, coach, cooking instructor, and recipe creator known as Hypothyroid Chef.

When I hit rock bottom with my health due to poorly managed hypothyroidism, I enlisted the help of a holistic medical practitioner: my beloved naturopath, who became my first true partner in healing. The first thing she talked to me about was food. She passed me a handout on anti-inflammatory eating, and it was like someone had handed me the keys to my healing journey.

After four years of suffering—even though I had a "normal" thyroid-stimulating hormone (TSH) level and was on medication—and being told there was nothing more I could do, I was beyond relieved. Hearing that it wasn't normal to feel tired all day, every day, was profoundly validating. I was thrilled that there were steps I could take, especially in the kitchen, to ease my lingering symptoms. On the heels of that relief came a tidal wave of grief. As a chef, food writer, and cooking instructor, food wasn't just sustenance: It was my world. How was I supposed to continue my work without staple ingredients like wheat flour or milk?

A week later, at one of my favorite restaurants, I found myself in tears, looking over the familiar menu through new eyes. I knew the freshly baked rolls and handmade pasta were no longer options if I wanted my health back, and not just because of what I'd learned about anti-inflammatory eating. I'd been clueing into my own food-triggered symptoms for years. Now, I'd finally found the missing explanation for them.

As someone who was born to cook, who'd dreamed of writing cookbooks since age nine, and who'd been creating recipes since she was tall enough to turn on the stove, my grief wasn't just about not being able to *eat* what I wanted; I couldn't *cook* what I wanted or *create* what I wanted either. If food were to remain my chosen medium, I would need to work with a more limited painter's palette.

When you discover that certain foods you love may not love you back, there's a very real grief process. Food is connection, celebration, comfort, and culture. But when some of those foods can cost you your health, change is required. The sadness, anger, and denial that follow can feel disorienting, especially when you find yourself mourning the foods that were making you sick in the first place! But there's no way around it. The only way out is through.

Not long after that tearful dinner, my husband, my son, and I found ourselves at another restaurant—our favorite pizza place. I was a month or two into my health turnaround and already feeling better. After four years of watching my inner flame dwindle to a smoldering ember, it was like a fresh breeze had sparked it back to life.

I ordered a chopped salad with vinaigrette—hold the cheese, hold the croutons. After the server walked away, my husband gave me a sympathetic look, sorry that I couldn't share in our favorite pizza.

"Don't feel sorry for me," I snapped. "I'm getting my life back."

The words came out with more force than I intended, but they marked a shift. A new version of me was emerging—one who was done with being sick. I wasn't going to let certain foods rob me of my joy, my dreams, or my ability to be the mother my son deserved.

Honestly, I didn't even want the pizza in that moment. It wasn't just a benign menu choice anymore: It came with a side order of clear, life-altering symptoms. Without gluten, my skin was clearing up. Without dairy, my bloating and joint pain were going away. Without grains, brain fog that had ruled my life for years lifted within days.

Changing my food choices—and my food career—was the price of admission for restored health. There was only one path forward.

I didn't become Hypothyroid Chef because I'm perfect at making food choices. I'm not. I became Hypothyroid Chef because this transition was *hard* for me, and I knew it must be hard for others too. *Maybe I have something to offer here,* I thought—and a new dream began to sparkle in the back of my mind.

My healing journey began that day in my naturopath's office. In the months that followed, I found myself back at my computer, writing about what I was going through: what I was eating, what I was learning, and how it was all starting to make sense. I knew I couldn't be the only one struggling to find thyroid-friendly, anti-inflammatory recipes. With my background and skill set, I felt called to help. In 2015, food gave me my life and health back, and Hypothyroid Chef was born.

Since then, I've created THYROID30, become a functional medicine health coach, and taught thousands of Thyroid Thrivers (which is what I call our community of health seekers) not just *what* thyroid-friendly food and lifestyle is, but *how* to make those changes in real life—where the results actually happen.

Before we dig in, dear Thriver, if you're feeling wary of—or weary from—your own transformation process, please know that it gets easier. Thyroid-friendly food choices are less about giving things up and more about gaining your vitality. You may always feel twinges of grief and frustration about having to limit or say goodbye to the foods that no longer support you, but believe me when I say that you learn not only to live with these changes but to love them for the energy, vitality, and relief they provide.

Health is our greatest wealth, and thyroid-friendly eating is like money in the bank. As you learn which foods help you thrive and which don't, those choices get easier to make—not because you have to, but because you *want to* feel your best.

This book will help you do just that. In the pages that follow, you'll start building a collection of favorite recipes, learn to fine-tune your food and lifestyle choices, discover your unique needs and sensitivities, and gain clarity around something many of us were never told: Food and lifestyle *do* make a difference for thyroid patients.

You'll learn life-changing skills and strategies—what to eat and what to avoid—not for the sake of restriction, but for the sake of feeling like *yourself* again. THYROID30 is like a time machine, helping you reach those milestones at warp speed.

I've come a long way from tear-stained restaurant menus. Today, I *love* my thyroid-friendly eating style and how it has restored my health and rippled out to help others. I wrote this book to do for you what my naturopath did for me: to hand you the keys to your healing journey and put *you* in the driver's seat. As your health coach, I'll be right beside you, riding shotgun with the water, the healthy snacks, the tunes, and the maps—ready to cheer you on and help you get where you want to go in a way that is tailor-made for *you.*

I've devoted my career to making this process as doable, empowering, positive, and fun as it can be. I know change can be challenging, but believe me when I tell you: If I can do this, *you* can too.

For me, it's been a process of metamorphosis from caterpillar to butterfly. Once I emerged from my chrysalis, I knew one thing for sure: I wouldn't trade these wings for all the pizza in the world.

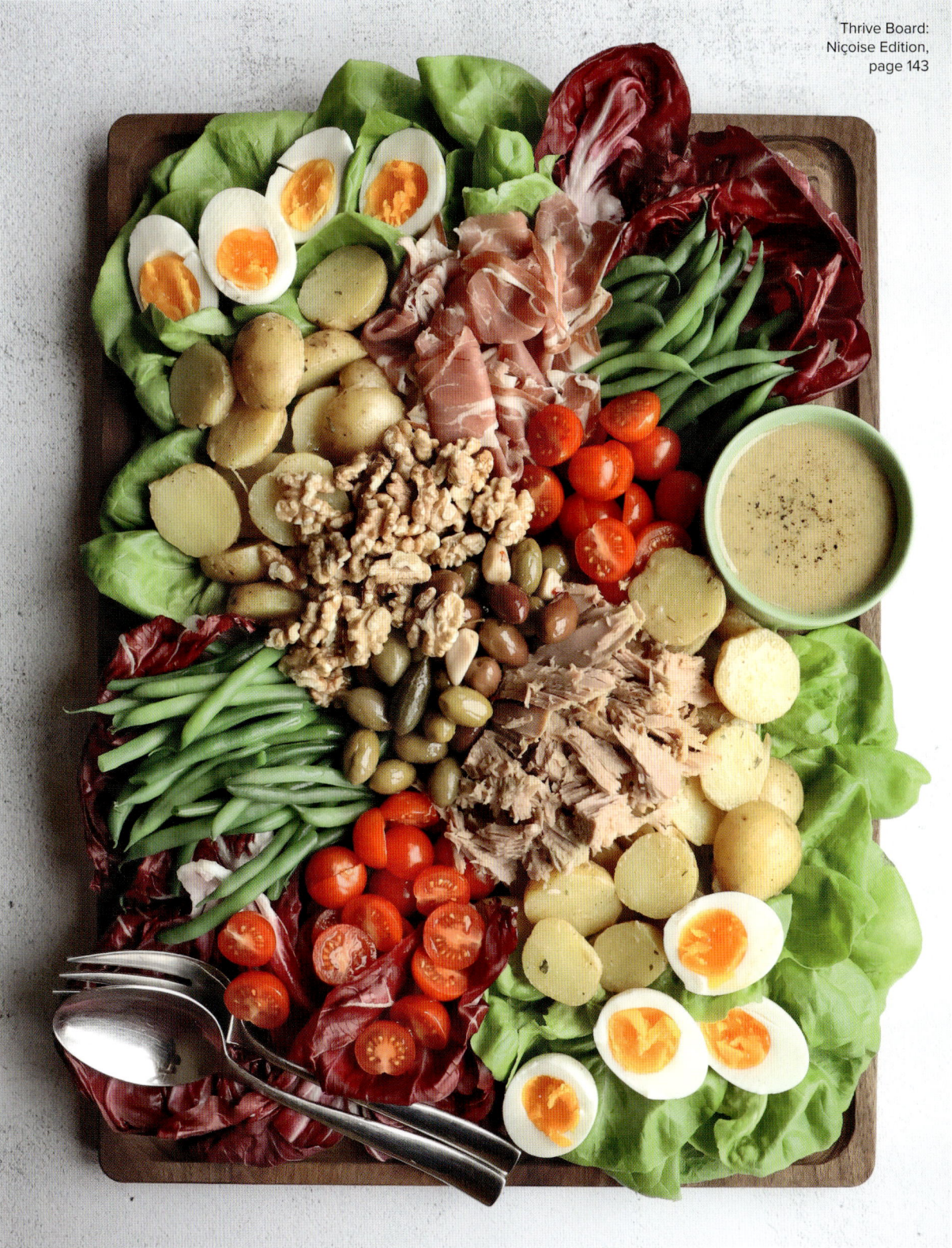

Thrive Board:
Niçoise Edition,
page 143

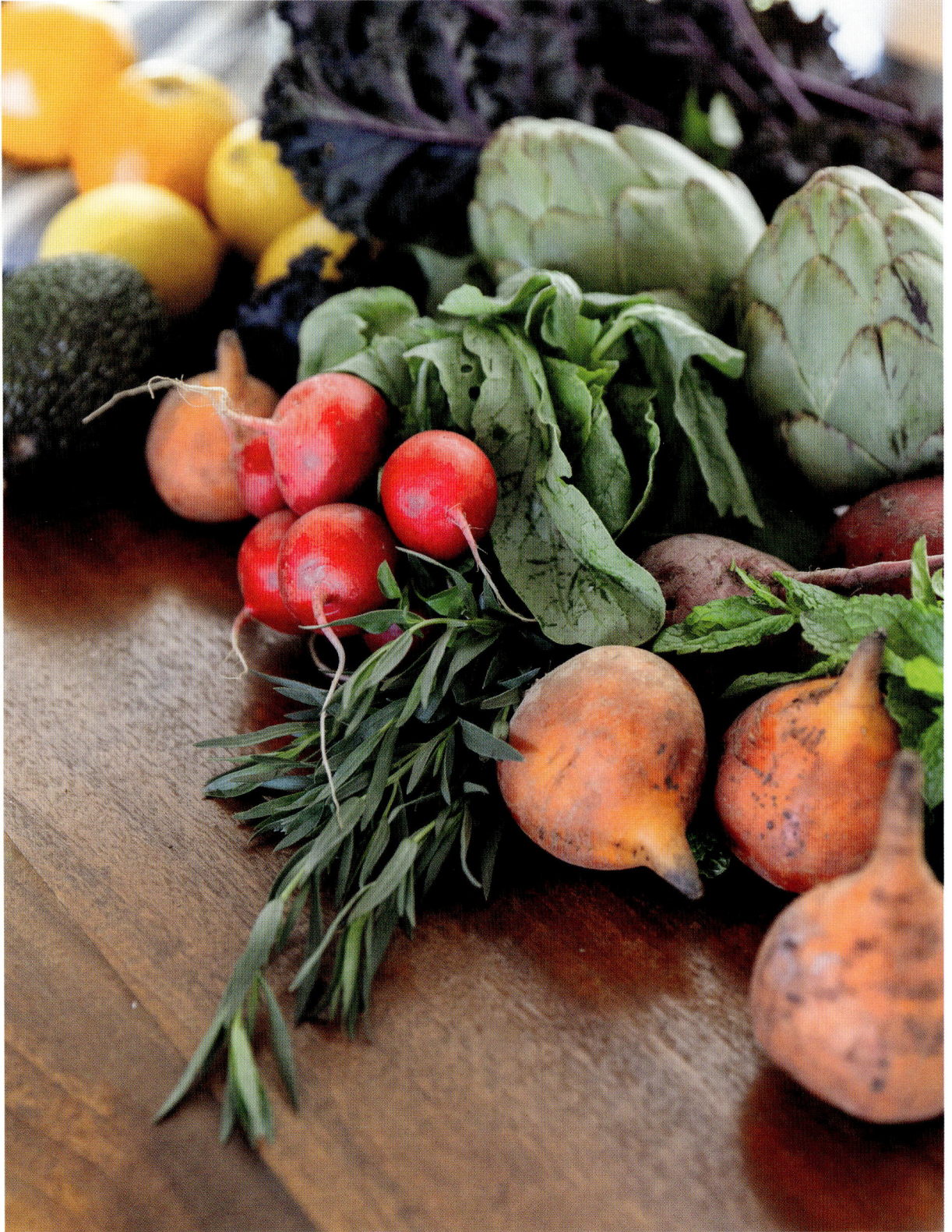

1

Welcome to *The THYROID30 Cookbook!*

If you can't remember what it's like to have energy, a clear mind, a lack of joint pain, a calm gut, or the simple ability to enjoy your life, you're not alone. I have both lived and woken up from that nightmare, as have many of the people who find their way to me. It's not an exaggeration to say that many thyroid patients have been compromised or even traumatized by years of debilitating thyroid-related symptoms we were told were "all in our heads."

I'm here to show you that there are several things you can do to reverse pesky thyroid symptoms and feel like you again. It's called thyroid-friendly food and lifestyle, and this book will teach you everything you need to know.

Because I've guided over a thousand people through my THYROID30 program, I've had a front-row seat to the life-changing power of thyroid-friendly food and lifestyle. I've seen symptoms reversed, dreams rekindled, pounds lost, strength gained, jobs recovered, relationships saved, and joy restored. I love what I do because I get to see the lights come back on inside of people. It's miraculous and heartening, and watching it happen never gets old. As one of my longtime community members put it, "I was ignorant even of my symptoms because I had lived with them for so long that they had become my new normal."

THYROID30 is a whole-life reset for your thyroid health and overall vitality, backed by the principles of functional medicine and real-world results. Our daily choices have a huge impact on how we feel and even on our markers for disease. When we learn to listen to what our bodies do and don't thrive on and then honor that feedback, we don't have to be doomed to our diagnoses, our genetics, or the residual thyroid symptoms that even proper thyroid medication sometimes leaves behind.

In the first part of this book, we'll cover the *what* of thyroid-friendly food and lifestyle. This will give you an essential understanding of the basic practices, the philosophy, and the evidence-backed *whys* behind them. But even if we know *what* to do, *how* do we actually do it? This is the question that the THYROID30 system answers.

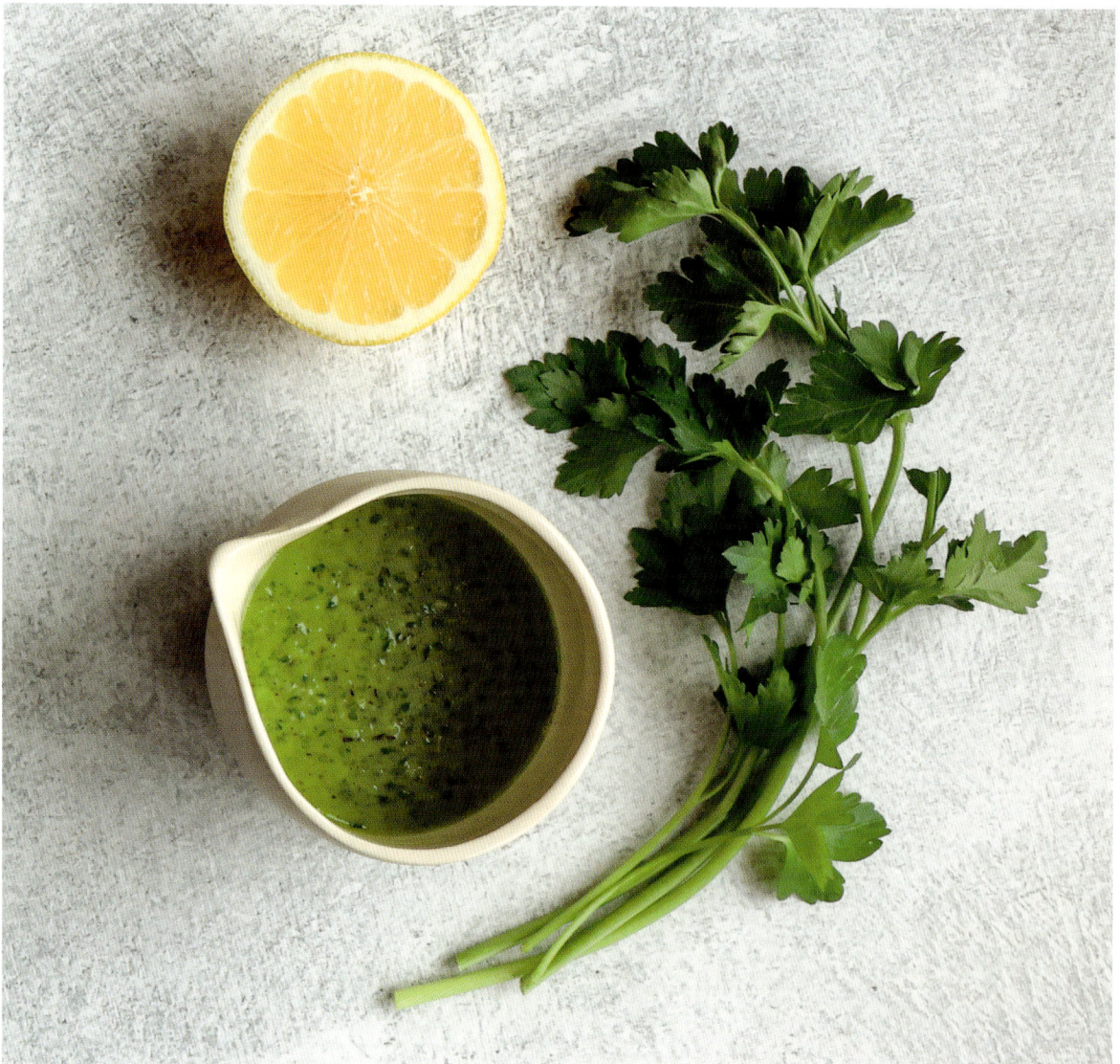

Even if you're incredibly well-informed, have lots of holistic and functional medical support, and are a biohacking wellness pro, applying healthy habits consistently in the real world can be a real challenge. Most of us go it alone, which often leaves us stuck in a yo-yo cycle of health spurts and stops that keeps us from achieving lasting results. Ultimately, this erodes our faith in ourselves and our ability to successfully make healthy changes. A support system that also offers community, like THYROID30, is often the missing piece of the puzzle.

What Is THYROID30?

The THYROID30 system is built on anti-inflammatory food and lifestyle practices. This includes things like eating anti-inflammatory foods, managing stress, getting regular exercise (but the right kind of exercise), avoiding toxins, prioritizing sleep, maintaining gut health, and remembering to take your daily medications and supplements (if needed).

That's a lot of plates to spin, right? And the truth is that even the experts have a hard time spinning them all at once. But what if you had a simple daily tracking system, designed to help you adopt these supportive food and lifestyle habits in a sustainable way, one small but doable step at a time? That's what THYROID30 is.

The 8 Rs

The backbone of THYROID30 is the 8 Daily Rituals of Thyroid-Healthy Living, or "The 8 Rs" for short.

We'll dig deeper into each of these in chapter 4.

Weaving the 8 Rs into your daily awareness and everyday lifestyle is the goal of THYROID30 and is what will enable you to move the needle on how you feel, including your energy, mood, skin, digestion, and even your ability to better use thyroid hormones (including thyroid hormone medication). We're talking about health and hypothyroidism management on a *cellular* level. Rather than being a 30-day quick fix or "diet," the THYROID30 system is a tool you can use again and again at any stage of your thyroid journey to uplevel or refresh those thyroid-healthy food choices and lifestyle habits. So, whether you're newly diagnosed or decades down the path, THYROID30 is for you.

The 8 Daily Rituals of Thyroid-Healthy Living

1. **REMEMBER** to take your medications and supplements.

2. **REFUEL** with the food and drink your body thrives on.

3. **REACTIVATE** by moving your body regularly.

4. **REPAIR** and care for your gut.

5. **REJUVENATE** with daily self-care and stress management.

6. **REDUCE** and avoid your exposure to toxins.

7. **RELISH** the journey, your wins, and your support system.

8. **RECHARGE** by prioritizing sleep and sleep hygiene.

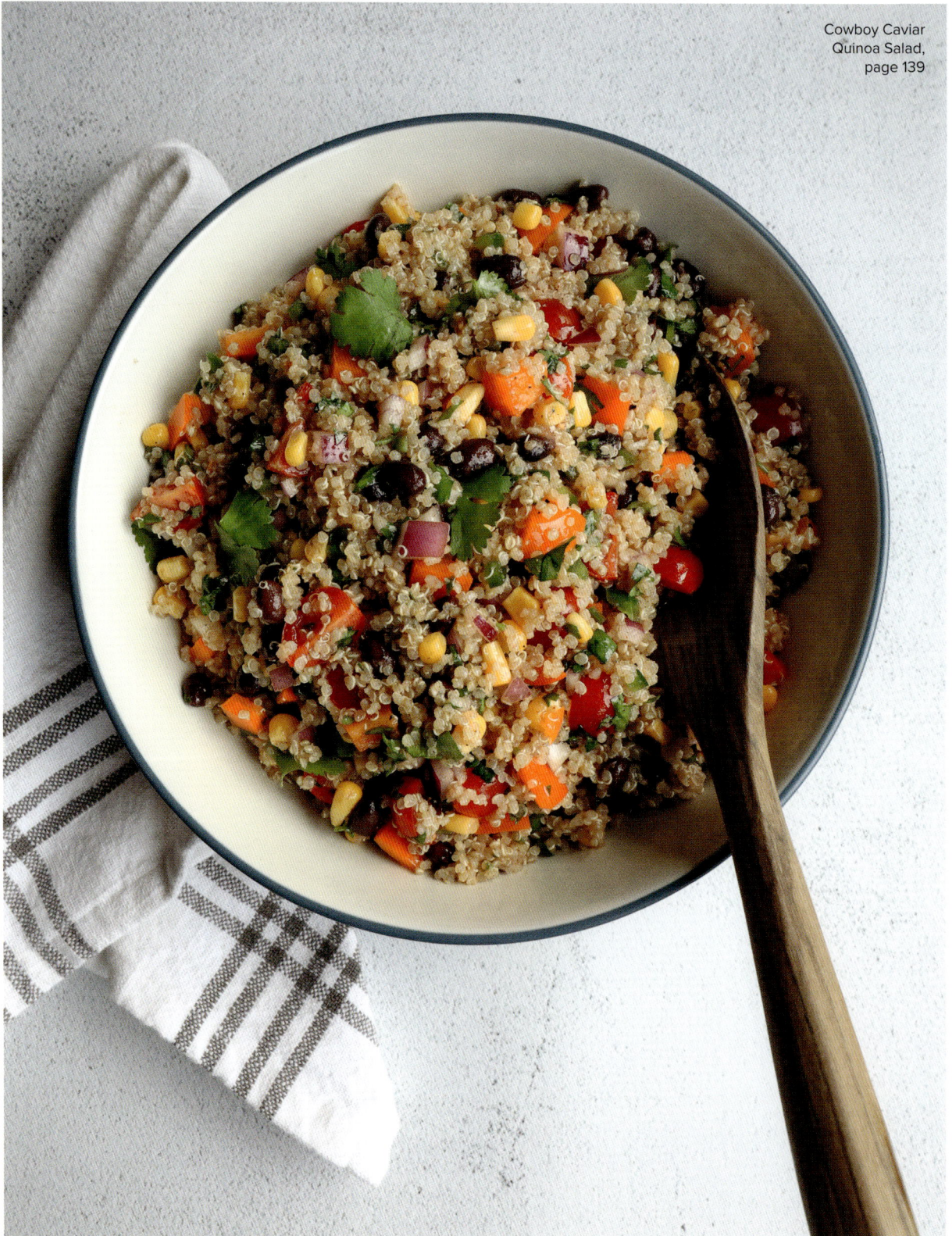

Cowboy Caviar
Quinoa Salad,
page 139

Let's Talk About the Recipes

The THRYOID30 Cookbook is a natural extension of the THYROID30 system, offering recipes that align with the 8 Daily Rituals and the principles of thyroid-friendly eating, which we'll cover in depth in chapter 3. Food isn't the only piece of the healing puzzle, but it is an essential piece. It's also the one people tend to need the most help with, so I've got you covered.

In the second part of this book you'll find 100 mouth-watering, colorful, easy-to-make recipes designed specifically for Thyroid Thrivers. While we each have unique dietary needs and sensitivities, you can choose from recipes that adhere to the most common dietary needs of Thyroid Thrivers. I've organized them into three levels, and you can choose from each during your THYROID30 experience:

- **Level 1:** Gluten-free/Dairy-free (also soy-free, refined sugar-free, and free of ultra-processed foods)

- **Level 2:** Paleo

- **Level 3:** AIP (The Autoimmune Protocol)

You'll also find done-for-you meal plans for each of these three levels, as well as other resources to help you reach your goals and make the process simple, clear, and fun. (We'll cover the meal plans in more detail, including how to choose the right one, in chapter 6.)

Because we're all at different points on the path and have unique needs, circumstances, and sensitivities, I encourage you to personalize the meal plans and recipes as needed. THYROID30 very intentionally offers a flexible framework that is customizable to *you*. It's not a set of rigid rules and restrictions: It's a system you can use to meet yourself where you are or to implement the personalized recommendations of your trusted health care professional(s).

Finally, you are invited to take your THYROID30 experience beyond the pages of this book and participate in a supportive community setting, with my personal coaching and guidance, inside my Thrivers Club community. It's a special place where everybody understands the unique set of challenges we face as thyroid patients. The 8 Rs and the THYROID30 model are the guiding principles of the Thrivers Club, helping you naturally build awareness, make successful and sustainable healthy-habit changes, overcome mindset roadblocks, find camaraderie and support, and use food as a powerful driver to reach your health goals—whether that's having the energy to play with your kids or grandkids, shedding unwanted weight, traveling the world, or being able to pursue your dreams again.

Who Is THYROID30 For?

THYROID30 is for anyone who needs a clear and effective starting point for, or an empowering refresher on, thyroid-friendly food and lifestyle habits. This 30-day plan is designed to guide you through a transformative journey to restore your energy and help you thrive.

As thyroid patients, we typically receive little to no guidance on food and lifestyle changes from conventional doctors, leading us to search for information ourselves. This can send us into a confusing online labyrinth of conflicting and outdated information plus sketchy internet ads promising unrealistic results.

Great information and experts are out there, but they're not always the first ones we come across. By the time people find their way to me, they're often in a state of *analysis paralysis*, so overwhelmed by information—much of it inaccurate—that they've lost all hope and don't know where to begin. This means that THYROID30 is for:

- Anyone who wants to harness the power of anti-inflammatory food and lifestyle changes

- Anyone who wants to know how they can better manage their hypothyroidism or Hashimoto's disease, beyond medication alone

- Anyone who wants to learn more about (and implement) thyroid-friendly food and lifestyle choices

- Thyroid patients at any phase of the journey, either newly diagnosed or decades down the path

- Thyroid patients who need support in implementing the recommendations of a doctor, nutritionist, or other health care professional

- Thyroid patients who are frustrated by ongoing symptoms despite proper medication or optimal thyroid levels

- Thyroid patients who are tired of feeling stuck and alone

What THYROID30 Is Not

Before we go any further, I want to state loud and clear that THYROID30 is not a replacement for proper medical care or necessary medication. Thriving with hypothyroidism or Hashimoto's requires what I call the "thyroid trifecta": proper medical care, including any needed medications and supplements; thyroid-friendly food choices; and thyroid-friendly lifestyle habits. While adding food and lifestyle enhancements to your overall treatment plan *may* lead to disease remission and even reduce medication needs, there are no guarantees. I emphasize this for two reasons:

1. **The growing mistrust of the medical/pharmaceutical industry has led some patients to refuse *necessary* thyroid medication at their own peril.** If left untreated, thyroid imbalances can be dangerous, even life-threatening.

THIS BOOK IS *NOT*:

- A replacement for proper medical care and treatment

- A substitute for needed thyroid medication

- Intended to treat serious, critical, or unmanaged health crises

- A cure for thyroid disease

- A quick or "magical" fix

- Intended for those with other health conditions that require medically tailored food or lifestyle interventions

- Aimed at people who aren't interested in taking an active role in their health journey

If you're unsure whether this approach is right for you, talk to your health care provider before making significant changes to your food or lifestyle.

2. **Dangerous online messaging promising disease remission (rather than disease *management*) gives patients false hope that can lead to food fear and disordered eating.** These guarantees lead patients to believe that if remission isn't achieved, it's because they didn't try hard enough or eat "perfectly" enough, which can be a slippery slope to orthorexia (an unhealthy obsession with eating only foods perceived as "safe" or healthy).

This may not be what you wanted to hear, but I care too much about your well-being to send you down a misleading path. I would probably have more followers if I made those "achieve remission" or "get off your meds" promises. They're alluring, hard to resist, and, unfortunately, not always possible. I'm not saying this to discourage you, but to keep you safe and to protect your mental and physical health.

The bottom line is that these things are not 100 percent within our control. Sometimes your thyroid gland has simply suffered too much damage to be able to produce the amount of thyroid hormone your body needs to function properly. So there is no shame in taking medication if you need it. If you can't get your Hashimoto's antibodies down, can't get off your thyroid meds, or can't achieve remission, it doesn't mean you "did it wrong" or didn't try hard enough. Sometimes it just is what it is.

This is why I advocate for an integrated approach. My advice is to start with a doctor's visit. Make the appointment and request a fresh round of thyroid labs, including TSH, free T3, free T4, and TPO antibodies. (I'll go into more detail about thyroid health and testing in chapter 2.) Make sure that you're on the right track with your thyroid meds, if needed. That way you'll have peace of mind and can benefit even more from the food and lifestyle journey we're about to embark on.

In implementing these thyroid-friendly food and lifestyle choices, the likelihood of you feeling much better is high, and you have a very good chance of reducing your symptoms and having more energy! Believe in that, but don't beat yourself up if you're unable to achieve the holy grail of disease remission.

Here are some key points to keep in mind:

- Start with proper medical care and testing (TSH, free T3, free T4, TPO antibodies).

- Recognize that food is powerful medicine, but it isn't a replacement for needed thyroid medication.

- Avoid the trap of over-restricting your diet in pursuit of "perfect" eating.

- Become an empowered, informed patient and advocate for yourself.

- Trust your own journey, your own body, and your chosen approach.

- If you're not seeing results, consider other factors like gut health, infections, or medication dosage.

The THYROID30 approach gives you agency over your health journey while acknowledging that medical partnership remains essential.

The THYROID30 Promise

There is no one-size-fits-all solution or cure for thyroid disease, but food and lifestyle are foundational to our health. For thyroid patients, they rarely replace the need for proper medication, but they sure can help us feel better, manage symptoms, and provide our bodies with the inputs they need to thrive.

THYROID30 is an invitation to take the driver's seat on your wellness journey through healthy food and lifestyle choices, and the recipes in this book are an invitation to start healing with your very next meal. It's not about restriction or willpower but about listening to and honoring your body's needs. Through this awareness you'll gain a deeper understanding of the choices that help you thrive—and those that don't.

Also, the principles outlined in this book aren't just "thyroid-healthy." They're built on the evidence-based principles of functional medicine and nutrition and were created to help patients prevent and manage chronic diseases of all kinds through supportive food and lifestyle choices.

Embarking on THYROID30 is a transformative personal journey that can take you from hopeless to thriving. While results may vary, the promise of THYROID30 is to set your internal stage for increased energy, reduced inflammation, less bloat, better mood, glowing skin, improved digestion, and a sustainable approach to healthy living.

The pursuit of health is a lifelong journey, one that occasionally requires hitting the refresh button on our choices. If you're lost and confused or simply uninspired, don't worry: This book can help you find your way to vibrant energy, clearer thinking, happier hormones, balanced blood sugar, better mood, improved gut health, and more.

Let's get started!

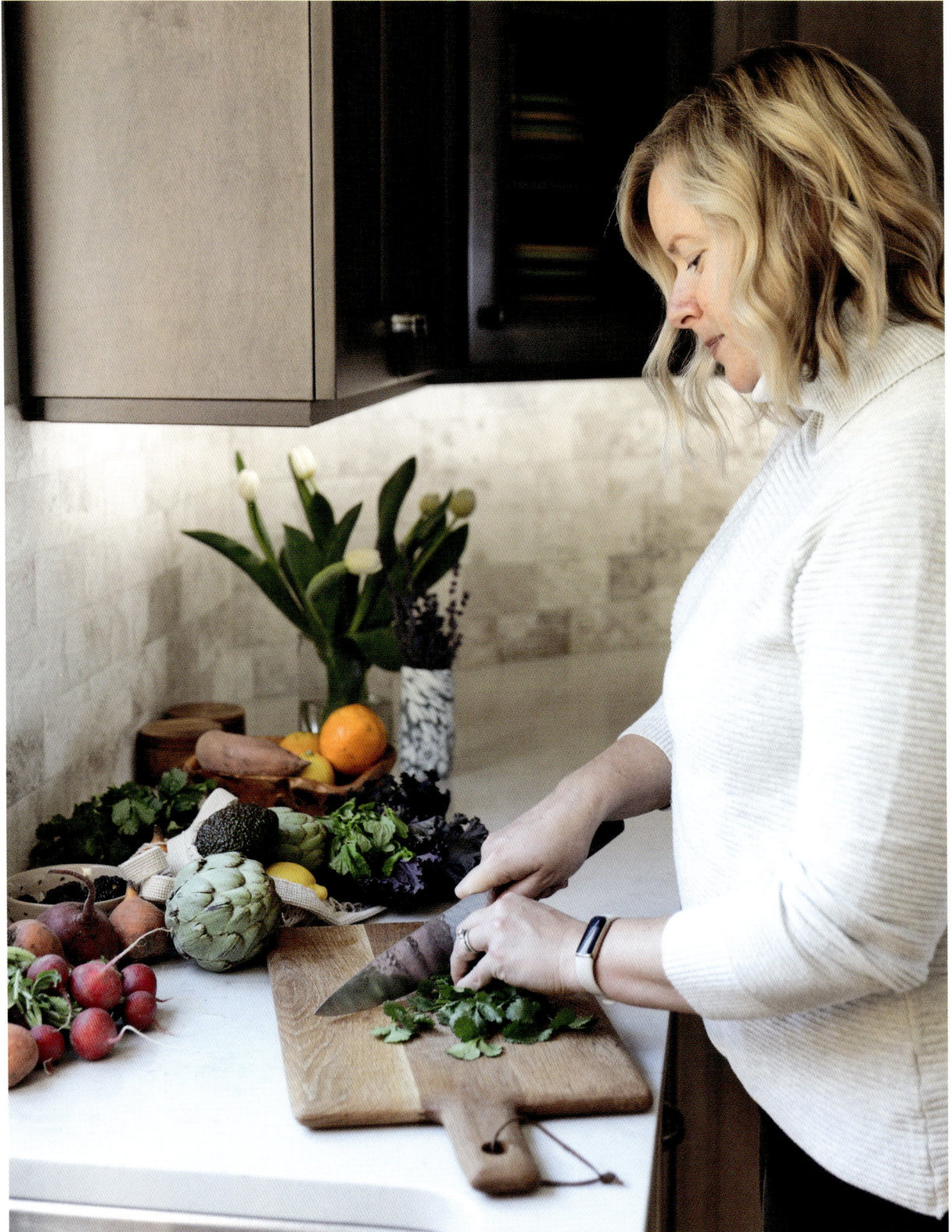

2

Understanding Your Thyroid

The first step in becoming an empowered thyroid patient is understanding what the thyroid is and what it does. In this chapter, we'll look at the vital role your thyroid plays in your overall health, including how it works and what happens when it doesn't. We'll explore the differences and overlap between hypothyroidism and Hashimoto's, how food and lifestyle can help, and why comprehensive testing and treatment options are essential to feeling your best. Most importantly, you'll come away with the foundational knowledge every Thyroid Thriver needs to advocate for the care they need and deserve and to finally start feeling better.

An Introduction to the Thyroid

Your thyroid is a small, butterfly-shaped gland located at the base of your neck that plays an enormous role in your overall health and well-being. Despite its modest size, the thyroid controls numerous vital functions, especially your metabolism. My dear friend and mentor, Mary Shomon, one of the world's leading thyroid advocates and experts and a *New York Times* bestselling author of over a dozen books on thyroid health, compares the thyroid to your body's gas pedal. You need just the right amount of fuel—or thyroid hormones—to move through life at a steady, healthy pace. This state is called **euthyroidism**—a normally functioning thyroid, producing the correct amount of thyroid hormone for a balanced metabolism.

Too much gas (or elevated levels of thyroid hormones) and you're racing along, revved up and burning through fuel too quickly. This state is called **hyperthyroidism**—a condition in which your thyroid is producing too much thyroid hormone, leading to an elevated metabolism. This can cause symptoms like rapid heart rate, weight loss, insomnia, tremors, bulging eyes, and heat intolerance.

Not enough pressure on the gas pedal (too little thyroid hormone) and you're dragging yourself through your days, putting along and running on empty. This state is called **hypothyroidism**—a condition in which your thyroid isn't producing enough thyroid hormone, leading to slowed metabolism.

Hypothyroidism can happen for a number of reasons, including the following:

- You were born without a thyroid gland or with a partially functioning one.
- Your thyroid has been damaged or removed through surgery, radiation, or disease.
- You're deficient in iodine or other nutrients essential for thyroid function.
- You're taking medications that slow down thyroid function (like lithium).
- You have an autoimmune condition attacking your thyroid (like Hashimoto's).

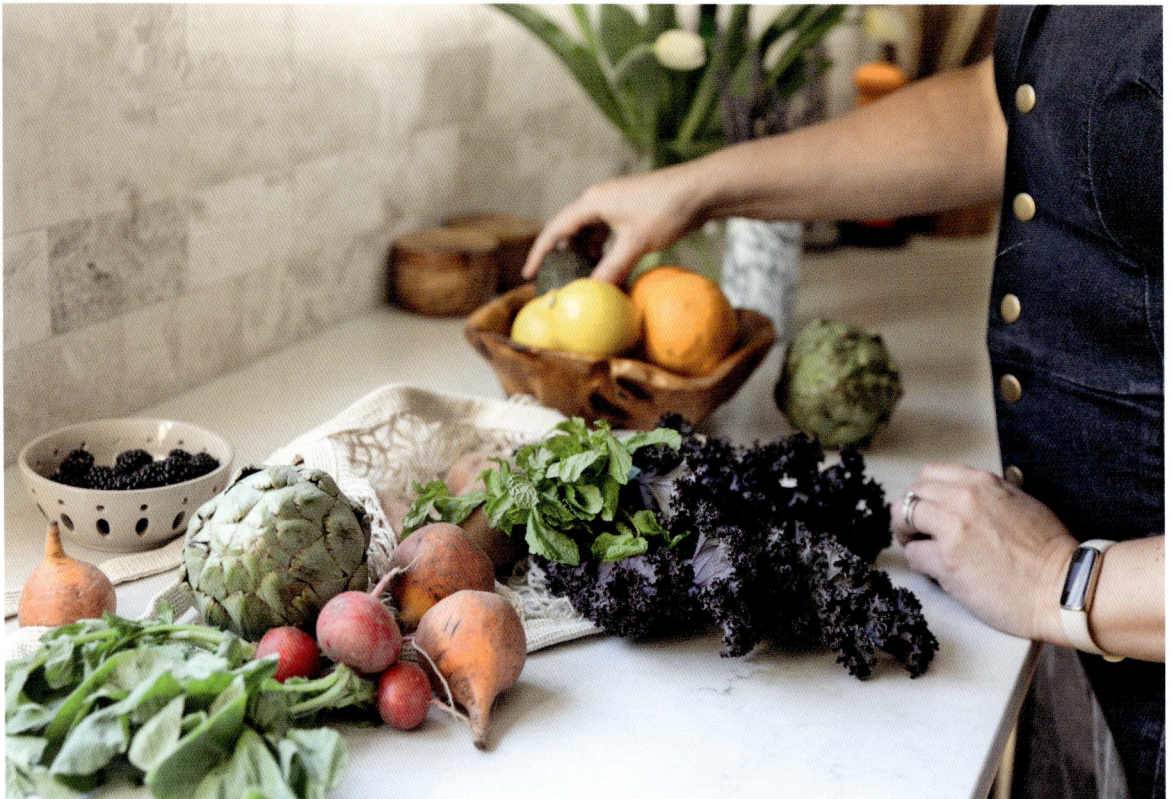

When thyroid hormone production is low, your body's processes slow down and change. The consequences of this extend far beyond your energy levels: Your metabolic rate influences your heart rate, breath rate, body temperature, weight, and even your mood.

Plus, nearly every cell in your body contains thyroid hormone receptors, so the thyroid affects virtually every physical system, including your brain, vision, hearing, digestion, muscles, ligaments, bones, lungs, hair growth, skin, heart, lungs, and hormonal balance.

How Hypothyroidism Affects the Body

Because the thyroid affects nearly all of the body's systems, the list of possible hypothyroidism symptoms is incredibly long: It's estimated that hypothyroidism may contribute to more than 300 potential symptoms. The list below highlights some of the most common ones:

- **Brain fog:** Difficulty concentrating, memory problems, mental fuzziness
- **Fatigue:** Persistent tiredness that isn't relieved by rest
- **Puffy face:** Facial swelling and puffiness, especially around the eyes and cheeks
- **Hearing issues:** Muffled hearing, ringing in the ears, or sound sensitivity
- **Voice changes:** Hoarseness, feelings of tightness in the throat
- **Weight gain:** Or the inability to lose weight despite diet and exercise
- **Cold intolerance:** Feeling cold when others are comfortable
- **Hair loss:** Thinning hair, including the outer third of the eyebrows

- **Dry skin:** Rough, scaly skin that may crack easily
- **Constipation:** Sluggish digestive function
- **Blood sugar imbalances:** Increased risk of hypoglycemia, insulin resistance, and type 2 diabetes
- **Joints and muscles:** Aches, weakness, and muscle loss
- **Depression:** Persistent low mood or sadness
- **Anxiety:** Ongoing feelings of worry, nervousness, and unease
- **Menstrual changes:** Heavier, more frequent, or irregular periods
- **Reproductive health:** Increased risk of infertility, miscarriage, and pregnancy complications
- **High cholesterol:** Particularly elevated LDL ("bad" cholesterol) levels
- **Heart issues:** Elevated blood pressure and increased risk of heart disease
- **Slowed metabolism:** Leading to fatigue, weight gain, and lower body temperature
- **Digestive issues:** Stomach bloating, heartburn, and increased risk of gallstones

NOTE
Many of these symptoms can be attributed to other conditions, which is why proper testing, including a complete thyroid panel, is essential for accurate diagnosis and effective treatment.

How the Thyroid Works

Your thyroid gland uses iodine, which must be obtained from your diet, to produce two key thyroid hormones:

- **Triiodothyronine (T3):** The active hormone that helps the delivery of oxygen and energy into your cells
- **Thyroxine (T4):** A storage hormone that gets converted to T3 in your body

There are other thyroid hormones, including T1 and T2, which have historically been considered relatively inert, but are now being studied for the roles they play in determining our metabolism.

Your pituitary gland regulates the production of thyroid hormones through TSH. When functioning properly, your pituitary senses when you need more thyroid hormone and releases TSH, which signals your thyroid to increase production. So, when your TSH level is high, it indicates that your pituitary is communicating more urgently with your thyroid, saying, "Hey, we're flagging here! It's time to produce more thyroid hormone!"

This is why TSH is the most common thyroid test patients get. If it's low, it could indicate hyperthyroidism; if it's high, it can indicate hypothyroidism.

Thyroid Disease by the Numbers

When I was first diagnosed with hypothyroidism, I had no idea just how common it was—or how misunderstood. I've since learned that thyroid disease affects 12 percent of the U.S. population, primarily women, who are five to eight times more likely than men to develop thyroid issues. What's truly mind-boggling is that more than half of patients are unaware of their condition. When left undiagnosed and untreated, thyroid disease can pose serious health risks like heart disease, infertility, dementia, and osteoporosis.

While iodine deficiency remains the leading cause of hypothyroidism worldwide (more so in developing countries), that's not the case for developed countries and regions like the United States, Canada, and Europe, where it's estimated that over 90 percent of hypothyroidism cases are caused by autoimmune disorders—usually a specific condition called Hashimoto's thyroiditis.

That's a very important statistic when it comes to disease management, but here's the kicker: Most patients are never told that they have autoimmunity. They're rarely tested for it, even though it's likely to be the root cause of their thyroid condition. Why? Because the conventional standard of treatment usually consists of TSH testing alone and a T4-only medication prescription (typically levothyroxine, one of the top three most commonly prescribed drugs in the United States). This one-size-fits-all approach leaves millions—especially women—struggling with unresolved symptoms like fatigue, weight gain, brain fog, hair loss, and depression. I know, because I was one of them. And if you're reading this, maybe you're one of them too.

IS THIS BOOK ONLY FOR PEOPLE DIAGNOSED WITH HYPOTHYROIDISM OR HASHIMOTO'S?

This is one of the most common questions I get, and the answer can bring some welcome clarity. Here's the scoop.

Many treatment paths lead to hypothyroidism, regardless of where your thyroid journey began. Even though we may have different health backgrounds, including Graves' disease, thyroid cancer, a history of surgery, or congenital conditions, many of us are, or end up, in the same place: relying on daily thyroid hormone replacement.

This book is for you if:

- You've been diagnosed with hypothyroidism or Hashimoto's.

- You've had radioactive iodine (RAI) treatment for Graves' or hyperthyroidism and now rely on supplemental thyroid hormone medication.

- You've had all or part of your thyroid removed due to cancer, nodules, goiter, or Graves', and now rely on supplemental thyroid hormone medication.

- You were born with a low-functioning thyroid or without a thyroid (congenital hypothyroidism) and rely on supplemental thyroid hormone medication.

If any of those describe you, you're probably familiar with the lingering symptoms many hypothyroid patients experience, even on medication. You deserve to know what truly effective treatment and whole-health management look like, because thriving with a sluggish or missing thyroid often takes more than medication alone.

Hashimoto's: A Closer Look

Hashimoto's thyroiditis—the most common cause of hypothyroidism in developed countries—is an autoimmune condition where your immune system attacks your thyroid gland instead of targeting harmful invaders.

In people with Hashimoto's, the immune system produces antibodies that gradually damage the thyroid, reducing its ability to produce hormones. This autoimmune process can unfold slowly over many years. In fact, many people have thyroid antibodies long before their thyroid hormone levels become abnormal. The two antibodies most often used for diagnosis are thyroid peroxidase antibodies (TPOAb) and thyroglobulin antibodies (TgAb).

Understanding whether your hypothyroidism is caused by Hashimoto's is crucial because it gives you insight into what's really going on in your body. If you've been diagnosed with hypothyroidism but never tested for Hashimoto's, it's important to advocate for yourself and ask for the test.

It's also important to understand that once autoimmunity is present, your risk of developing additional autoimmune diseases triples. This is a compelling reason to educate yourself about the mechanisms of autoimmunity and how gut health, food triggers, and chronic stress can all play a significant role.

Dr. Alessio Fasano is a leading celiac researcher, pediatric gastroenterologist, and Harvard Medical School professor. According to his Autoimmune Triad Theory, three key factors must be present for autoimmunity to develop:

1. A genetic predisposition

2. An environmental trigger (like infection, toxin exposure, or stress)

3. Increased intestinal permeability, also known as "leaky gut"

This triad helps explain why autoimmune diseases like Hashimoto's don't just appear out of nowhere and why addressing gut health, food, and lifestyle factors can be so powerful in managing them.

The T4 Problem: Why Standard Thyroid Care Often Falls Short

Before we dive into thyroid testing, it's important to understand another fundamental issue with conventional thyroid treatment. As mentioned previously, the standard approach for hypothyroidism is prescribing a synthetic T4-only hormone like levothyroxine (some brand names include Synthroid, Levoxyl, and Tirosint) and then monitoring TSH levels. For many patients, TSH testing is the only test they're offered or given.

However, there's a glaring oversight in this approach. T4 is an inactive hormone: To use it, your body must convert it into T3, the primary active thyroid hormone. TSH testing does not tell us if that conversion is happening as efficiently as it should.

T4 to T3 conversion primarily happens in the liver and gut, two areas that are often compromised in people with thyroid disease, especially when autoimmunity is involved. Hypothyroidism impacts the liver's ability to process hormones, toxins, fat, and cholesterol, and also makes us more prone to gut health issues like dysbiosis and intestinal permeability, or "leaky gut."

Due to factors including genetic predisposition, poor health, chronic stress, disease, age, inflammation, diet, gut health, liver health, and nutrient deficiencies, some thyroid patients (myself included) don't convert T4 to T3 efficiently, which means that even with "normal" TSH levels, they may continue to experience hypothyroid symptoms like fatigue, weight gain, brain fog, and high cholesterol.

When thyroid patients report these ongoing symptoms to their doctors, they're often told that because they are on medication and their TSH is normal, they're actually fine—as if their symptoms are imagined or unrelated to their thyroid. This form of medical gaslighting is unfortunately all too common, particularly for women with hypothyroidism, who may live with debilitating symptoms for years or even decades without validation or receiving truly effective thyroid treatment. I know because I was one of those patients.

The good news is that awareness is growing about conversion issues, and more doctors are recognizing that some patients need T3 medication in addition to T4. T3 is often administered via combination therapy, in which a patient is given a T4 medication plus a T3 medication, or through natural desiccated thyroid (NDT) medications, like Armour (more about this shortly), which contain T1, T2, T3, and T4. Dr. Antonio C. Bianco, author of *Rethinking Hypothyroidism* and former head of the American Thyroid Association, is one of those doctors. He is a pioneer in this crusade and an expert on the very real science behind it. Thankfully, tides are shifting for thyroid patients as a result of books like his—although most of the medical establishment still has some catching up to do.

The key takeaway here is that identifying these issues may require your doctor's help in tinkering with different types, dosages, ratios, and brands of medication (in addition to regular testing and monitoring) to find the optimal formula for you.

Essential Testing for Hypothyroidism

Let's break down the key thyroid tests every Thyroid Thriver should know about.

1. **TSH (Thyroid-Stimulating Hormone)**
    - Measures the amount of TSH
    - Reference range: 0.5–5.0 mIU/L
    - Optimal range (functional medicine): 0.75–2.0 mIU/L
    - Elevated levels indicate hypothyroidism.

2. **Free T4 (Free Thyroxine)**
    - Measures levels of available, circulating T4 hormone
    - Reference range: 0.8–1.8 ng/dL
    - Optimal range: 1.3–1.6 ng/dL
    - Low levels may indicate hypothyroidism.

3. **Free T3 (Free Triiodothyronine)**
    - Measures levels of available, active thyroid hormone
    - Reference range: 2.3–4.2 pg/mL
    - Optimal range: 3.5–4.0 pg/mL
    - Low levels may indicate hypothyroidism.

4. **TPOAb (Thyroid Peroxidase Antibodies)**
    - Found in about 90 percent of individuals with Hashimoto's
    - Reference range: 0–35 IU/mL
    - Elevated levels suggest autoimmune activity.

5. **TgAb (Thyroglobulin Antibodies)**
    - Found in 50–80 percent of individuals with Hashimoto's
    - Often tested alongside TPOAb antibodies
    - Elevated levels suggest autoimmune activity.

6. **Reverse T3**
    - When the body is under stress, it may not effectively convert T4 to T3. Instead, it produces more reverse T3, which blocks active T3.
    - High levels can indicate "cellular hypothyroidism," a condition in which the body's cells are unable to properly use thyroid hormone, even when blood levels appear normal.
    - Reference range: 10–24 ng/dL
    - Optimal: Below 15 ng/dL

Tests 1 through 3 are essential for regular thyroid testing, which you should undergo at least twice a year and more often if you've made any changes to your medication, symptoms, or food and lifestyle.

Test 4 is also essential for individuals who have Hashimoto's because it assesses how high the autoimmune activity is. Ideally, TPOAb testing should be performed on all patients diagnosed with hypothyroidism to determine if autoimmunity is present.

Tests 5 and 6 are also helpful, especially when establishing baselines, but may not be required at every regular round of testing.

Understanding Your Test Results

It's important to recognize that "normal" lab values are not necessarily optimal ones. Many thyroid patients continue to experience symptoms even when their results fall within the standard reference ranges. This is why many functional and holistic practitioners interpret labs using narrower, optimal ranges rather than relying on what's simply considered "normal."

For example, a TSH of 4.5 might be labeled "normal" by conventional standards, but many patients feel significantly better when their TSH is below 2.0. The truth is that it depends on the individual: We all have our sweet spot. Remember that the goal of lab testing isn't just to hit a number; it's to help you feel your best.

Your practitioner will ultimately help you interpret your test results. But one test worth understanding is free T3, your biologically active thyroid hormone. If your free T3 is low—even when your T4 is high or normal—it could mean your body isn't getting enough T3, or isn't converting T4 into T3 efficiently.

That's why a complete thyroid panel is essential when trying to optimize your medication and thyroid levels. TSH alone is simply not enough. Partnering with your doctor to run a full panel of tests and fine-tune your treatment is a foundational step toward better energy, mood, and overall wellness.

How Often Should You Get Tested?

That depends. If you've been relatively stable on your thyroid medication, haven't experienced notable changes in your symptoms or health status, or made significant modifications to your diet or lifestyle, then testing every six months is typically sufficient. (Some doctors may test only once every twelve months, but as a thyroid patient advocate, I feel that's a long time to go unchecked.)

However, if you've noticed changes in your symptoms—even a gradual return of the tireds or the foggies—it's a good idea to get tested right away.

When making food and lifestyle changes that support thyroid or autoimmune health, more frequent monitoring can help track how your body is responding, especially if these are long-term changes you're planning to maintain. And finally, if you're adjusting your thyroid medication—whether changing the dose or switching medications—it's important to get retested approximately six weeks after you first make the change. That gives your body time to adjust and ensures you're still within your optimal range for symptom relief.

Root Cause Testing

Beyond standard thyroid labs, testing for potential root causes of thyroid dysfunction can bring major relief and insight, especially if you're still struggling with symptoms despite having addressed medication, food, and lifestyle factors. Many of these tests go beyond what conventional doctors typically order, so you may need to work with a functional or holistic practitioner to access them.

Here are some of the most common root cause factors to consider testing for:

- **Food sensitivities:** Especially gluten, dairy, and other common immune triggers
- **Gut health:** Including leaky gut, digestive imbalances, infections, and dysbiosis
- **Underlying infections:** Various bacterial, viral, or parasitic infections including Epstein-Barr (EBV), herpes simplex 1 and 2, hepatitis C, Blastocystis hominis, and Lyme disease
- **Hormonal imbalances:** Including sex hormones and adrenal (cortisol) function
- **Nutrient deficiencies:** Especially vitamin D, ferritin, B12, magnesium, zinc, and selenium
- **Environmental toxins:** Mold, heavy metals, and chemical exposures
- **Genetic variations:** Such as MTHFR mutation and other methylation-related variants
- **Inflammatory markers:** To assess systemic inflammation or immune system activation

Work with your health care provider to determine which of these tests are most appropriate for your specific symptoms and health history.

Types of Thyroid Hormone Replacement Medication

There are several types of thyroid medication, and finding the right one for you can be a game-changer when it comes to managing symptoms. There's no single best option: It's really about finding the right medication, at the right dosage, for *you*. Working with your doctor to optimize your thyroid medication can take time, trial, and error, but is a worthwhile endeavor.

Keep in mind that what works beautifully for one person might not work as well for another. Also, some patients find that a certain brand of medication agrees with them better than other brands or generics, so it's important to stay in communication with your doctor and advocate for yourself if you're not feeling well on your current medication.

The main types of medication include:

- **Levothyroxine (T4-only medication):** Synthetic T4 is the most commonly prescribed thyroid medication and includes brands like Synthroid, Levoxyl, and Euthyrox. It contains synthetic T4, which your body must convert into the active form, T3.

- **Tirosint:** This is also a synthetic T4-only medication (levothyroxine) like the ones mentioned above, but comes in a gel cap or liquid form with minimal fillers. This option is ideal for those with sensitivities, allergies, or absorption issues.

- **Liothyronine (T3-only medication):** This is synthetic T3, available as Cytomel or generic liothyronine. It is sometimes added to T4 when patients don't convert it efficiently on their own.

- **Combination therapy (T4 + T3):** Some doctors prescribe a combination of synthetic T4 and T3—either as separate medications or through a compounded formula—to better match your body's natural hormone production.

- **Natural desiccated thyroid (NDT):** Made from the dried thyroid glands of pigs, NDT includes naturally occurring ratios of T4 and T3, as well as T2, T1, and T0. Brand names include Armour Thyroid and NP Thyroid. Some patients feel their best on NDT, though it's not for everyone.

What matters most is how *you* feel on your medication. Lab results are helpful, but if you're still experiencing symptoms despite being "in range," it may be time to explore other medication options with a thyroid-savvy practitioner.

Finding the Right Doctor

As both a thyroid patient and advocate, I can attest to the valid frustration so many of us feel in trying to get comprehensive testing and effective treatment. Too often, patients are dismissed and invalidated by conventional providers who insist that TSH is the only test that's needed, medications other than synthetic T4 are unsafe, or their patients' ongoing symptoms have nothing to do with their thyroid because the patient is on levothyroxine with a "normal" TSH.

It's not uncommon for a patient to wait months to see an endocrinologist—hoping for more advanced care—only to find that many hormone specialists follow the same outdated standard of care as their GP.

Of course, all of this depends on the doctor. There are general practitioners and endocrinologists out there who dig deeper, offer additional testing, and are open to alternative thyroid medications. Some of them are living with thyroid issues themselves and have learned firsthand that there's more to effective treatment than what they may have been taught in medical school. But it can take persistence to find the right fit.

If you're not being taken seriously or your concerns are being brushed off, it may be time to find a new doctor.

What to Look for in a Thyroid Provider

Seek out a practitioner who:

- Is a prescribing physician who can provide needed thyroid medication

- Listens to your symptoms and takes them seriously

- Is willing to order comprehensive thyroid labs, not just TSH

- Looks for and addresses root causes, not just symptoms

- Is knowledgeable about multiple medication options, including T3 or NDT

- Treats you as a whole person, not just the sum of your lab results

- Evaluates for nutrient deficiencies, gut health, and other contributing factors

Finding all of these qualities in a conventional provider is rare—not impossible, but rare. That's because conventional and functional medicine differ fundamentally. Conventional medicine primarily focuses on treating disease, while functional/holistic medicine focuses on preventing disease and restoring optimal function using a food- and lifestyle-based approach. Both systems have value—and hopefully, someday, they'll work together more seamlessly. But until that becomes more common, you may benefit from expanding your health care team to include a practitioner trained in functional or holistic medicine.

In short, both conventional and holistic care are important for thyroid patients—but don't bark up the wrong tree. I wouldn't see my naturopath for a broken arm, for instance, and I don't expect my conventional doctor to help me manage my Hashimoto's using food and lifestyle.

Other Practitioners to Consider

While conventional thyroid care may be standardized, any thyroid patient will tell you that living with thyroid disease is anything but standard. What works for one person may not work for another. Optimal treatment often requires a whole-body, individualized approach—one that takes time, seeks root causes, and doesn't simply fit into a 10-minute appointment slot. For this reason, you may benefit from adding one of the following practitioners to your health care team:

- **Naturopathic doctors (ND or NMD):** Trained in both conventional and natural medicine

- **Functional medicine physicians:** Focus on identifying underlying causes of disease, and managing or preventing disease with food and lifestyle

- **Integrative medicine doctors:** Blend conventional care with holistic therapies

- **Osteopathic physicians (DO):** Trained in whole-body healing, including structural and lifestyle factors

Remember, if you're struggling with symptoms, you deserve to be seen, heard, and validated. You're not crazy. Having symptoms despite normal lab results doesn't make you a hypochondriac. It's not "all in your head."

So, if your doctor isn't addressing your health concerns, you deserve to find one who will. Keep searching. The right doctor is out there, and finding them is worth every ounce of effort. (Check out THYROID30 Support and Resources on page 246 for finding a doctor.)

NOTE

The prescribing physician bullet is especially important for thyroid patients. Practitioners who are not licensed to prescribe medication may attempt to treat thyroid imbalances with supplements such as thyroid glandulars or biologics. These unregulated products are not recommended and may cause unpredictable thyroid levels. For safe treatment, it's essential to have a prescribing physician on your team.

Remember: Your Thyroid Is Looking Out for You

Thyroid issues can impact every single aspect of your life. They can leave you feeling like your body has failed you—or even betrayed you. But here's a question that might spark a powerful shift in perspective: What if your body isn't failing you, but protecting you?

That's the essence of the Safety Theory, especially as it relates to the Cell Danger Response, a concept beautifully explained in *The Thyroid Debacle* by Dr. Eric Balcavage and Dr. Kelly Halderman. According to this theory, the body may sometimes intentionally suppress thyroid function—or reduce how thyroid hormone is used at the cellular level—as a protective mechanism. When you're under extreme stress, your body may slow your metabolism to conserve energy, promote healing, and keep you alive. That's not dysfunction: It's a biologically intelligent survival strategy.

In terms of the thyroid, this protective response can be triggered by:

- Chronic dieting or under-eating (which the body perceives as famine)
- Physical or emotional trauma
- Chronic stress
- Overtraining or burnout
- Environmental toxins
- Chronic infections

This doesn't mean hypothyroidism should go untreated: far from it. But it does mean that healing requires more than just a prescription. It means supporting your body as it works to return to balance—a natural state known as homeostasis. Your body is always striving for homeostasis, but it needs you, as its caretaker, to help it get there. That means addressing the deeper stressors that may be signaling your system to slow down.

Hypothyroidism and Hashimoto's aren't failures. Sometimes they're your body's way of telling you, "Hey, slow down. You need care. You need rest. You need nourishment. You need safety and joy."

In fact, history suggests that hypothyroidism has helped humans survive extreme conditions like famine. Some experts have noted that caloric deficiency during widespread famines like Ireland's Great Potato Famine of 1845–1852 triggered hypothyroidism in some individuals, whose consequent lower metabolic rate helped them to stay alive. This is evidence that your body remembers how to protect you. That's not betrayal: It's resilience. So, instead of scolding your body for letting you down, try offering it some tender loving care. Give it good nutrition, deep rest, joyful movement, quality sleep, and space to destress.

Understanding how your thyroid works is the first step toward healing. With the THYROID30 approach, you have a proven, whole-life framework that makes the process doable, empowering, and even fun. You're not just managing symptoms here: You're learning how to support your body, reclaim your vitality, and truly thrive.

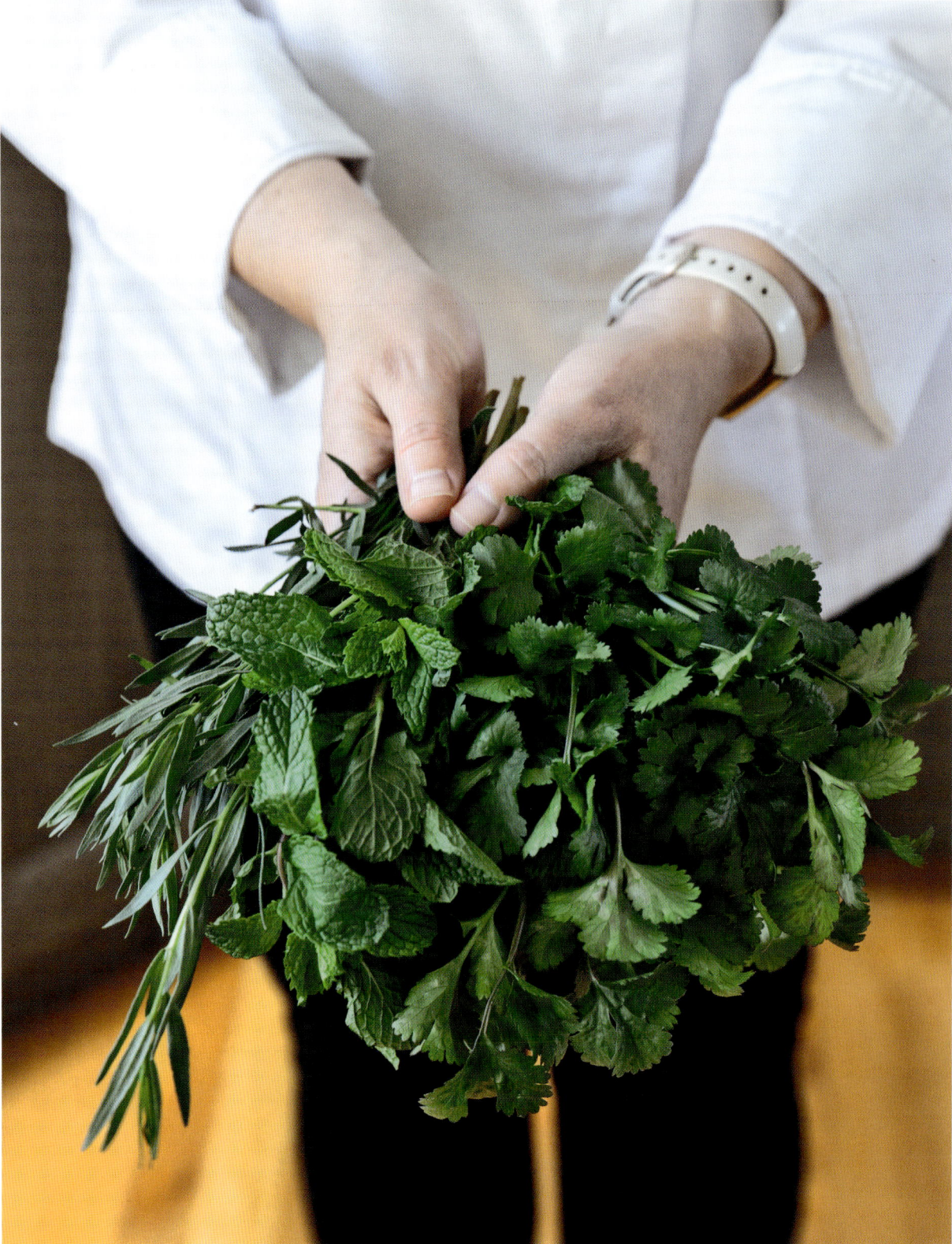

3

The Why, What, and How of Thyroid-Friendly Eating

Whether you're eating a processed, sugar-laden standard American diet (SAD) or a whole-food, colorful, health-supportive diet like the one outlined in this book, food is powerful stuff. The way we nourish our bodies is the foundation of healthy living—for everyone! For Thyroid Thrivers, it can also help us reverse symptoms and get our lives back. You've heard the saying, "Food is medicine," but for us, that's more than just a trending phrase: It's a science-backed reality.

One thing that may surprise you is that thyroid-healthy eating isn't just thyroid-healthy; it's also gut-healthy, hormone-healthy, and blood sugar–healthy. It's based on the foundations of functional nutrition, which is designed to help us both prevent and manage chronic illness. This means that everyone at your table can benefit from the principles, skills, and shifts you'll learn about in this chapter. In short, this chapter is all about how we can use food to combat inflammation—a root cause factor of so many diseases.

Food is foundational to our health, and learning how it can help or harm you as a thyroid patient is essential knowledge. In this chapter, I'll walk you through the principles and pillars of thyroid-friendly eating, outline key thyroid-supporting nutrients, and share the secrets to personalizing your approach.

Before we dive in, let me assure you that thyroid-healthy eating isn't about restriction or deprivation. It's about healing. It's about understanding which foods your body thrives on and which foods it doesn't. It's about empowering you with a personalized road map of your body's dietary needs and sensitivities.

Thyroid-friendly eating does *not* require you to make "perfect" food choices 100 percent of the time or to cut out more and more foods to experience benefits. Finding a balance is built right into it: You'll learn which foods you must completely avoid and which you have some wiggle room with. This enables you to live your life with as much food freedom as possible, especially when you're traveling, dining out, or sharing communal meals. I'll teach you not only how to *thrive* using food but also how to *live well* with whatever dietary restrictions you may have.

Functional Nutrition: The Language of Thyroid-Friendly Eating

Think of thyroid-friendly eating as learning a new language, one that your body already speaks but that you may have forgotten how to interpret.

In functional nutrition, one of the guiding principles of this book, food is regarded as:

- Medicine
- Energy
- Connection
- Information

Every meal, every forkful, sends signals to the body that go far beyond calories and nutrients. Food promotes your well-being at a cellular level: When you consider the fact that every single cell in your body has thyroid hormone receptors, you can start to understand how our food choices can influence our thyroid health and overall well-being on a foundational level.

Think of THYROID30 as your immersion course and this chapter as your essential vocabulary guide as you learn this new language. Some words might feel new and awkward at first, but remember, this language is already inside you. Gaining fluency in thyroid-friendly eating will open up a whole new line of communication between you and your body.

As we explore the principles and pillars of thyroid-friendly eating, you'll notice how seamlessly this approach integrates with the 8 Daily Rituals Framework. While the "Refuel" ritual focuses specifically on nourishing your body, what you eat impacts all aspects of your health, from how well your medications work ("Remember") to how well you sleep ("Recharge"). This interconnected framework is what makes THYROID30 so powerful.

WHAT THYROID-HEALTHY EATING CAN DO FOR YOU

In chapter 1, I introduced you to the 8 Daily Rituals of Thyroid-Healthy Living, or the 8 Rs. Here are a few examples of how thyroid-healthy eating can support them—and improve your health in the process. Thyroid-healthy eating can help:

Refuel Your Body:
- Regulate blood sugar and metabolism
- Support proper thyroid hormone production and conversion
- Balance other hormones that interact with thyroid function
- Reach your body's natural, healthy weight

Repair Your Gut Health:
- Heal your gut lining and seal intestinal "leaks"
- Cultivate a diverse and balanced gut microbiome
- Strengthen your immune defenses against infections

Rejuvenate Your Well-Being:
- Dramatically reduce whole-body inflammation
- Calm overactive immune responses in autoimmunity
- Lift persistent brain fog
- Sharpen memory and focus
- Stabilize mood swings and relieve depression

Recharge Your Energy:
- Improve sleep quality
- Support mitochondria, your cellular power plants
- Improve cellular energy production
- Enhance nutrient delivery to tired tissues

Reduce Your Risks:
- Lower your elevated risk of developing additional autoimmune diseases
- Reduce your consumption of toxic, ultra-processed foods
- Minimize your consumption of thyroid-disrupting pesticides and herbicides
- Protect against common thyroid-related complications like heart disease
- Decrease risk factors for prevalent diseases like diabetes, obesity, and cognitive decline

Why Thyroid-Healthy Eating Matters

If your doctor has told you that diet won't make a difference to your thyroid disease, you're not alone. Despite mounting evidence to the contrary, many conventional practitioners still believe that as long as you're taking your thyroid medication, what you eat is irrelevant to thyroid function.

There are several reasons why that's not true. Let's take a closer look at each.

Thyroid hormone production and conversion: Your thyroid gland requires specific nutrients to produce thyroid hormones. Additionally, about 80 percent of the thyroid hormone your body produces is in the inactive form (T4) which must be converted to the active form (T3) to be used by your cells. If you depend on synthetic T4-only medications like levothyroxine, your body also has to convert that T4 into T3. This conversion process is influenced by nutrition status (how well-nourished you are), gut health, and liver health, all of which can be directly impacted by the food we eat.

Inflammation and autoimmunity: Chronic inflammation is regarded as one of the primary drivers of disease, and hypothyroidism can lead to chronically elevated systemic inflammation. Inflammation is especially prominent in people with Hashimoto's, which is an autoimmune disease and the leading cause of hypothyroidism in developed countries. With Hashimoto's, your immune system attacks the thyroid tissue, causing inflammation in the thyroid gland itself and disrupting thyroid function, which can then lead to further inflammation. That autoimmune attack on the thyroid can be triggered by certain foods (like those containing gluten). On the flip side, certain anti-inflammatory foods can help calm inflammation, making food a powerful factor in managing thyroid-related inflammation and autoimmunity.

Gut health and nutrient absorption: Thyroid patients are more likely to experience gut health issues: According to some studies, their risk is five times higher than the general population's. Hypothyroidism also affects our digestive system, including how well we break down and process both the food we eat and our medications. When gut health and digestion are compromised, so is our ability to absorb and assimilate nutrients. This means that excellent nutrition and gut-supportive food choices are of the utmost importance for thyroid patients.

Energy and metabolism: Beyond direct effects on your thyroid function, your food is the fuel your body uses for energy. The quality of this fuel directly impacts your mitochondria, which are like the powerhouses of your cells. Fatigue is one of the most common and plaguing symptoms for thyroid patients, so supporting our energy with optimal food choices is essential.

Thyroid medication isn't a cure-all: While thyroid hormone replacement medications like levothyroxine are an essential part of treatment for most of us, they often leave behind residual symptoms. While medication helps, it doesn't always solve everything, as both patients and doctors may be led to believe, nor does it address underlying root cause factors that may have led to thyroid dysfunction in the first place, like dietary sensitivities, chronic stress, or gut health issues.

This is why feeling your best requires tackling the thyroid trifecta: medical treatment, lifestyle, and diet. Food and lifestyle *do* matter for Thyroid Thrivers. I know this beyond the shadow of a doubt, not only because of the many evidence-based reasons previously mentioned, but also because of my training and my experience working with this community. And, finally, because I'm living proof.

The 5 Principles of Thyroid-Friendly Eating

Put simply, thyroid-friendly eating is:

1. Anti-inflammatory
2. Nutrient-dense
3. Gut-healing
4. Blood sugar–friendly
5. Personalized

These are the five principles that guide all of my recipes and resources, including the ones in this book.

Thyroid-friendly eating is not a diet but a new perspective on food and the power it has over our health—for better or worse. When we make the shift to a thyroid-friendly style of eating, we pass our food choices through an upgraded filter: Will this food serve and support my well-being or diminish it?

There's a lot to learn when you're new to this eating approach, and finding your ideal, sustainable path will take time. That's okay. Give yourself the gift of letting this process take the time it takes: Trying to do too much at once tends to set people back. Every small step adds up, and eventually you will master the skills of learning to control symptoms and manage inflammation, and will have the energy you need to live and love your life to the fullest.

While THYROID30 makes a great springboard into thyroid-friendly eating, the long-term goal is long-term results. That's why these nutritional principles are timeless, rooted in functional nutrition, recommended by the leading thyroid and autoimmune experts, and have been proven effective by thousands of thyroid patients. They have also stood the tests of time, scrutiny, and emerging research, and can support anyone's ongoing health and vitality. Let's take a closer look at what each of these five nutritional principles means.

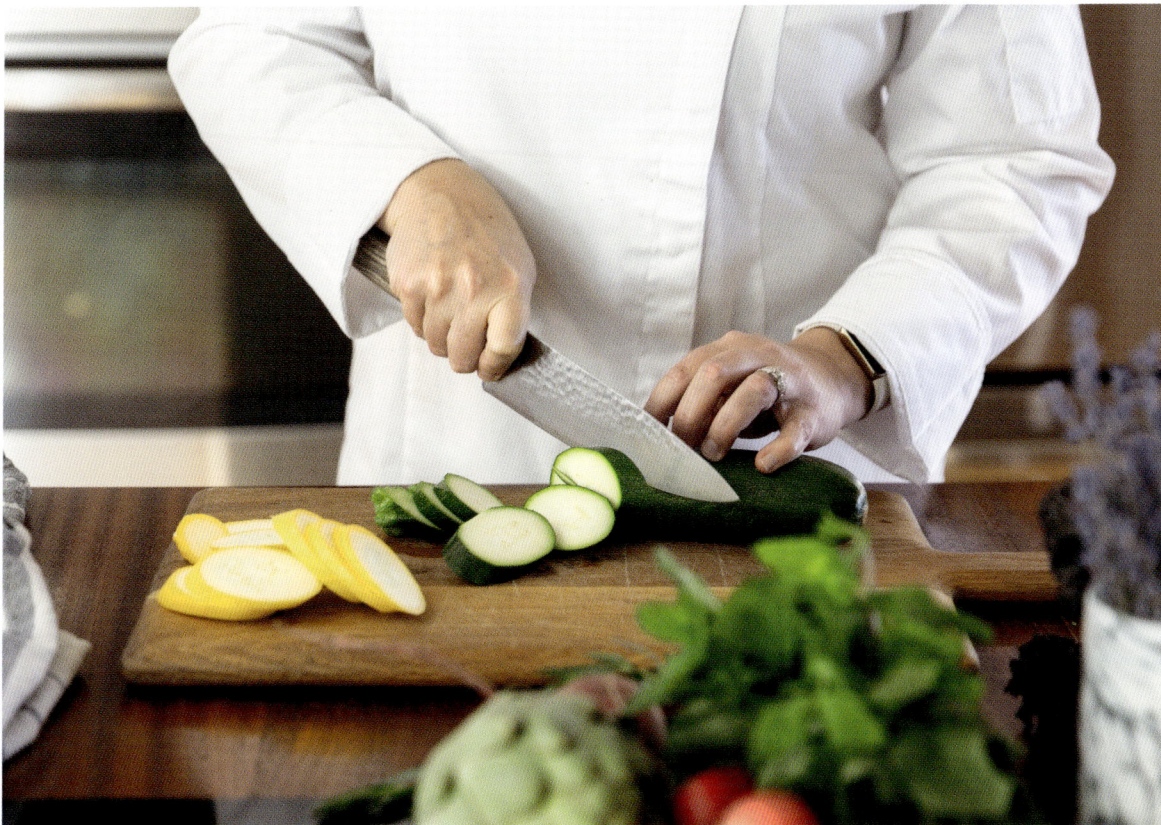

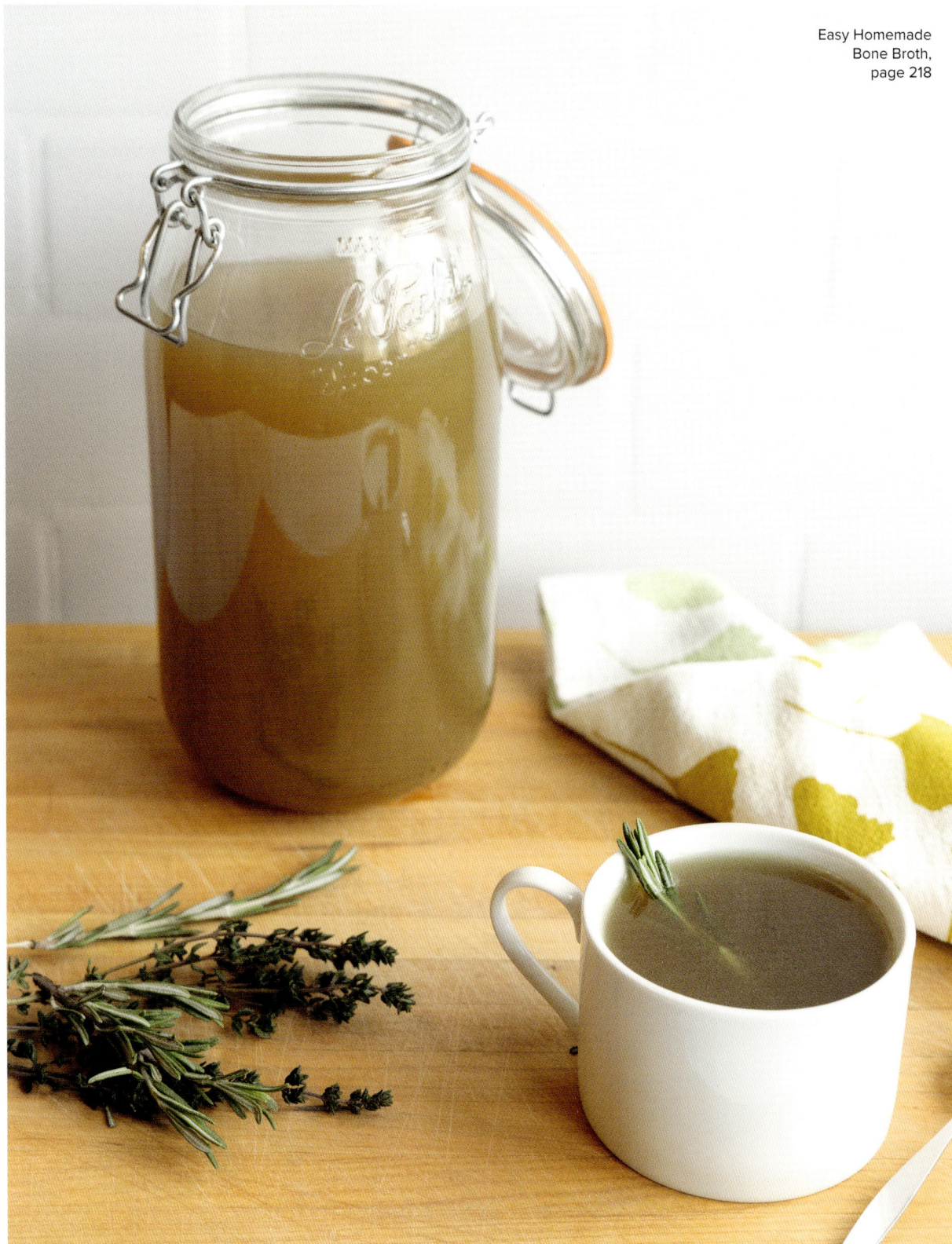

Easy Homemade
Bone Broth,
page 218

1 An Anti-inflammatory Approach

I often hear thyroid patients say things like, "I feel ten years older than my actual age." That's inflammation at work, and it's at the root of many thyroid-related struggles.

Inflammation is a natural and necessary part of your body's healing and defense system. It's when inflammation becomes chronic and systemic that it creates serious problems, especially for thyroid patients.

Here's why. Inflammation can:

- Disrupt the hypothalamic-pituitary-thyroid signals (the HPT-axis), which regulates thyroid function and hormone levels
- Damage thyroid tissue, leading to reduced hormone production and impaired thyroid function
- Block thyroid hormone receptors, reducing the body's ability to use thyroid hormones
- Inhibit the conversion of T4 to active T3
- Increase production of reverse T3 (rT3), potentially reducing thyroid hormone uptake by the cells

While we may not have complete control over our body's inflammatory responses, one of the best ways to dial it down is the food on our plates. Anti-inflammatory eating approaches like the Mediterranean diet have emerged as an effective way to manage and prevent inflammation and disease.

There are three key aspects of anti-inflammatory eating:

1. **Avoiding inflammatory foods:** Many unhealthy and highly processed foods can contribute to inflammation. To reduce inflammation, we want to avoid foods that are generally considered inflammatory, including highly refined white flour, gluten, sugar, trans fats, fried foods, industrially refined cooking oils (such as soybean and canola oil), artificial ingredients, and ultra-processed foods (UPFs). These foods can promote oxidative stress, disrupt hormone balance, and contribute to gut health issues.

2. **Avoiding foods we are personally sensitive to:** While some foods are generally considered inflammatory, others depend on individual sensitivities. Common culprits for Thyroid Thrivers include dairy, grains, soy, legumes, nightshades, nuts, and eggs. Identifying and eliminating personal trigger foods is baked right into thyroid-friendly eating and can help reduce symptoms and improve overall well-being.

3. **Incorporating anti-inflammatory foods:** It's not just about what we remove from our diets; it's about adding in more of the good stuff! Whole, nutrient-dense, anti-inflammatory foods help calm the immune system, support gut health, and reduce oxidative stress.

The Takeaway: Your daily food choices have tremendous power to either promote or reduce inflammation. The standard American diet (SAD)—high in refined carbohydrates, industrial seed oils, and ultra-processed foods—creates the perfect inflammatory storm. By contrast, a thyroid-healthy diet built on colorful plant foods, high-quality proteins, and healthy fats is naturally anti-inflammatory.

ANTI-INFLAMMATORY FOODS

- **Healthy fats:** Avocados, extra-virgin olive oil, coconut oil, nuts, and seeds (if tolerated)
- **Fatty fish:** Wild-caught salmon, sardines, mackerel, and other omega-3-rich seafood
- **Anti-inflammatory spices:** Ginger, turmeric, garlic, cinnamon, and many more
- **Leafy greens and cruciferous vegetables:** Kale, spinach, broccoli, and Brussels sprouts (preferably cooked to reduce goitrogens)
- **Colorful fruits and vegetables:** Foods like berries, sweet potatoes, carrots, and bell peppers, among many others, provide antioxidants that combat oxidative stress.
- **Gut-healing foods:** Foods like bone broth, fermented vegetables, and collagen, among many others, support gut health and immune function.

2 Maximizing Nutrient Density

When it comes to your food choices, it's not just about quantity: It's about quality. While conventional diets focus primarily on calories and macronutrients—protein, fat, and fiber—thyroid-friendly eating puts added focus on micronutrients, the vitamins, minerals, phytonutrients, and other compounds that support your overall health, boost your energy, foster mental clarity, prevent aging and disease, and help to optimize your overall thyroid function on a cellular level.

Your thyroid depends on key nutrients to:

- Produce thyroid hormones
- Convert T4 into active T3
- Transport and regulate hormones in the bloodstream
- Protect against oxidative stress
- Support thyroid hormone receptor function on a cellular level

The Takeaway: By consistently choosing nutrient-dense whole foods, you provide your body with essential nutrients, often in their most bioavailable and effective forms. These foods also contain synergistic compounds that can enhance nutrient absorption and utilization, helping both you and your thyroid function at their best.

3 A Gut-Supportive Focus

The relationship between your gut and your thyroid is a critical piece of the puzzle for Thyroid Thrivers. It's called the thyroid-gut axis, and it's a powerful two-way line of communication between your gut and your thyroid. They constantly influence one another, meaning that what's going on with one affects the other—for better or worse!

Here's what the thyroid-gut axis means for you:

- **Twenty percent of thyroid hormone conversion happens in the gut.** This means that even if you're properly medicated, gut imbalances can limit how much active T3 your body can access and use.

- **Thyroid hormones regulate digestion.** This impacts gut motility, digestive enzyme production, and stomach acid levels. Hypothyroidism is strongly linked to hypochlorhydria, or low stomach acid, which can lead to poor digestion and nutrient absorption, as well as dysbiosis.

- **Autoimmune thyroid patients are more prone to leaky gut.** There is a well-established connection between intestinal permeability and autoimmune thyroid disease. When the intestinal lining becomes compromised, tight junctions between cells loosen, allowing food particles, toxins, and bacteria to enter the bloodstream. The immune system then launches an attack, which can trigger or worsen thyroid autoimmunity.

- **Poor gut health affects your overall health.** Because 70 percent of your immune system is housed in your gut, an unhealthy gut means compromised immunity. There's also a strong gut-brain axis, so your brain and mental health can also be significantly impacted.

So, how can thyroid-friendly eating support gut health? So many ways! By focusing on the 5 Pillars of Thyroid-Friendly Eating (which we'll discuss in the next section), we can:

- Reduce our exposure to gut-disrupting foods and toxins
- Support healthy digestion with plenty of colorful plant foods
- Maintain a healthy and balanced gut biome
- Promote beneficial bacteria with probiotic foods
- Feed beneficial gut bacteria with prebiotic fiber
- Calm, heal, and seal an inflamed or leaky gut with amino acids like glycine, glutamine, and proline found in collagen-rich foods like bone broth

The Takeaway: Thyroid-friendly eating is gut-friendly eating: The two go hand in hand. And by supporting our gut health with our food choices, we are, in turn, supporting our thyroid function.

FOODS TO SUPPORT A HEALTHY GUT (AND THYROID!)

FOODS TO AVOID	PROBIOTIC FOODS	PREBIOTIC FOODS	ANTI-INFLAMMATORY AND DIGESTIVE FOODS	GUT-HEALING FOODS
Alcohol	Cultured buttermilk (for those who tolerate dairy)	Blackberries	Asparagus	Bone broth (one of the richest sources of collagen)
Artificial additives	Fermented pickles	Blueberries	Avocado	Bone-in pastured poultry (including skin)
Artificial preservatives	Fermented sauerkraut	Cacao/dark chocolate	Berries	Canned salmon (especially with skin and bones included)
Artificial sweeteners (aspartame, sucralose, saccharine)	Fermented soy products in moderation if tolerated (for example, tempeh, natto, soybean-based miso)	Chicory root	Bitter greens (for example, dandelion, radicchio)	Eggs (if tolerated)
Cured and processed meats (hot dogs, salami, deli meat with added nitrates)	Kefir (try coconut or water-based for dairy-free)	Cooked, cooled, and reheated potatoes	Bone broth	Gelatin
Foods you are personally intolerant to (for example, dairy, nightshades, eggs, nuts, beans, grains, super-spicy foods, and so on)	Kimchi	Cooked, cooled, and reheated rice or rice pasta	Broccoli	Grass-fed beef collagen peptides (a.k.a. collagen hydrolysate)
Fried foods	Kombucha (consume in moderation due to sugar content)	Dandelion greens	Cabbage	Grass-fed beef shanks, short ribs, oxtails, or tongue
Gluten (wheat, barley, rye)	Kvass	Flaxseeds	Cacao/dark chocolate	Lamb shanks
Industrially refined fats	Miso (chickpea miso is gluten-free and soy-free)	Garlic	Cherries	Liver and other organ meats
Refined or excessive sugar	Traditionally fermented olives	Globe artichokes	Cinnamon	Pork shanks or ribs
Trans fats and partially hydrogenated oils	Unfiltered apple cider vinegar (ACV)	Green bananas	Cumin	Shellfish (for example, shrimp, crab, lobster)
Ultra-processed snacks	Yogurt (choose low- or no-sugar brands with simple, recognizable ingredients and live and active cultures; try coconut or nut-based for dairy-free)	Green plantains	Extra-virgin olive oil	Whole sardines (with skin and bones)
		Jerusalem artichokes	Fatty fish	
		Jicama	Fennel	
		Leeks	Flaxseeds	
		Legumes (if tolerated, properly soaked and cooked for better digestibility)	Garlic	
		Mushrooms	Globe artichokes	
		Nuts	Green tea	
		Onions	Kiwi	
		Pomegranate	Leafy greens	
		Raspberries	Lemons	
		Seaweed (nori-style is a good choice to avoid excessive iodine)	Limes	
		Strawberries	Mushrooms	
		Sweet potatoes	Papaya (fruit and seeds)	
			Pineapple	
			Quinoa, rinsed to remove saponins	
			Sweet potatoes	
			Turmeric	
			Unfiltered ACV	
			Walnuts (spaced away from thyroid meds)	

4 A Blood Sugar–Balancing Eating Style

One of the most overlooked aspects of thyroid health is blood sugar balance. Many thyroid patients find themselves caught in a frustrating cycle of energy crashes, cravings, and weight struggles without realizing that unstable blood sugar may be a contributing factor, or that simple changes can end this cycle.

Your thyroid gland plays a central role in regulating metabolism and energy production, processes that are tightly intertwined with blood sugar regulation. When thyroid function is impaired, metabolic processes slow down, which can affect how your body uses insulin, the hormone that helps move glucose from your bloodstream into your cells. In some cases, this can lead to increased insulin resistance, blood sugar imbalances, and a greater risk of developing type 2 diabetes over time.

Common habits that keep you trapped on the blood sugar roller coaster:

- Morning coffee on an empty stomach
- Carb-heavy breakfasts with little to no protein
- No protein with meals and snacks
- Chronically high stress levels that go unchecked and unmanaged
- Regular consumption of soft drinks, sugary foods, processed snacks, and refined carbs
- Alcohol consumption, especially before bed
- Frequent marijuana use
- Poor sleep hygiene

These habits can trigger a cascade of hormonal responses, including:

- Increased inflammation throughout your body
- Impaired thyroid hormone conversion (T4 to T3)
- Stress on your adrenal glands, affecting cortisol production
- Disrupted sleep patterns
- Worsening fatigue and brain fog
- Strong cravings that derail your best intentions

Blood sugar is supposed to fluctuate to some degree: It's never going to be a flat line, but thyroid-friendly eating is designed to prevent the erratic highs and lows that can zap your energy, crash your mood, mess up your sleep, and lead to unwanted weight gain. By emphasizing protein, healthy fats, and fiber-rich produce, you'll help your body maintain steadier energy levels throughout the day. This balanced approach prevents the dramatic spikes and crashes that come from consuming quick-burning refined carbohydrates.

Many THYROID30 participants report that one of the first benefits they notice is "more even energy" or "no more afternoon crashes." One participant in particular comes to mind: We'll call her Jackie. Jackie loved to bake for her family, but traditional baked goods are often loaded with quick-burning refined carbohydrates like white flour and sugar. Blood sugar balance wasn't really on Jackie's radar. She often started her day with oatmeal topped with berries, which is a meal with many nutritional pros (for those who tolerate gluten-free grains), but lacks protein. She participated in THYROID30 to learn more about thyroid-friendly eating.

Not everyone chooses to follow the meal plans, but Jackie followed them to the letter. When we hopped on a group coaching call at the one-week mark, she was beaming. "I feel like a whole new person," she told me. "I have so much more energy, I'm happier, my energy isn't so up and down, and I feel so much calmer."

That newfound energy and sense of calm stuck with Jackie because she now understood how and why to balance her blood sugar with simple, healthy eating habits. These are the kinds of lifelong skills I absolutely love to empower people with.

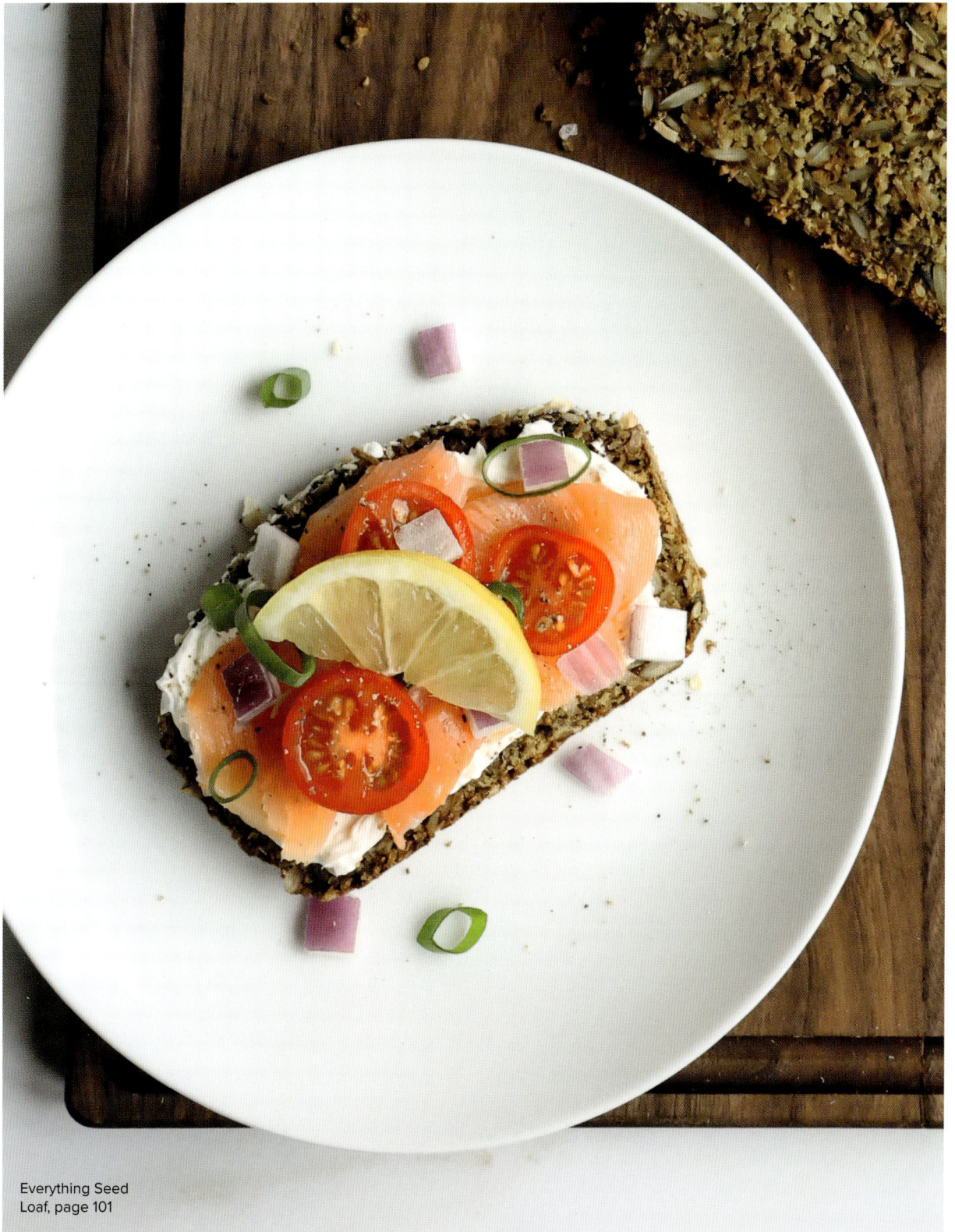

Everything Seed
Loaf, page 101

ONE IMPORTANT NOTE ABOUT SUGAR

Don't fall into the trap of trading sugary foods or soft drinks for sugar-free versions made with artificial sweeteners. These come with a host of health risks, and studies have shown they may even lead to the development of Hashimoto's!

What habits shifted things for Jackie?

- Enjoying a savory, protein-rich breakfast
- Eating breakfast *before* having coffee
- Including protein with every meal and snack
- Getting most of her carbs from nutrient-dense whole plant foods
- Satisfying her sweet tooth with low-sugar, high-fiber fruits like berries
- Swapping traditional baking for paleo-style recipes made with more protein, fiber, and healthy-fat-rich ingredients, and just a small amount of natural sweeteners like honey or maple syrup

Jackie's energy transformation happened *without* giving up her love of baking or making her feel deprived.

What's even more encouraging is that studies have found that balancing blood sugar can help reduce thyroid antibodies in Hashimoto's patients, directly affecting the autoimmune process. This makes blood sugar regulation not just a symptom management strategy but a potential root cause approach.

Unlike highly restrictive or extremely low-carb diets, THYROID30 offers a balanced, sustainable way to regulate blood sugar while supporting all aspects of thyroid health.

The Takeaway: By focusing on whole foods and the right balance of macronutrients—high-quality protein, healthy fats, complex carbs, and fiber—you, like Jackie, may finally be able to get off the blood sugar roller coaster you've been riding for years.

5 Personalization Is Paramount

Perhaps the most important principle of thyroid-friendly eating is recognizing that we are all unique, with unique dietary needs and sensitivities. That's why there is no one-size-fits-all approach. Your optimal way of eating may look different from mine—or anyone else's, for that matter.

This nutritional concept of personalization is called *bio-individuality,* meaning that your optimal diet should consist of foods that work *for you* personally and should avoid foods that work against you. I often field comments on social media like, "I thought nightshades were bad for the thyroid" or "I thought we were supposed to avoid all grains." My answer is simple and almost always the same: It depends on the individual.

A food might be generally considered "healthy," but if you are sensitive to it, it's likely to contribute to inflammation and gut health issues and won't be healthy for *you.* Conversely, just because paleo and AIP both eliminate gluten-free grains and legumes, for example, doesn't mean that *all* Thyroid Thrivers need to eliminate gluten-free grains and legumes. The goal isn't to eliminate as many foods as possible: It's not a competition to see who can withstand the most limited diet, and there are no prizes awarded for having the most dietary restrictions. The goal is to *heal* and eventually to reintroduce as many foods as possible—even with AIP!

We may need to avoid some foods permanently and entirely, while we may find we can tolerate certain amounts of others. And we may be able to successfully introduce still other foods after root cause factors are addressed and healing has occurred (especially when it comes to healing the gut). So, not only is our ideal bio-individual diet personalized, but it can also change over time.

My experience, both personally and in working with my community, has shown me that once root cause factors are addressed and thyroid issues are well managed, Thrivers are often able to tolerate more foods rather than fewer. The development of new food sensitivities can be an indication that new root cause factors have arisen, like gut dysbiosis, for example.

The good news is that as you tune in, learn these skills, and add these tools to your toolbox, it will become easier to recognize and address new dietary sensitivities (if they arise). Again, just like learning a new language, you will become more fluent and confident with practice.

The Takeaway: Dietary diversity and food freedom are important, as is meeting yourself where you are. Personalizing your eating approach is not just about food sensitivities: It's about what is and isn't sustainable for you, and what is and isn't appropriate for you at this time. That's why the THYROID30 community is a judgment-free zone. Just because one person is thriving on the AIP, for example, doesn't mean it's the right approach for everyone. That's why the meal plans offered here can be tweaked and adjusted to fit your needs. The THYROID30 framework both welcomes your unique dietary needs and teaches you how to identify them.

HOW NOT TO DO THE AUTOIMMUNE PROTOCOL

The first time I embarked on the Autoimmune Protocol (AIP), at the recommendation of my naturopath, I didn't know what to expect, so I neglected to tell her that we had just gutted our 1979 kitchen and would be cooking on a hot plate in the garage for the next five months.

I white-knuckled it and stuck to the elimination phase of AIP for 30 days as per her recommendation. It helped with the gut healing we were working on, but there was a *lot* of cooking involved, which wasn't ideal when we were doing our dishes by hand in the laundry room sink and dining out two or three nights a week! Nonetheless, I managed (barely) and did feel better.

At the end of those 30 days, when I was *supposed* to start the systematic reintroduction phases, I was so burned out by trying to do all that cooking under all those restrictions under less-than-ideal circumstances that I blew it. I went right back to eating nightshades, nuts, eggs, seeds, spices, and basically everything but gluten and dairy within a few days. In doing so, I also blew my opportunity to reintroduce these foods one by one (with a few days in between each) to isolate reactions and see what symptoms, if any, each of these foods was causing.

If I could turn back time, I would have mentioned our kitchen renovation to my doctor. I imagine she would have said something like, "Okay, let's talk about a less restrictive approach (like paleo, perhaps) that will help calm inflammation and give you the opportunity to identify some common food sensitivities without having to cook for a full-blown elimination diet on the workbench between your skis and scuba gear!" Lesson learned.

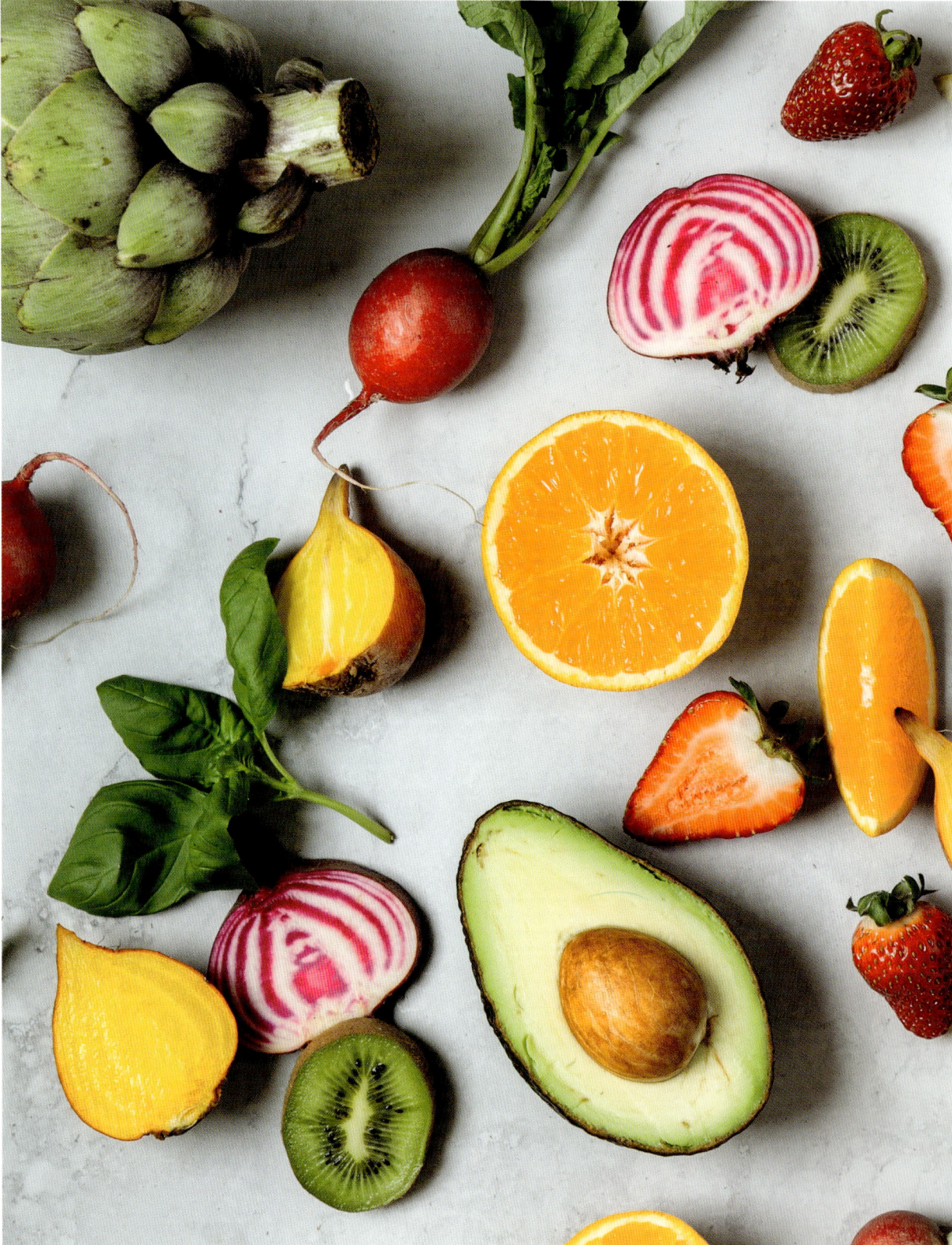

The 5 Pillars of Thyroid-Friendly Eating

Now that you understand the principles behind thyroid-healthy eating, let's take a look at what thyroid-friendly meals are made of. These five pillars translate the five principles you just learned into the thyroid-friendly meals on your plate.

The 5 Pillars of Thyroid-Friendly Eating are:

1. Lots of colorful produce (organic if possible)
2. High-quality protein
3. Thyroid-supportive foods
4. Healthy fats
5. Adequate hydration using filtered water

Let's explore each of these pillars in a little more detail.

Pillar 1: Lots of Colorful Produce

"Eat the rainbow" is more than just a nutrition trend: It's an evidence-backed concept with staying power. Scientists have categorized over 25,000 different phytonutrients found in plant-based foods, many of which also have antioxidant properties. For Thyroid Thrivers, eating the rainbow supports thyroid health by reducing inflammation, enhancing natural detox pathways, and protecting against oxidative stress—all of which play a role in hormone balance and immune function.

The goal is to include a variety of vegetables, fruits, herbs, and spices in your meals while adhering to your personal dietary requirements. This dietary diversity delivers a broad spectrum of nutrients that support metabolism at a cellular level and promote overall well-being.

A diverse diet is especially helpful in nourishing a diverse gut microbiome. Fiber-rich plant foods play a vital role in supporting gut health, especially by delivering prebiotic fiber, which feeds the beneficial bacteria in your gut.

Is buying only organic produce absolutely essential? No. While organic produce can help "reduce" exposure to pesticides and agricultural chemicals, the best produce is the produce on your plate. Conventional produce is better than no produce, and it provides a net-positive nutritional benefit.

Pillar 2: High-Quality Protein

Protein plays a vital role in balancing blood sugar, maintaining and building lean muscle mass, supporting the body's natural detoxification pathways, and promoting steady energy levels. Protein is essential for the thyroid because it provides key amino acids and minerals needed for thyroid hormone production. For example, your body uses tyrosine—an amino acid found in meat, fish, eggs, nuts, and seeds—along with iodine to make T4, the primary thyroid hormone.

Many animal proteins are also rich in selenium, zinc, iron, and B vitamins, all of which are crucial to thyroid function. While animal proteins are typically complete proteins (that is, they contain all nine essential amino acids), plant proteins can also be excellent sources, especially when a variety of plant foods are included in the diet throughout the day to provide all nine essential amino acids.

In terms of quantity, a good general target is 20 to 30 grams of protein per meal, depending on your body size, activity level, and health goals. Some sources recommend 30 to 50 grams per meal for those focused on blood sugar balance, muscle maintenance, or fat loss. The quality of the animal protein you consume—meaning how the animals were raised, fed, and harvested—can make a significant difference in what the protein can offer you nutritionally, so it's a good idea to opt for certified organic animal products whenever possible. While organic guidelines can vary, meat and eggs with the USDA organic label, for example, come from animals that have received 100 percent organic feed and forage and access to pasture and outdoor space, and have not been given antibiotics or added hormones.

Best choices for high-quality animal protein:

- Wild-caught fish, especially those low in mercury and high in omega-3s, such as salmon, sardines, and trout
- Organic, grass-fed or grass-finished beef and lamb
- Organic, pasture-raised poultry and eggs
- Organic, pasture-raised pork

Best choices for plant-based proteins (soy-free options):

- Legumes (chickpeas, black beans, kidney beans, lentils): Rich in fiber, iron, and protein
- Quinoa: A complete plant protein with all nine essential amino acids
- Buckwheat: Another complete plant protein with all nine essential amino acids
- Hemp seeds: High in protein, omega-3s, and magnesium; yet another complete plant protein
- Pumpkin seeds: Rich in zinc, a key thyroid-supporting nutrient
- Chia seeds: Contain protein, fiber, and anti-inflammatory omega-3s
- Tree nuts (almonds, walnuts, cashews): Contain protein and healthy fats

While many plant-based proteins are lower in certain essential amino acids than animal-based proteins, combining a variety of sources can provide a complete protein profile. Examples include:

- Rice + beans
- Sweet potatoes + lentils + tahini
- Corn + black beans
- Oats + pumpkin seeds

FAQ: WHAT ABOUT PLANT-BASED DIETS?

Plant-based diets work well for some people, but not for others. Some Thyroid Thrivers feel great on a plant-based diet, while others may experience fatigue, hair thinning, blood sugar instability, weakness, or difficulty maintaining lean muscle mass. If you're following a plant-based approach and not feeling your best, it may be time to evaluate whether your body's unique nutritional needs are being met.

Several key thyroid-supportive nutrients are more abundant and bioavailable in animal-based foods, which can make plant-based diets more challenging for those with thyroid issues, especially when food sensitivities or gut health concerns limit your ability to eat legumes, nuts, or seeds.

Meeting your protein and micronutrient needs—particularly vitamin B12, iron, zinc, and the amino acid tyrosine—on a plant-based diet requires more intentional planning, but it is possible. My best advice is to work one-on-one with a thyroid-savvy nutritionist or dietitian to ensure you're getting the full spectrum of nutrients your thyroid needs, whether through food, fortified sources, or targeted supplementation.

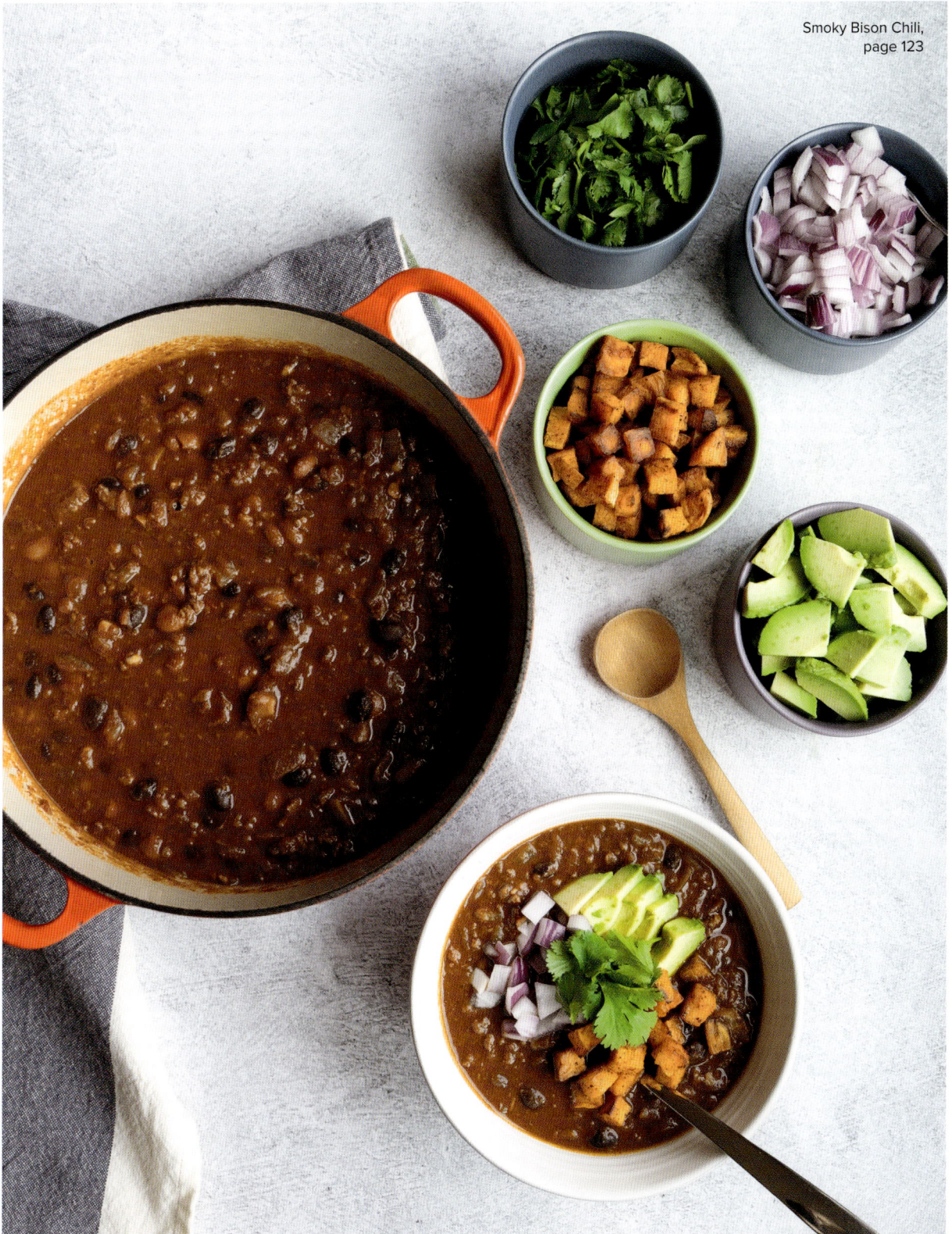

Smoky Bison Chili,
page 123

Pillar 3: Thyroid-Supportive Foods

While thyroid-friendly eating is based on the foundations of functional nutrition, this is the point at which we consider how we can support the thyroid more specifically with food. There are three main ways to do this:

1. Include foods in our diets that provide key thyroid-supporting nutrients

2. Include detoxifying foods in our diets to help protect the thyroid from environmental toxins and improve overall thyroid hormone function

3. Include foods in our diets that heal, protect, and maintain gut health so we can positively influence our thyroid health through better gut health

We talked about the importance of gut-healthy foods on pages 38 to 39, so now I'll talk you through the other two aspects of Pillar 3.

1. Key Thyroid-Supporting Nutrients in Food

While the thyroid relies on many nutrients, these are some of the most important and influential for thyroid function.

- **Tyrosine** is an amino acid that combines with iodine to form thyroid hormones. **Sources:** Grass-fed beef, lamb, poultry, pork, wild-caught fish, oats, lentils, beans

- **Vitamin A** is necessary for thyroid hormone activation, especially the conversion of T4 to active T3. **Sources:** Liver, ghee, egg yolks, and wild-caught fish

- **Vitamin C** is an antioxidant that supports iron absorption, collagen synthesis, and thyroid hormone balance. **Sources:** Citrus fruits, bell peppers, strawberries, kiwi, tomatoes, and cruciferous vegetables

- **Vitamin D** plays a crucial role in immune regulation, especially for those with autoimmune thyroid disease. Studies show that over 70 percent of Hashimoto's patients are vitamin D deficient. **Dairy-free sources:** Sardines, salmon, tuna, egg yolks, and sunlight!

- **Iodine** is required for thyroid hormone production. It's an essential nutrient that the body cannot produce on its own. **Sources:** Eggs, meat, poultry, seafood, cranberries, potatoes (with skin), and select seaweed varieties

IODIZED SALT VS. NATURAL SALT: WHAT'S BEST FOR YOUR THYROID?

Many people wonder whether iodized salt is essential for thyroid health. The short answer is no. While iodine is crucial for thyroid hormone production, iodized table salt is highly processed: It is stripped of its natural minerals and then fortified with iodine. In contrast, unrefined salts like Celtic sea salt and Himalayan salt contain a broad spectrum of trace minerals, which can support overall health. (See THYROID30 Support and Resources on page 246 for mineral-rich salt recommendations.) However, these natural salts contain little to no iodine, so you may need to ensure adequate intake from other food sources, like seafood, eggs, dairy (if tolerated), nori or wakame seaweed, turkey, or potatoes with skin. The RDA for iodine is 150 mcg per day. Remember, balance is key: Both too much and too little iodine can disrupt thyroid function.

- **Iron** is essential for thyroid hormone production. Deficiency can contribute to hypothyroidism, and hypothyroidism can impair iron absorption, creating a vicious cycle. **Sources:** Grass-fed beef, liver, shellfish, eggs, legumes, and dark leafy greens

- **Selenium** helps regulate thyroid hormones and supports antioxidant activity, protecting the thyroid from oxidative stress. **Sources:** Brazil nuts, wild-caught salmon, sardines, oysters, shrimp, and mushrooms

- **Zinc** helps reduce thyroid-related inflammation and supports cognitive function. **Sources:** Oysters, beef, lamb, pumpkin seeds, pork, mushrooms, spinach, cashews, and cacao

2. Thyroid-Supporting Detoxifying Foods

The thyroid is highly sensitive to environmental toxins, making detoxification a key factor in thyroid health. Toxins can disrupt thyroid function, interfere with how we metabolize thyroid medication, and impair the conversion of inactive T4 into active T3.

The body's built-in detox pathways are highly effective at handling toxins, so harsh detoxes are not needed—and can even do more harm than good. That said, we're also bombarded with an unprecedented amount of toxins in the modern world, so we can benefit from gently supporting our natural detoxification systems. Luckily, many foods have detoxifying properties or support the body's ability to detoxify in direct and indirect ways. Here are some of the MVPs:

- **Blueberries** have the highest antioxidant levels of any commonly consumed fruit or vegetable, and wild blueberries, in particular, have twice the antioxidants of cultivated blueberries. These high levels of antioxidants, particularly anthocyanins, help protect and support the liver by neutralizing free radicals and reducing inflammation, while their high fiber content promotes healthy digestion and the excretion of toxins.

- **Cilantro** is a natural chelator, meaning that it helps bind and remove heavy metals from the body. Because heavy metals have been linked to thyroid disease and increased thyroid antibodies, incorporating chelating foods like cilantro can provide gentle, natural detox support.

- **Turmeric** is another natural chelator with detox-supportive properties. It helps regulate liver enzymes and protects against glutathione depletion (glutathione is one of the body's most powerful antioxidants and detoxifiers).

- **Artichokes** promote bile flow, protect the liver from damage, and even support the regeneration of liver tissue. They help prevent fat buildup and reduce inflammation in the liver, both of which are key for optimal liver function.

- **Beets** support liver detoxification, aid in eliminating toxins, and provide cellular protection against oxidative stress.

- **Lemon** stimulates digestive juices, aiding in digestion and nutrient absorption while promoting waste elimination. Drinking warm lemon water with a pinch of sea salt in the morning can help support digestion, reduce bloating, and nourish the adrenals.

You'll find these detoxifying superfoods woven throughout the recipes in this cookbook.

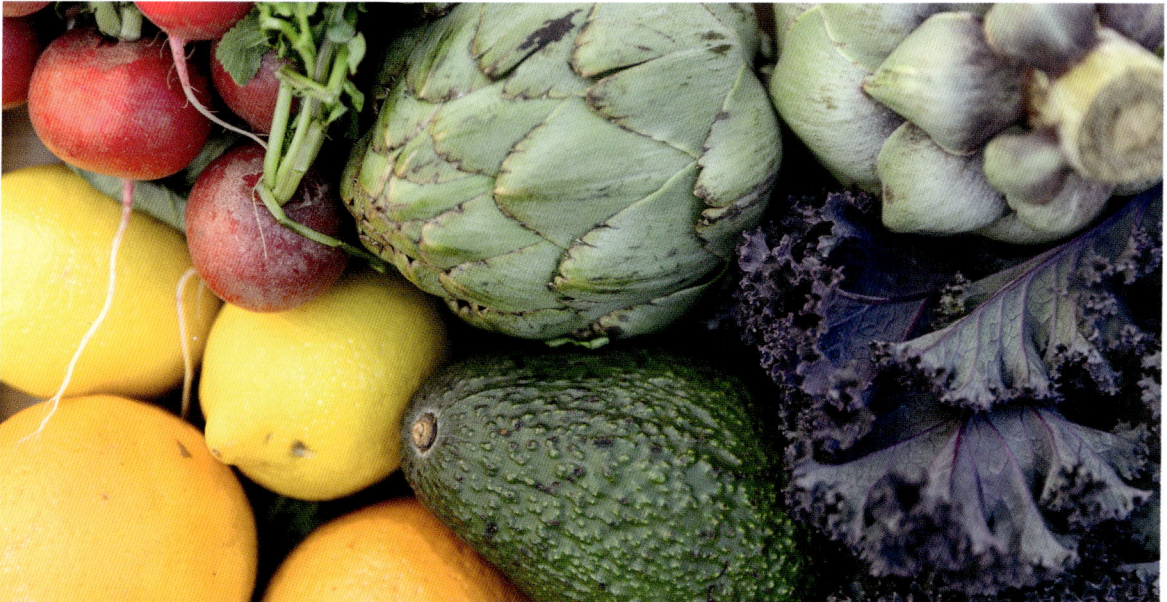

Pillar 4: Healthy Fats

Healthy fats are a cornerstone of thyroid-friendly eating, playing a vital role in overall wellness. They are essential for hormone production, brain function, and reduction of inflammation. They promote satiety, enhance mitochondrial and cellular function, boost energy levels, and help the body absorb fat-soluble vitamins like A, D, E, and K.

Some of my favorite thyroid-supportive cooking fats include:

- **Avocado oil:** A heart-healthy oil with a very high smoke point and ideal for just about any cooking purpose

- **Extra-virgin olive oil:** Rich in antioxidants and anti-inflammatory compounds; contrary to popular belief, extra-virgin olive oil can be a great cooking oil for temperatures as high as 400°F (204°C). It's because of those high levels of antioxidants that extra-virgin olive oil is more resistant to heat-related oxidation than previously believed. Look for the words "extra virgin" on the label to be sure you're getting the most health-supportive, antioxidant-rich, and unrefined olive oil available.

- **Unrefined coconut oil:** Contains medium-chain triglycerides (MCTs) that can support energy production and metabolism; note that you want unrefined coconut oil, not refined.

- **Ghee:** A clarified butter that's easy to digest, packed with fat-soluble vitamins, and free of lactose and casein (two components that cause inflammation for many Thyroid Thrivers)

Equally as important as incorporating healthy fats into your diet is avoiding inflammatory, industrially refined oils like vegetable, canola, soybean, corn, and sunflower. These oils are often chemically processed and high in omega-6 fatty acids, which can contribute to systemic inflammation and disrupt hormonal balance. By prioritizing healthy fats, you're giving your thyroid—and your whole body—the fuel it needs to function optimally.

Pillar 5: Adequate Hydration Using Filtered Water

Hydration is essential for every system in the body, but it plays a particularly important role for those with hypothyroidism. Proper hydration supports digestion, energy levels, cognitive function, and metabolism while also helping to support our built-in detoxification systems and flush out toxins that could otherwise interfere with thyroid function. Studies have also shown that drinking around 68 ounces (2 L) of water per day can slightly boost calorie burning, supporting weight management.

How much water should you drink? While individual needs vary, a good rule of thumb is a minimum of 64 ounces (1.9 L), or eight 8-ounce (240 ml) glasses, per day, increasing accordingly for factors like activity level, climate, and other bio-individual considerations.

What happens when we don't drink enough water? Dehydration can exacerbate common thyroid symptoms such as fatigue, brain fog, dry skin, constipation, and sluggish digestion.

The quality of water you drink also matters. Tap water often contains fluoride and chlorine, both of which can block thyroid receptors and interfere with the absorption of iodine, a critical nutrient for thyroid hormone production. (In fact, fluoride was once used medicinally to suppress an overactive thyroid!) Heavy metals and microplastics, which can accumulate in the thyroid, are another concern in some water sources.

Drinking filtered or purified water is the best way to avoid these thyroid-disrupting toxins; however, not all filters remove fluoride and chlorine, so it's important to choose one that does. By making hydration a priority and choosing the right water filter, you'll be supporting your thyroid, your metabolism, and your overall health and vitality. (See THYROID30 Support and Resources on page 246 for my favorite thyroid-friendly water filter recommendation.)

Common Dietary Trigger Foods for Thyroid Thrivers

While there's no one-size-fits-all "thyroid diet," many Thyroid Thrivers share common dietary triggers that can spark symptoms, cause autoimmune flares, or even contribute to the root cause of thyroid disease. Identifying your unique triggers often involves an elimination and reintroduction process, which we'll cover in the next section.

First, let's cover the most common dietary trigger foods for Thyroid Thrivers.

Things to keep in mind before we dive into the trigger foods:
The inclusion of a food on this list doesn't necessarily mean that it's an "unhealthy" food. Many of these foods offer very beneficial nutrients, and not every Thyroid Thriver needs to avoid all of them.

All-or-nothing thinking, like putting foods into "bad" versus "good" categories based on these lists, is one of the most common pitfalls for those embarking on a thyroid-friendly, anti-inflammatory, or autoimmune-friendly eating approach. Vilifying these foods can contribute to unnecessary dietary eliminations, food fear, loss of the ability to tolerate these foods, and even disordered eating. So, I invite you to lean into the nuance around these potential trigger foods. Be mindful, not fearful. Know that just because a food might be inflammatory for one person doesn't mean it will be inflammatory for you. And if a food isn't right for you right now, that might not be the case forever. As our bodies heal and change over time, our dietary triggers may also change.

Gluten

Gluten is the top dietary trigger for thyroid patients. Even in people without a celiac or gluten sensitivity diagnosis, gluten can drive chronic illness, autoimmunity, and gut issues. Research shows that even tiny amounts can provoke an inflammatory response that lasts for months. Many thyroid nutrition experts recommend completely and permanently eliminating gluten. While not everyone notices a difference by eliminating gluten, many do, making it well worth a trial elimination.

Dairy

Dairy is second on the list of the most common dietary trigger foods for Thyroid Thrivers. Compounds like lactose and casein can spark inflammation and contribute to leaky gut in sensitive individuals. According to thyroid specialist Dr. Izabella Wentz, going dairy-free often reduces symptoms and antibodies in those with Hashimoto's.

It's important to note that lactose-free products won't help those who are reactive to casein, the primary protein in milk. And alternatives like goat or sheep dairy aren't necessarily safe substitutes, either: Studies show that 60 to 75 percent of people who react to cow's milk also experience cross-reactivity to these products.

That said, some Thrivers—myself included—find that certain types or amounts of dairy may be better tolerated once the gut is healed and inflammation is under control. Factors that can influence tolerance include:

- Cultured versus uncultured dairy
- Aged raw-milk cheeses versus mass-produced cheese
- Goat's or sheep's milk products versus cow's milk products
- Milk from grass-fed cows versus conventional dairy cows
- A2 milk, which contains a different form of casein and may be better tolerated by people who are reactive to casein

Everyone is different, and reintroducing dairy takes time, patience, and trial and error. Listen to your body, and don't rush the process.

Soy

Soy is a controversial topic in the world of thyroid-friendly eating. Some experts caution against its consumption due to its goitrogenic and estrogenic effects, while others consider it safe for those without a sensitivity, especially in moderation and in less processed forms like tofu, tempeh, tamari, or edamame.

Because soy intolerance is common—and because it retains its thyroid-inhibiting properties even when cooked—it's best to be mindful and keep soy on your radar. The greatest risk lies in overconsumption, especially when it comes to highly processed soy products or plant-based eating styles that are heavily reliant on soy.

Refined or Excessive Sugar

Excess consumption of sugar, especially added and refined sugars, can disrupt the gut microbiome, increase inflammation, and impair immune function. It's also associated with an increased risk of insulin resistance, heart disease, and certain types of cancer. While natural sweeteners like maple syrup or coconut sugar are slightly better options, they can still have negative effects if consumed in excess and should be used sparingly. Added sugar, especially in processed form, is one food that should be avoided or at least minimized for optimal health.

Ultra-Processed Foods (UPFs)

Foods with artificial ingredients, preservatives, trans fats, refined oils, added sugars (see above), or artificial sweeteners typically offer little nutritional value, lots of empty calories, and may contribute to thyroid-related symptoms. Like excess sugar, UPFs are best avoided if you're prioritizing your health. Sticking to whole, real foods is the ground zero foundation of thyroid-friendly eating. Shopping the perimeter of the grocery store, where whole foods like fresh produce and meats are likely to be found, is a helpful strategy for avoiding these inflammatory items.

Grains (Especially Refined Grains)

Particularly due to their lectins and phytates, which may interfere with nutrient absorption or irritate the gut lining in sensitive individuals, grains like wheat, corn, rice, oats, and rye can be inflammatory for some people. Even a short-term grain-free trial can bring symptom relief for many.

Eggs

Eggs are a nutrient-dense food rich in protein, choline, and healthy fats, but they can also be a hidden trigger for some Thyroid Thrivers, particularly those with autoimmune conditions. Egg white contains several proteins that may provoke an immune response, including albumin and lysozyme. Lysozyme is an enzyme that helps protect the egg from bacteria, but in sensitive individuals, it can be difficult to break down and may contribute to intestinal permeability, or "leaky gut."

Egg yolk tends to be less reactive, and during the reintroduction phases of the AIP, it is reintroduced first, before egg whites or whole eggs. If you suspect eggs may be contributing to your symptoms, try eliminating them for thirty days, then reintroduce them one part at a time (yolk first, white later) to assess your body's response.

Legumes

This family of foods includes beans, lentils, peas, and peanuts. Legumes, while high in fiber, plant-based protein, and other beneficial nutrients, can be difficult for some individuals to digest and may contribute to gut issues. Presoaking and cooking can make these foods easier to digest and less likely to cause symptoms while also increasing the bioavailability of the nutrients they contain.

Nightshades

This family of plants includes tomatoes, tomatillos, potatoes (excluding sweet potatoes), peppers (such as bell peppers, banana peppers, and hot chiles), eggplant, goji berries, and the adaptogenic herb ashwagandha. Spices made from nightshades, such as paprika, chile powder, cayenne, and crushed red pepper flakes, also fall into this category.

Nightshades contain naturally occurring chemical compounds such as alkaloids (like solanine and capsaicin), saponins, and lectins. These compounds serve as a natural defense system for the plant, helping protect it from pests and pathogens. In sensitive individuals, these substances may irritate the gut lining, trigger immune responses, and contribute to increased inflammation.

Oxalates, Salicylates, Histamine, and Sulfur

These lesser-known food sensitivities are caused by naturally occurring chemical compounds found in otherwise healthy foods. While most people tolerate these substances without issue, some individuals—especially those with chronic inflammation, gut issues, or impaired detoxification pathways—may experience adverse reactions.

- **Oxalates** are found in high amounts in foods like spinach, almonds, beets, and sweet potatoes. In sensitive individuals, they can contribute to joint pain, bladder irritation, skin reactions, or kidney stone formation.

- **Salicylates** are natural plant chemicals found in strawberries, apples, herbs, spices, and some teas. Reactions may include skin rashes, headaches, or asthma-like symptoms.

- **Histamine** is produced during the fermentation or aging process of foods like bone broth (if cooked for extended periods), aged cheeses, cured meats, leftovers, and fermented vegetables. If your body doesn't break down histamine effectively (due to DAO [diamine oxidase] enzyme deficiency or gut imbalance), it can cause headaches, flushing, hives, digestive distress, or anxiety.

- **Sulfur compounds,** including sulfites, are found in garlic, onions, cruciferous vegetables (like broccoli and cabbage), eggs, and wine. Some people may experience fatigue, skin issues, or gastrointestinal (GI) symptoms when they can't tolerate or properly metabolize sulfur-rich foods.

These sensitivities can be especially confusing for Thyroid Thrivers who are making healthy changes, like increasing their intake of colorful produce or bone broth, yet find that they feel worse instead of better.

I was one of those people! It took me months to figure out that I was reacting to sulfur and then months more to figure out how to manage it. With the help of my naturopath and some targeted supplements to help me process sulfur, today I can enjoy delicious, detoxifying, sulfur-rich foods (like garlic, onions, and kale) without issue!

If one of the compounds noted seems to be affecting you, consider working with a trusted holistic or functional health care provider. With their guidance, symptoms can often be reduced through moderation, strategic food preparation, targeted supplementation, or gut-healing protocols, helping you restore your tolerance for these nutrient-rich foods.

FODMAPs

FODMAPs, which stands for Fermentable Oligo-saccharides, Disaccharides, Monosaccharides, and Polyols, are a group of fermentable carbohydrates found in many otherwise healthy foods, including garlic, onions, apples, asparagus, and legumes.

For some Thyroid Thrivers, especially those with IBS or small intestinal bacterial overgrowth (SIBO), FODMAPs can cause bloating, gas, cramping, and other digestive issues. If you're struggling with IBS-like symptoms or find that you have uncomfortable bloating, belching, and gas 20 to 30 minutes after eating, talk to your doctor right away about testing for SIBO.

SIBO is surprisingly common within the thyroid community and can go undiagnosed for years. Studies have shown that up to 50 percent of hypothyroid patients may have SIBO, and up to 80 percent of IBS sufferers test positive for SIBO. Why is it so common? Low stomach acid, which is commonly associated with hypothyroidism, as well as the use of antacids, can increase our risk of bacterial overgrowth.

The good news? SIBO is treatable! While the low-FODMAP diet is not a cure for SIBO or IBS or a permanent way of eating, it can be used as a short-term strategy to help reduce symptoms while root cause treatments are being applied (like antibiotics, herbs, or antifungals). Working with a qualified practitioner, such as a functional or holistic provider, is essential to safely navigating testing, treatment, and reintroduction. When SIBO is properly diagnosed and effectively treated, many people experience significant improvements in digestion, energy, and overall well-being. I've supported many Thyroid Thrivers through SIBO and IBS, and once it's addressed, they feel so much better!

Goitrogens and the Truth About Cruciferous Vegetables

You may have heard that cruciferous vegetables—like broccoli, cabbage, or cauliflower—are harmful for thyroid patients because they're "goitrogenic." This concern comes from early animal studies showing that these vegetables contain compounds called glucosinolates, which can interfere with iodine uptake and potentially contribute to goiter (an enlarged thyroid gland), especially in cases of iodine deficiency.

As a result, many thyroid patients have been told to avoid cruciferous vegetables altogether. But today's thyroid experts largely agree that this warning is outdated and overblown. While the science behind goitrogens isn't entirely a myth, it's been misinterpreted and exaggerated, often by uninformed practitioners. Sadly, this has led many thyroid patients to avoid some of the most nutrient-dense, detoxifying, and healing foods available—all for no good reason.

Goitrogens aren't limited to cruciferous vegetables. In fact, several different mechanisms—not just the presence of glucosinolates—can make a food goitrogenic. That's why the list of goitrogens includes a surprisingly wide range of foods.

The truth is, unless you're consuming massive amounts of raw goitrogens daily—like juicing a bunch of raw kale every morning—it's highly unlikely to be an issue for you, especially if your iodine and selenium levels are adequate.

Practical guidelines for eating goitrogenic foods safely:

- **Cook them:** Light steaming, roasting, or sautéing reduces goitrogenic compounds significantly.

- **Ferment them:** Fermentation (as in sauerkraut or kimchi) breaks down goitrogens and adds gut-supportive probiotics.

- **Raw is okay in moderation:** Occasional consumption of raw crucifers and most other goitrogenic foods (like stone fruits or strawberries) isn't a problem for most thyroid patients.

- **For smoothies, use cooked or frozen greens:** If you love a green smoothie like I do, you can keep adding those energy-boosting greens. Just steam them beforehand or use frozen greens, which are conveniently washed, chopped, and preblanched before packaging.

- **Practice dietary diversity:** Avoid eating the same foods over and over to ensure varied nutrients while avoiding an overload of various goitrogenic compounds

Be cautious with these goitrogenic foods:

- **Soy** contains isoflavones that may affect thyroid function, especially when iodine intake is low. Cooking does not destroy the goitrogenic substances in soy.

- **Millet** has been shown to suppress thyroid function even with adequate iodine, especially when consumed in large quantities.

- **Canola oil** is derived from rapeseed, a cruciferous plant. While much of the goitrogenic compounds in canola oil are removed through refining, you should still approach it with caution.

- **Cassava,** especially in raw form, contains cyanogenic compounds that can interfere with iodine uptake. Cooking and soaking reduce this risk. I do include cassava in a few recipes in this book, but I recommend cooking it fully and enjoying it in moderation for safety.

My philosophy: Be *aware* of these foods, not *afraid* of these foods.

You may see some of these goitrogenic ingredients peppered throughout the recipes in this book. If you have known iodine deficiency or feel particularly sensitive to goitrogenic foods, you are always welcome to make substitutions, but for most of us, it's simply not necessary.

GOITROGENIC FOODS

Goitrogenic foods include, but are not limited to:

- Almonds
- Arugula
- Bamboo shoots
- Bok choy
- Broccoli
- Brussels sprouts
- Cabbage
- Canola
- Cassava
- Cauliflower
- Cherries
- Collard greens
- Corn
- Flaxseed
- Horseradish
- Kale
- Kohlrabi
- Lima beans
- Millet
- Mizuna
- Mustard greens
- Nectarines
- Peaches
- Peanuts
- Pears
- Pine nuts
- Plums
- Radishes
- Rutabagas
- Soy
- Spinach
- Strawberries
- Sweet potatoes
- Turnips
- Walnuts
- Watercress

What About Caffeine and Alcohol?

Thyroid-healthy eating isn't just about what's on your plate: It includes what's in your glass or cup too. While food gets most of the attention, beverages can also play a significant role in how you feel and how your thyroid functions.

Caffeine affects the body's stress response by increasing adrenaline and cortisol levels—even when you're at rest. This can be a concern for those with thyroid conditions, as chronic stress and overworked adrenals can contribute to thyroid imbalance. While caffeine doesn't directly harm the thyroid gland itself, overconsumption has the potential to significantly impact your thyroid and adrenal health.

That doesn't mean everyone needs to give up coffee forever. However, if you're struggling with symptoms like fatigue, anxiety, poor sleep, or adrenal burnout, reducing caffeine consumption or taking a break from it can be a powerful step in supporting your healing.

Alcohol can also present challenges for Thyroid Thrivers, particularly because of the way it impacts the liver and the gut, two key areas involved in hormone metabolism and immune regulation.

Your liver plays a vital role in converting inactive T4 into active T3. When you consume alcohol, your liver produces a byproduct called acetaldehyde, a toxin that can damage liver cells over time and impair the liver's ability to do its job—including supporting healthy thyroid hormone conversion.

In terms of gut health, alcohol can contribute to disruption of the gut microbiome, intestinal permeability ("leaky gut"), inflammation, and autoimmunity. It can also contribute to hormonal imbalances, blood sugar imbalances, and weight gain, and significantly diminishes the quality and restfulness of your sleep.

The Takeaway: Taking steps to minimize caffeine and alcohol can offer big payoffs, but these are deeply personal choices. If you're not ready to give them up entirely, taking a break from them during your THYROID30 wellness adventure can be a great way to see how your body responds.

Foods That Can Affect Your Thyroid Medication

No discussion of thyroid-friendly eating is complete without addressing medication absorption. Certain nutrients, especially calcium, magnesium, iron, and fiber, can affect how well your thyroid medication works in your body. This is why most thyroid medications recommend waiting at least 30 to 60 minutes before consuming anything other than water after taking your medication (with a full glass of water).

Key Timing Considerations

Timing food consumption with your thyroid medications depends on *when* you take them, which can vary based on your individual needs and preferences:

- Most thyroid patients are advised to take their thyroid medication immediately upon waking and to wait 30 to 60 minutes before consuming anything other than water.

- Some patients take their medication at bedtime. Research suggests that this may improve absorption. Plus, some people prefer not to have to wait an hour after waking before eating breakfast.

- Some people may take multiple doses throughout the day, especially with T3 medications.

- Some individuals with absorption issues might need to strictly avoid consuming calcium, iron, and fiber within four hours of medication.

Supplements: For best results, wait four hours after taking your medication before you take supplements containing iron, calcium, magnesium, or fiber, as these nutrients can inhibit thyroid medication absorption. If you take your thyroid medication upon waking in the morning (by 8 a.m.), an easy workaround is to take your supplements with lunch (around noon) or dinner.

Food sources: Recommendations vary on whether to avoid the naturally occurring amounts of calcium, iron, magnesium, and fiber in whole foods. High doses are typically the primary concern. Here are some general guidelines:

- **Most important to avoid:** Calcium, iron, magnesium, and fiber-fortified foods (calcium-fortified orange juice, nutrient-fortified cereals, fiber-fortified yogurts and snack bars, and so on) can contain relatively high doses of these nutrients.

- **May also have an effect:** Natural amounts of calcium, magnesium, iron, and fiber in foods may have an effect. Also, soy, grapefruit, and walnuts may interfere with the absorption of thyroid medication. Recommended waiting times are typically 1 hour, but some sources recommend waiting up to four hours to consume these foods after you take your medication. Check with your doctor if unsure.

- **When in doubt:** Follow your health care provider's guidance on what's best for you.

Coffee and tea: Some studies suggest that these beverages can impact medication absorption. If you're a morning coffee drinker, waiting at least 1 hour after taking thyroid meds helps ensure optimal absorption.

Those small but *consistent* habits can influence your thyroid medication needs over time. For example, adding cream to your coffee every morning an hour after taking medication may slightly affect its absorption. But if you feel well, your labs are stable, and the routine works for you, it may not be worth stressing over.

The Takeaway: Some individuals need to be more cautious about food and supplement timing than others. The best approach is to read your medication instructions carefully, be consistent with your medication timing to ensure stable thyroid levels, consult your doctor for personalized guidance, and do what's right for you. Some of the recipes in this book (including some breakfast recipes) contain calcium, magnesium, iron, or fiber. As you follow the THYROID30 plan, adapt the timing of your meals and medication to suit your unique needs. The goal is not perfection but awareness and consistency.

Discovering Your Unique Dietary Needs and Sensitivities

Built right into THYROID30 is the opportunity to discover your unique dietary needs and sensitivities. This allows you to personalize your eating style by avoiding the foods that are inflammatory to you as an individual—not based on trends or generalizations, but on your own body's feedback.

This concept is rooted in what's known as an elimination and reintroduction process, or an elimination diet. By temporarily removing potentially inflammatory foods from your diet and tracking how your symptoms change, you can gather powerful personal data.

For some foods, the improvement may be so marked that you won't want to reintroduce them at all. For others, reintroduction helps pinpoint exactly what symptoms the food may trigger. By reintroducing foods one at a time and carefully observing your body's response, you can begin to connect the dots between foods and symptoms.

This kind of self-discovery is incredibly empowering, and it's a skill many Thyroid Thrivers use again and again on their healing journey. Giving up favorite foods can be hard—but not as hard as suffering from unexplained symptoms when simple dietary changes could bring relief.

What About Missing Out on Healthy Foods or Nutrients?

This is a valid concern when making dietary eliminations, and one reason why we want to develop our skills of discernment here is to keep us from avoiding healthy foods and the nutrients they contain for no good reason.

That said, here's the bottom line: If a food—even a "healthy" one—is causing inflammation, gut disruption, or triggering your autoimmune condition, then it's not a healthy food for you at this time. When we feed that inflammatory cycle by consuming foods we are sensitive to, we are feeding a cycle of disease.

If you do end up with long-term dietary restrictions, getting the nutrients you need can often be accomplished via other foods or targeted supplementation. Consulting with a thyroid-savvy nutritionist or dietitian to help you fill any nutritional gaps is a smart idea.

Brazil Nut
"Parmesan,"
page 225

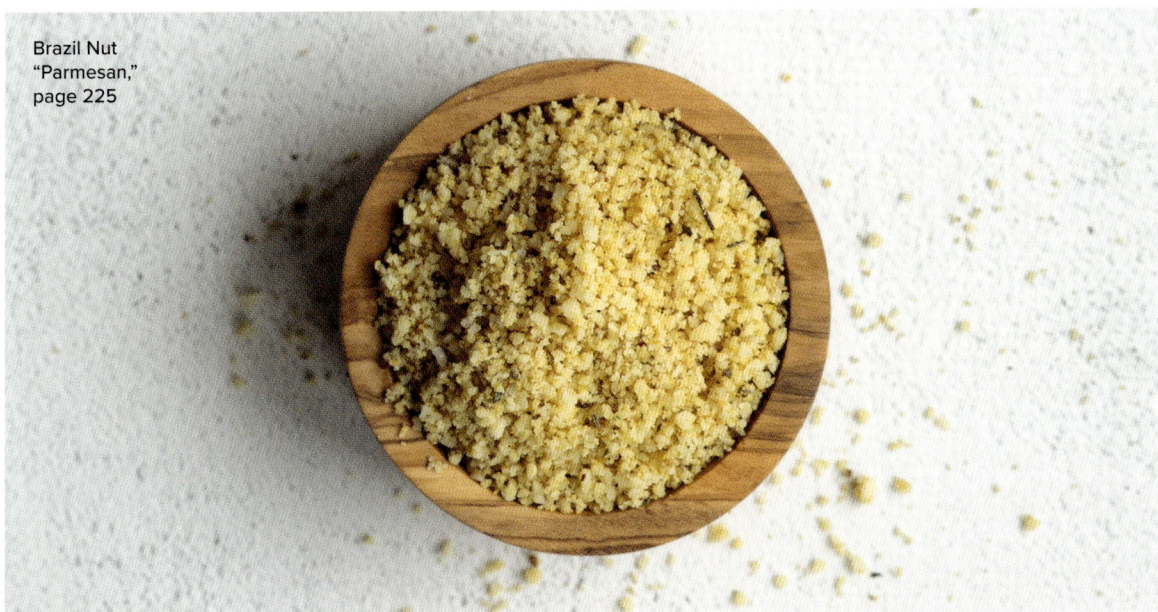

How the Elimination and Reintroduction Process Works

The simple three-step process I'm about to walk you through is considered the gold standard for identifying food sensitivities—ranking even above food sensitivity testing, which can sometimes produce false positives or negatives and inconsistent results.

Step 1: Establish Your Baseline

Before you begin your THYROID30 and before you eliminate any foods, take time to record your baseline symptoms. Grab a notebook or open a digital document and write down what you're currently experiencing physically, mentally, and emotionally.

Remember that not all food sensitivity symptoms are digestive. Food can affect the body in surprising ways and may cause a variety of nondigestive symptoms from anxiety to acne.

Here are some areas to note before you make any changes to your lifestyle:

- General physical feeling
- Mood, including anxiety or depression
- Bloating (or lack of)
- Joint pain (or lack of)
- Energy levels
- Sleep quality
- Memory and focus
- Brain fog
- Headaches
- Skin, hair, and nail health
- Digestive symptoms (constipation, diarrhea, gas, bloating)

Recording your starting point in this way helps you accurately track improvements and identify patterns once foods are eliminated and later reintroduced.

Step 2: Eliminate Food(s) and Track Symptoms

You can eliminate one food (like gluten) or several foods at a time, as in elimination diets like paleo or AIP. THYROID30 includes three dietary levels to choose from, all of which can guide you through this process:

- Level 1 (Gluten and Dairy-Free): Eliminates gluten, dairy, refined sugar, soy, and ultra-processed foods
- Level 2 (Paleo): Eliminates all of Level 1, plus grains and legumes
- Level 3 (AIP): Eliminates all of Level 2, plus eggs, nightshades, nuts, and seeds

During the elimination phase, be sure to track any symptom changes or improvements in your food journal. Note dates and key milestones: Some people begin to feel better within a week, while it may take longer for others. While thirty days (or more) is commonly recommended for the elimination phase, the Institute for Functional Medicine (IFM) has found that a twenty-one-day period is often sufficient to reduce inflammation and calm symptoms while also improving completion rates and making the process more sustainable for participants. THYROID30 incorporates a twenty-one-day elimination window based on this evidence-informed approach.

IMPORTANT NOTE

The elimination and reintroduction process is not intended to diagnose or manage food allergies, which can be severe or life-threatening. Always consult with your health care provider regarding potential allergies.

Finding Substitutions

With so many varying dietary needs and restrictions, sourcing products that don't contain ingredients you're trying to avoid can feel a little tricky at first, but the good news is, we're lucky to live in a time when those products are out there! Because I know how helpful recommendations can be, I've included a list of some of my favorite GF/DF, paleo, and AIP products in THYROID30 Support and Resources (page 246). For more severe issues like celiac or severe gluten sensitivity, an app like the Eat! Gluten-free App from the Celiac Disease Foundation is the best way to ensure you're buying foods that meet your requirements.

Step 3: Reintroduce Food(s)

Once your elimination trial is complete and your body has had time to reset, it's time to reintroduce foods. There are three important rules to follow here so that you get clear results and avoid common mistakes.

Rule #1: Only reintroduce one food at a time. This helps isolate your body's reaction to individual foods. Reintroducing multiple foods at once makes it impossible to tell which one is responsible for a reaction.

Rule #2: Wait three to five days between reintroductions. Some reactions take days to show up. Give your body time to register any reactions to a food before introducing another food.

Rule #3: Eat enough of the reintroduced food (if possible). When you're reintroducing foods that are highly reactive for you, you may want to start with a single bite or ease yourself in gradually, giving yourself weeks rather than days to reintroduce a single food. With other foods, though, a single bite may not be enough to trigger a noticeable reaction. If possible (and safe), eat a normal serving, then observe. If no adverse reactions occur, eat additional servings to ensure a confident understanding of how (and if) that food affects you.

Throughout the process, pay attention to any symptoms that pop up, return, or worsen. Be a good scientist and write everything down in your food journal. You'll be glad you did when you come away with definitive answers about which foods cause which symptoms.

After the Trial: Analyzing Your Results

When your reintroduction phase is complete, review your notes. Which foods caused a clear reaction? Which felt fine, causing no reaction at all? Which were unclear, perhaps requiring a second test later?

Reactions may be subtle or dramatic. Some foods may be tolerated in small doses, while others may be "off-limits" for now, but that can change. With time and healing, many people become able to reintroduce foods they once reacted to.

What's the payoff for all this? Understanding your unique dietary needs and sensitivities. This process will also help you uncover your ideal bio-individual diet—the pinnacle of personalized nutrition. You'll no longer be guessing or relying on a list of foods from a cookie-cutter dietary template. You'll have *your own* custom-tailored plan.

Calming inflammation and removing problem foods can lead to reduced symptoms, improved gut health, more energy, better mental clarity, easier weight management, and greater overall vitality—not to mention disease prevention. Best of all, you'll gain confidence in your ability to care for your body because you'll have this powerful elimination-reintroduction tool in your Thriver's toolkit and can reach for it anytime you need it. Our dietary needs and sensitivities can change over time, so you'll likely come back to this particular tool again and again.

Putting It All Together

Kudos to you for empowering yourself with a better understanding of thyroid-friendly eating: what it is, what it isn't, how it works, and common myths surrounding it. Now, let's talk about how to put it all together and make it doable in real life.

There's a lot of support, understanding, and empathy in the thyroid community around dietary restrictions and food sensitivities. But go out into the real world for five minutes and you're bombarded with flashy fast-food ads and hyperpalatable processed foods that are lab-designed to make them hard to put down. At restaurants or social gatherings, there may or may not be options you can eat (without sparking symptoms). When you're traveling, you'll quickly learn the importance of bringing along your own snacks and staples.

Many of us *need* to stick to our dietary restrictions to feel well and be able to function, so we have to learn to navigate these things. The good news is that it is absolutely possible—with a little practice and finesse—to live (and love) your life, share family meals, enjoy holiday celebrations, travel, and dine out, even if staples like gluten and dairy just don't work for you anymore. Let's talk about how.

Establish Your Hard Lines and Wiggle Room

Hard lines: These are your nonnegotiable foods, the ones that consistently trigger symptoms or inflammation. For many Thyroid Thrivers, this includes gluten. For others, it might also include dairy, grains, or something else. Maybe you're currently on a strict gut-healing protocol and need to adhere to a set diet like paleo or AIP. What are the foods you *must* avoid at this time? These hard-line foods are worth the extra effort to avoid, even when it's inconvenient.

Wiggle room: Just as important as identifying your hard lines is knowing where you have flexibility. What foods can you tolerate occasionally, or in small amounts? For example, maybe you can enjoy a sprinkle of cheese on a salad, but not a cheese-heavy plate of nachos. This wiggle room allows for more food freedom, which makes it easier to socialize and dine out without derailing your health. Traveling, socializing, celebrating, or dining out can be good opportunities to leverage your wiggle room. Identifying both your hard lines and your wiggle room makes dining away from your own kitchen much easier. Remember that your hard lines and wiggle room may change over time as healing occurs or as your body's needs shift.

Planning Ahead Makes Everything Easier

Whether you're dining out, traveling, or attending social gatherings, a little planning goes a long way.

Here are a few tips:

- **For restaurants:** Review menus online beforehand, call ahead with special requests, or have simple meal suggestions ready (like grilled protein and steamed vegetables drizzled with extra-virgin olive oil).

- **For travel:** Pack thyroid-friendly snacks and easy meal components in case you can't find options that work for you. If you're on a strict protocol like AIP, consider bringing frozen prepared meals or researching grocery stores at your destination.

- **For social events:** Eat something before attending if you're unsure about what food options will be available for you, or offer to bring a shareable dish that meets your unique needs.

The more restricted your current diet, the more essential planning becomes. But with each successful experience, you build confidence and develop strategies that make the balancing act easier.

Speak Up About Your Needs

Take it from me: Trying to ignore or hide your dietary needs from friends, family, and coworkers because you don't want to be *that person* will slow your healing journey way down. Many of us hesitate to "make a fuss" about our dietary needs, but your health matters. These are *needs* (not just *wants*), and when you can speak up about them clearly, you'll be amazed at how much easier life can be. It's a skill many of us must develop over time. The alternative is, quite literally, making yourself sick to spare someone else a minor inconvenience.

Most restaurants and hosts are happy to be accommodating when given clear information and *advance* notice. As a former restaurant chef, I can attest to that—but do keep it simple. Rather than sharing your entire health history and listing everything you can't eat, focus on simple dishes that work for you. For example, "I have dietary restrictions for medical reasons. Could the chef prepare some grilled fish with steamed vegetables using only olive oil and salt?"

Remember: You're not being difficult; you're taking care of your health so that you can be there for the people and purposes you care about.

Bottom line: If you don't *tell them* about your dietary needs, they can't possibly accommodate them.

Balance Is Key

Don't let perfect be the enemy of good enough. If you're doing well with your thyroid health, occasional compromises while traveling or celebrating special occasions won't completely undo your progress. There are exceptions here, though, for instance, if you're celiac or highly reactive to gluten. In cases like these, even microexposures truly must be avoided. But in many cases, and with many foods, we do have some wiggle room.

Besides, sometimes the stress of trying to maintain dietary perfection can actually do more harm to your well-being than those minor dietary deviations.

So, know your nonnegotiables, use your wiggle room wisely, lean on the 8 Daily Rituals to support your body in bouncing back from slipups, and remember that thyroid-friendly eating isn't about restriction: It's about supporting your body so you can live life to the fullest.

With time, these choices become second nature, and what once felt overwhelming becomes your new normal. And you don't have to do this alone! The THYROID30 system will walk you through this process step-by-step. You'll start building a collection of go-to meals with the cookbook you're holding in your hands right now. With the right support and a proven system, thriving can happen faster—and feel easier—than you ever thought possible.

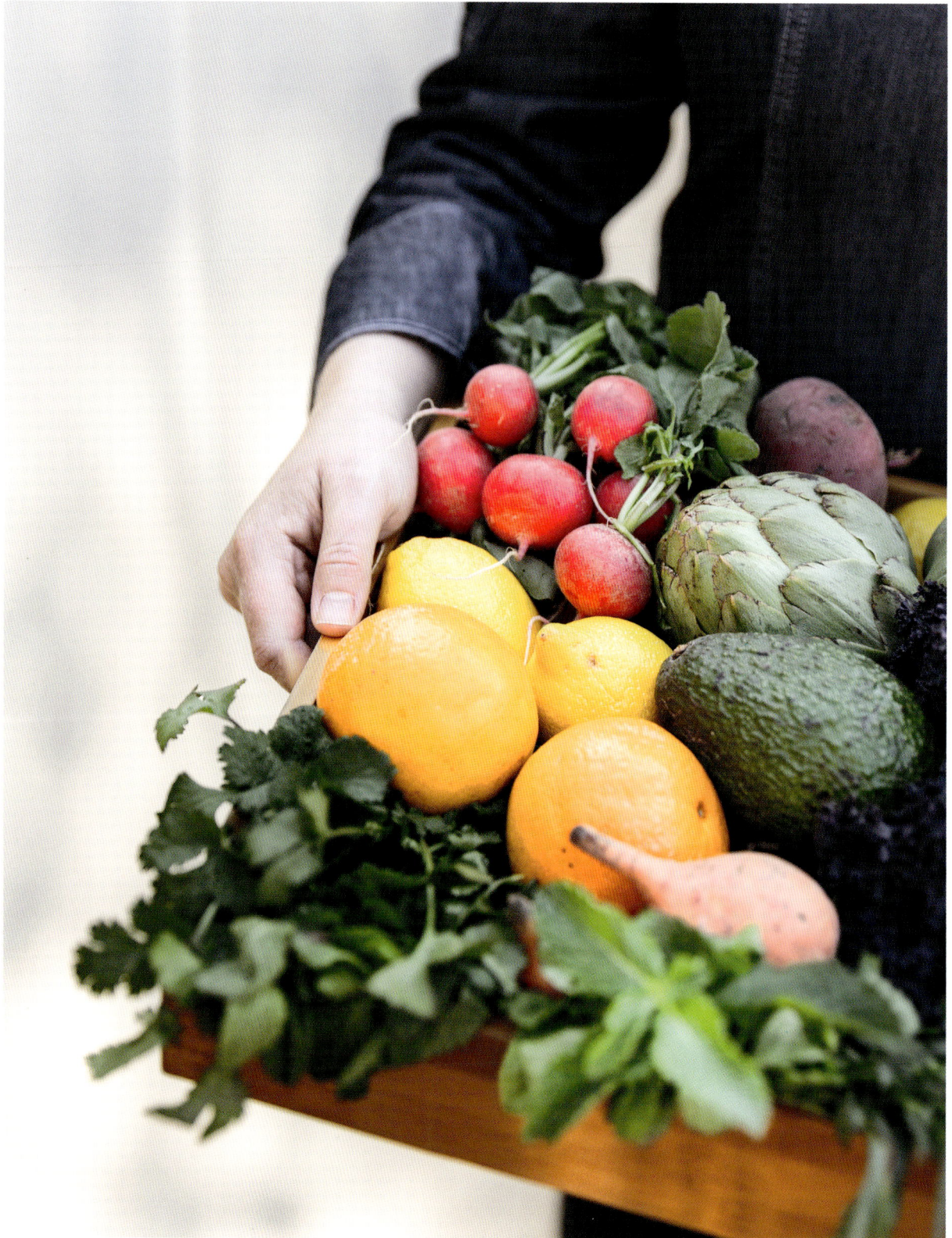

4

The 8 Daily Rituals of Thyroid-Healthy Living

Welcome to the core framework that guides THYROID30. While these rituals were developed with the specific needs of thyroid patients in mind, they're also universal principles that benefit anyone seeking vibrant health. Based on the pillars of functional medicine—which is essentially food and lifestyle medicine—these simple, sustainable practices can help prevent disease and support people living with hypothyroidism, Hashimoto's, or any of the hundreds of chronic, autoimmune, or "lifestyle" diseases of our time. Chapter 1 already introduced you to the 8 Daily Rituals, or the 8 Rs, but we'll go into more detail on them in this chapter.

To refresh your memory, the 8 Rs are:

1. **REMEMBER** to take your medications and supplements.

2. **REFUEL** with the food and drink your body thrives on.

3. **REACTIVATE** by moving your body regularly.

4. **REPAIR** and care for your gut.

5. **REJUVENATE** with daily self-care and stress management.

6. **REDUCE** and avoid your exposure to toxins.

7. **RELISH** the journey, your wins, and your support system.

8. **RECHARGE** by prioritizing sleep and sleep hygiene.

The Origin of the 8 Daily Rituals

When I was just starting out on my own thyroid-healing journey, I remember thinking, "Okay, now what? Where do I begin? *How* am I supposed to implement all of these recommendations in a way that will actually make a difference to my health?"

If you're a thyroid patient searching for ways to feel optimal, you've probably heard a *lot* of recommendations about topics like food, exercise, gut health, self-care, toxin avoidance, sleep, community support, and more. These recommendations may make sense on paper, but when it comes to applying them in real life, the overwhelm quickly sets in. It's easy to get lost in the sea of advice. With so much information to process, it's no wonder we sometimes freeze instead of moving forward.

One day, in the shower (where I do my best thinking), the idea for a codified thirty-day wellness adventure to help thyroid patients implement the practices of thyroid-healthy living hit me like a lightning bolt. It could be called . . . THYROID30.

I immediately called my friend and former business partner, Danna Bowman, and shared my lightning-bolt idea. It sparked a wildfire of inspiration for us. As fellow thyroid advocates and patients who had lived this struggle, we both knew we were onto something. This was the solution *we needed* as thyroid patients. We didn't just pull the 8 Rs out of thin air. These were the consistent recommendations echoed by thyroid, autoimmune, and gut health experts everywhere. We took what was an overwhelming jumble of expert directives and boiled them down to their essence—to something that could fit on an index card (or scorecard). That's how the 8 Rs became the framework for THYROID30. Our mission was to simplify thyroid-healthy living and make it doable and fun, incorporating the proven power of community into the process.

We put the 8 Rs to the test when we officially launched THYROID30 in 2017. From day one, the 8 Daily Rituals became a beloved road map for Thyroid Thrivers to follow on the path to fewer symptoms, more energy, and better health.

The 8 Rs have stood the test of time and were further validated during my certification as a Functional Medicine Health Coach, when I realized that these same principles also make up the pillars of functional medicine. Over the years, the body of scientific evidence backing up these principles—like the importance of gut health, sleep, and stress management—has ballooned, along with anecdotal proof from thousands of health warriors who are using these daily habits to prevent and manage chronic disease. What makes these rituals so powerful is their timeless, flexible nature. They're adaptable habits anyone can follow, regardless of where they are on their health journey. The THYROID30 game plan presents them in a digestible, easy-to-follow format: simple, daily practices you can incorporate into your life, supported by delicious recipes designed to nourish and heal.

Let's walk through each of the 8 Daily Rituals and the *whys* behind them.

1 Remember

Remember to take your daily medications and supplements.

Remembering to take your medications and supplements is an important step in feeling better. Most thyroid medication must be taken daily, at the same time and on an empty stomach. Missing doses or taking your thyroid meds at inconsistent times and in inconsistent ways can diminish the benefit you get from them. It can also affect the accuracy of your thyroid lab results, making truly accurate dosing more difficult. Many of us are also taking targeted supplements (chosen with the help of our health care providers), adding another thing for us to remember. For some, "Remember" is the easiest daily ritual there is. For others, it's a very real struggle that can have a significant impact on how you feel. Incorporating tools like pill caddies, sticky notes, or automated reminders can help, but the first step is tracking and identifying how consistent you are in taking your medications and supplements on time so that you can make any necessary changes to help you get on track.

2 Refuel

Refuel with the food and drink your body thrives on.

As we saw in chapter 3, what we eat and drink has a massive impact on our overall well-being. While there is no one-size-fits-all thyroid diet, the common goal is to eliminate foods that cause reactions and inflammation in those with thyroid disease while incorporating more nutrient-dense, anti-inflammatory foods, including foods with key thyroid-supporting nutrients.

The foods you may need to eliminate and the foods your body thrives on will depend on you and your unique dietary needs and sensitivities, as well as your individual health factors. Dietary levels 1, 2, and 3, outlined in this book on page 79, make helpful starting points for those who wish to calm inflammation, support gut health and healing, and need a place to begin.

In choosing your approach, it's important to factor in where you are on your healing journey. If you're newly diagnosed and currently eating the standard American diet (SAD), you may do well to start with Level 1 (Gluten and Dairy-Free [GF/DF]). Another Thyroid Thriver may be ready for a bigger step like Level 2 (Paleo) or Level 3 (AIP). Choose the approach that's right for you, right now.

3 Reactivate

Reactivate by moving your body regularly.
Physical activity has numerous benefits for those with thyroid disease. It can help boost energy levels, improve emotional and mental health, and support weight management. However, finding your exercise "sweet spot"—neither overdoing it nor underdoing it—is crucial.

For thyroid patients who feel like they can't get results no matter how much they work out, less is sometimes more. The conventional advice to "just eat less and exercise more" can actually contribute to hypothyroidism if done in excess or for too long. So, if you're just starting out, start slowly and focus on mobility first, and then gradually incorporate resistance training before adding cardio. This progression can help avoid exercise-induced symptom flares. In general, the thyroid-friendly approach to movement emphasizes strength training over excessive cardio, as muscle is more metabolically active and provides receptors for thyroid hormones.

Listen carefully to your body's feedback to avoid pushing yourself into exhaustion and exercise-induced symptom flare-ups that can last for days and undermine your efforts. You should feel energized thirty minutes after a workout, not desperate for a nap. Both regular movement and building up your routine slowly at a level that's appropriate for you will help you stay active without triggering the inflammation, joint injuries, or autoimmune flares that can come from overexertion.

4 Repair

Repair and care for your gut health.
Good health begins in the gut. Beyond digesting food and absorbing nutrients, your gut is home to about 70 percent of your immune system, so it plays a critical role in whole-body wellness.

For thyroid patients, healing the gut is often a foundational step in reducing symptoms and restoring energy. In fact, lingering gut issues—like leaky gut, SIBO, or *H. pylori*—can stand in the way of real progress until they're addressed.

As you learned in chapter 3, leaky gut (also called intestinal permeability) is particularly common in thyroid patients. The good news is that there are many ways to support gut repair. Start by eliminating inflammatory foods and toxins, then focus on adding in healing foods: probiotic-rich foods (review the table on page 39), fiber-rich foods (as tolerated), collagen, bone broth, and foods with targeted nutrients like L-glutamine and zinc. Think of your gut microbiome as a garden: Weed out what harms it (sugar, alcohol, toxins, stress), seed it with beneficial bacteria, feed it with fiber (especially prebiotic fiber) and anti-inflammatory foods, and create the right environment to heal and seal your gut lining.

With consistency and care, gut repair can help reduce thyroid antibodies, improve hormone conversion, boost nutrient absorption, and restore a healthier, more resilient you.

5 Rejuvenate

Rejuvenate with daily self-care and stress management practices.
Self-care isn't a luxury: When it comes to thyroid health, it's nonnegotiable. Chronic stress can disrupt the adrenal-thyroid connection, throwing off hormone balance and triggering symptom flares like fatigue, brain fog, anxiety, and poor sleep. By nurturing your nervous system daily, you're also supporting your thyroid, your hormonal balance, your adrenals, and your ability to heal.

Rejuvenation looks different for everyone, and it's all about finding the practices you enjoy and benefit from the most. It might look like ten minutes of mindful breathing; a slow walk in nature; an Epsom salt bath; or a few moments of journaling with a warm cup of tea. It might also mean setting healthy boundaries, practicing gratitude, dancing to your favorite music, or simply saying no to something that drains you. The key is to find what genuinely restores you and to give yourself the time, space, and permission to prioritize it.

Research shows that simple self-care practices like mindfulness, rest, joyful movement, connection, and sleep can lower cortisol, reduce inflammation, and improve both mental and physical health. The more joy and intention you bring into your daily routine, the better you'll feel. And remember, even one deep breath can make a difference in your day.

6 Reduce

Reduce and avoid exposure to toxins.

Reducing your exposure to everyday toxins is one of the most overlooked aspects of thyroid-healthy living. We're not aiming for perfection here, though: We're aiming for progress. While it's impossible to avoid all environmental toxins, we can take small, meaningful steps to lower our total toxic load and support our body's natural detox systems.

Why does this matter for thyroid patients? Environmental toxins like pesticides, plastics, heavy metals, and endocrine-disrupting chemicals (EDCs) have been linked to thyroid dysfunction, autoimmunity, metabolic issues, and more. They're what functional medicine practitioners call "drivers of disease."

But here's the good news: Reducing your toxic burden doesn't have to be overwhelming. Start where you are, and layer in small changes over time. That might mean choosing organic produce when possible, using a stainless-steel water bottle, swapping plastic food storage containers for glass, switching to low-tox personal care products, or upgrading your cookware to avoid nonstick coatings. Even tiny shifts—like opening your windows to let in fresh air or filtering your water—can make a big difference over time.

The goal isn't zero exposure. It's about becoming more informed, empowered, and intentional about what you bring into your home and your body. Every reduction counts.

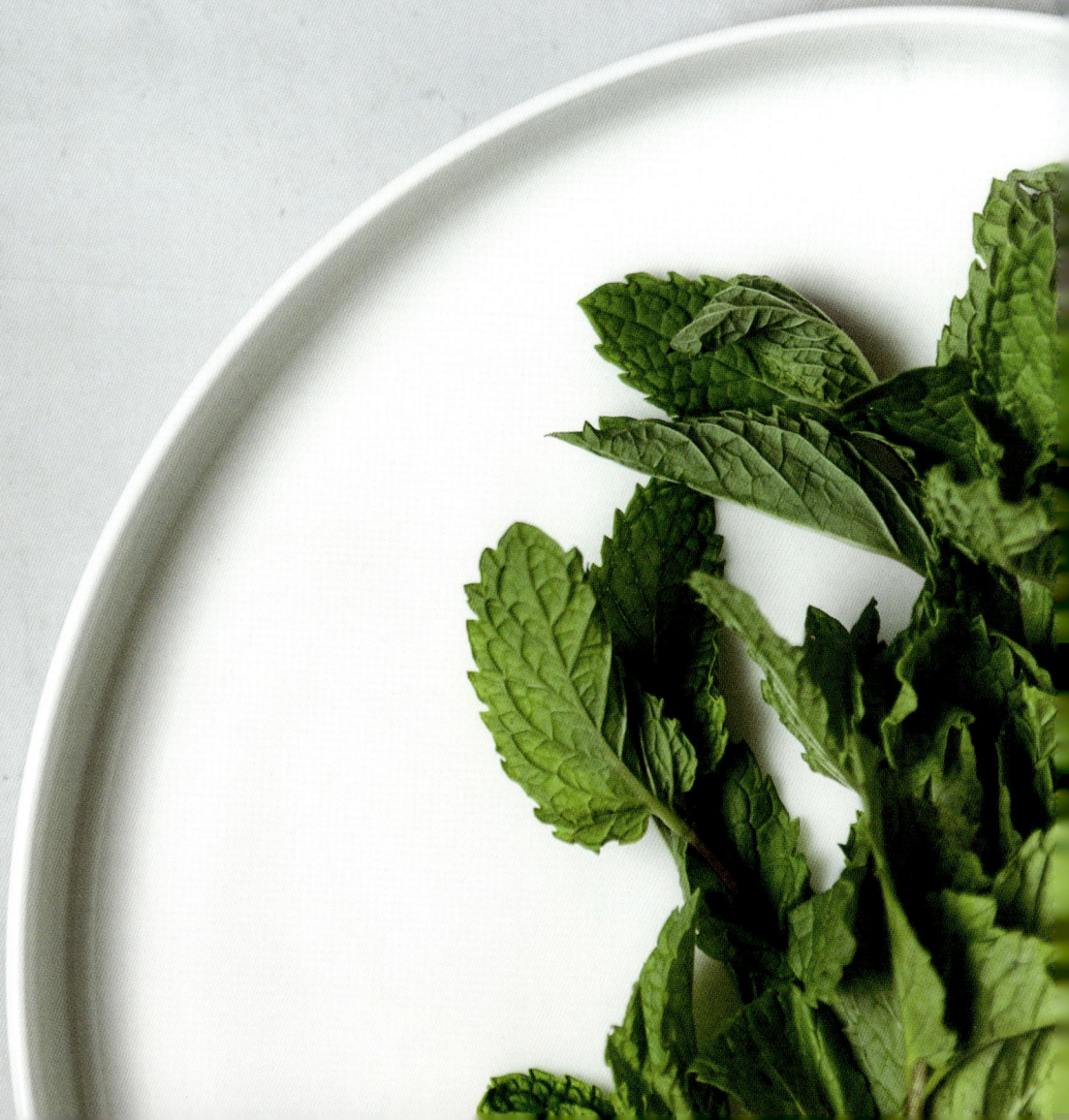

THYROID-FRIENDLY FOOD STORAGE TIPS

- Choose glass or ceramic containers, which are nontoxic, freezer-safe, microwave-safe, and oven-safe, over plastic. Bonus: With glass containers, you're more likely to eat your leftovers when you can see them!

- Avoid freezing, storing, cooking, or reheating foods in plastic. Even BPA-free plastic can leach thyroid and endocrine-disrupting chemicals (EDCs).

- Use silicone bags selectively. Resealable silicone bags can be great for storing dry snacks, produce, or freezer items. While silicone is generally considered safer than plastic, some leaching may still occur, so avoid using these with hot or acidic foods, or anything that will sit in long-term surface-to-surface contact (like soups or other liquid foods), to minimize chemical exposure.

- Label and date leftovers. Remember: The freezer is not a cryogenic time capsule. Foods perish more slowly when frozen, but they do still perish. Use masking tape and a permanent marker to label and date that freezer treasure, and discard anything that's past its prime.

Every small swap makes a difference when avoiding toxins, and a onetime investment in thyroid-safe food storage can provide years of health-supporting returns.

7 Relish

Relish the journey, your wins, and your support system.

This one's all about celebrating your wins and connecting with others. By intentionally noticing and acknowledging each victory on your thyroid-healing journey—no matter how small—you'll create powerful momentum toward lasting health transformation.

Tiny celebrations—like a fist pump or high-fiving yourself in the mirror—may seem silly, but they have a powerful neurological effect that is backed by behavioral science. These moments of joy help rewire your brain to associate healthy habits with positive emotions, making you more likely to stick with them. *Relishing* your wins is one of the core principles baked into THYROID30 and is one of the reasons THYROID30 consistently produces results.

This ritual also encompasses the importance of connection and community. Healing can be isolating and difficult, especially when symptoms linger or progress feels slow. Having a space where you're met with understanding as you share your wins and reflect on your struggles is a surefire way to overcome common health hurdles like inconsistency.

It's possible to do THYROID30 on your own, but you'll get way more out of it if you do it in a community setting. In my Thrivers Club community, we practice the 8 Daily Rituals and celebrate our wins together using the THYROID30 model. We remind each other of how far we've come, help each other through the low moments, and keep the focus on growth, self-acceptance, and progress—not perfection, dogma, or shame.

Relishing the journey and fostering a positive mindset doesn't mean ignoring the hard stuff. It means giving yourself the support to meet and overcome challenges with compassion and clarity. Whether you're celebrating a consistent week of morning walks or simply remembering to take your medications every day, take a moment to pause and recognize your progress. You deserve that. And you don't have to do it alone.

8 Recharge

Recharge by prioritizing sleep and sleep hygiene.

Sleep is one of the most important ways to create a strong foundation for thyroid health, hormonal balance, metabolism, immunity, and emotional resilience. Unfortunately, many thyroid patients struggle to get enough restorative rest due to issues like insomnia, adrenal dysfunction, or disrupted circadian rhythms.

Sleep challenges are common in both hypothyroid and autoimmune thyroid conditions and can worsen fatigue, brain fog, weight gain, depression, and other symptoms.

Getting enough quality sleep—ideally between 7 and 9 hours a night—can reduce inflammation, boost immunity, regulate hunger hormones, support weight management, and improve mood, memory, and energy. After all, your thyroid hormones convert and replenish, your brain detoxifies, and your body heals while you're sleeping.

So, if you're skipping out on sleep, you're skipping out on healing.

Start by assessing your sleep patterns and identifying obstacles to better rest. It's also important to practice good sleep hygiene: Maintain a consistent sleep schedule, limit evening screen exposure, create a cool and dark sleeping environment, and develop calming bedtime rituals like gratitude journaling, warm baths, or meditation. Additional strategies include avoiding alcohol and late meals, managing stress effectively, and supporting your thyroid and adrenal function through appropriate testing and treatment.

Sleep amplifies every other healing effort. Improving sleep quality can transform your thyroid health journey, often producing noticeable results within days. If sleep remains challenging for you, approach it with curiosity rather than frustration, and remember that practical solutions exist.

Reflection Time

Before moving on to the next chapter, take a moment to consider these questions:

- **Which of the 8 Rs are you crushing right now?**
- **Which of the 8 Rs do you most need to work on?**

The answer to those questions will be different for everyone and may change over time. They can also provide you with some direction as you embark on your THYROID30 journey.

As we gradually peel back the layers of our health and habits, we can sustainably and successfully adopt a thyroid-friendly lifestyle. Success doesn't mean that we do everything perfectly and have impeccable willpower and self-discipline 100 percent of the time. It means that we keep going and stay committed to our health, even when those inevitable hurdles and road bumps pop up.

We can learn a lot about ourselves by following the 8 Rs, including the areas in which we're already strong and those in which we have room to grow. Building self-awareness and then leaning in and embracing all of it is how we can get our lives back, reduce symptoms, and thrive—for good!

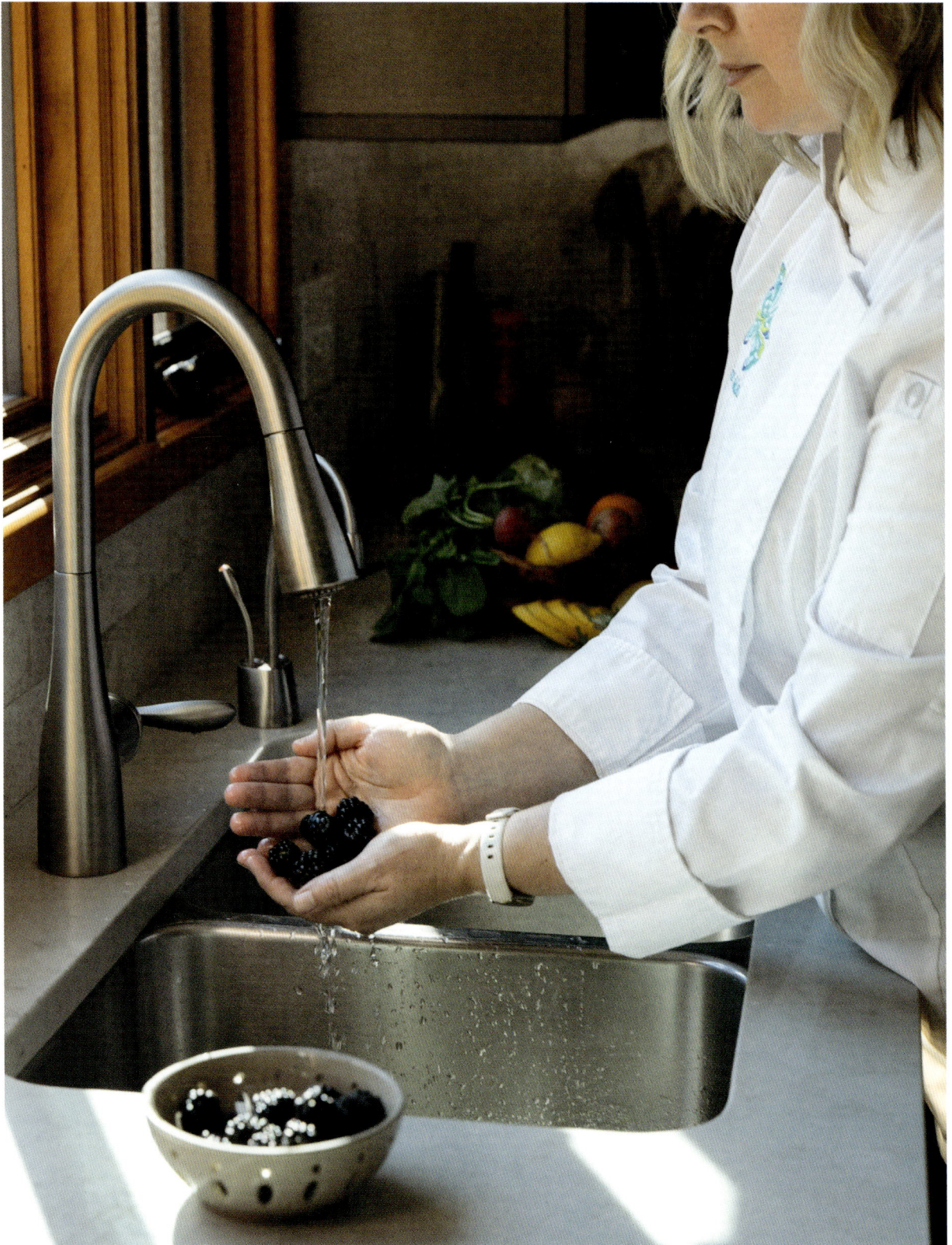

5

Embracing a Thyroid Thriver's Mindset

One thing I've learned from both leading and living the THYROID30 program is this: When it comes to thriving with thyroid challenges, mindset is more than half the battle. The way we think about our health, our bodies, and our ability to change can either empower or sabotage us.

Those who get the most out of THYROID30 embrace what I call a Thyroid Thriver's Mindset. Many of them didn't start with one, but they cultivated it along the way. So, before we dive into how the 30-day experience works, let's lay some foundations for it with a few essential mindset shifts.

Meet Yourself Where You Are

Each person comes to this journey from a different place and with different needs. That's why THYROID30 is fully customizable. You're encouraged to:

- Tailor the program to fit your current goals and capacity

- Take small, consistent steps rather than big leaps

- Focus on progress, not perfection

Whether you're just dipping a toe into the water or ready to dive right in to the deep end of the pool, it's all progress. This is *your* journey. Own and honor that. Tailoring your approach to fit your life isn't cheating: It's essential for success. As a wise person once said, "Don't compare your chapter 1 to someone else's chapter 20." For someone who's just starting out, THYROID30 might mean skimming this book, trying a few recipes, and beginning to imagine what feeling better could look like. For someone who's further along, it might mean doubling down on the AIP or focusing on specific lifestyle factors like sleep ("Recharge"). Neither of those individuals is "doing it better." They're both on the path—just in different places along the cycle of change.

Understanding the Cycle of Change

Behavioral change isn't a single decision followed by a rigid adherence to a new behavior (like quitting smoking): It's a process and a science. Psychologists James Prochaska and Carlo DiClemente identified six phases in what's called the Transtheoretical Model of Change, or, as we'll call it, the Change Cycle:

1. **Precontemplation:** You're not thinking about change yet.

2. **Contemplation:** You're considering a change but haven't committed to it.

3. **Preparation:** You're gearing up for the change—researching, planning, gathering support.

4. **Action:** You're making the change.

5. **Maintenance:** You're working to sustain it.

6. **Relapse:** The changes you've made have become your "new normal," and no longer require much effort. This often includes cycles of relapse or temporarily returning to old, unwanted behaviors.

Take a look at that last one again. **Relapse isn't failure: It's part of the change process.** It is part of the cyclic nature of change in which, after reverting to those old, unwanted behaviors, you are given the opportunity to resume your beneficial behaviors and reaffirm your commitment to them. In fact, when you make the choice to keep going, to recommit to your health and well-being after a relapse, you're strengthening your path forward. Making healthy changes isn't a linear upward ramp; it's more like a spiral staircase. You may circle back to old patterns now and then, but you're still moving upward, deepening your resilience and resolve with each turn.

This doesn't mean that we intentionally relapse. It means we don't let one slipup take us entirely off course. What THYROID30 offers is a road map through these phases, helping you avoid common pitfalls, bust through barriers, and keep going—farther and faster toward your healthiest, best life. The key is to trust the process and know that wherever you are, you're still engaged in the cycle of change. You'll know when it's time to move on to the next phase.

Speak Kindly to Yourself

THYROID30 isn't about willpower or perfection: It's about leveraging self-awareness and self-acceptance to find the path that works for you. It's about listening to your body and choosing to respond with care instead of criticism.

We often think that we need someone else to tell us what to eat and what to do, but what we really need is an approach that helps us understand and own who we are and how we thrive as individuals. That means that we are accountable and responsible for our choices, which is the true path to personal freedom, fulfillment, and, in this case, unshakeable health. So, when we "relapse" or fall offtrack, it's not a sign to quit. It's a sign to recommit. Each so-called failure is a choice point: Will I give up entirely, or will I choose my health once again?

True success doesn't mean a perfect THYROID30 score sheet. It means that we keep going and develop a long-term commitment to our health. Every step forward builds self-trust and momentum, and even the so-called failures and the smallest steps count.

Say Goodbye to Diet Culture

We've been conditioned by diet culture to believe that success requires restriction, discipline, and perfection. We've also been told that it requires following a cookie-cutter set of rules that someone else came up with and that don't acknowledge your bio-individuality.

That's not what we're doing here. What we're doing is getting empowered, building awareness, tuning in to our bodies, and learning to trust our own choices, especially around food.

Diet culture says:

- You need someone else to tell you what to eat.

- You have to follow the rules perfectly.

- If you fail, it's your fault.

- If it doesn't work, there must be something wrong with you.

Let's toss all of that into the firepit. (*Flick.* There goes the match.)

You are not broken. You do not need fixing. You simply need the support, tools, and freedom to create an approach to health that works for *you*. While THYROID30 is not a weight-loss program, participants often do lose unwanted weight as a result of *supporting* (rather than depriving) their bodies. See the fundamental difference?

It's All About Listening to Your Body

Healthy habits don't stick because we force them to: They stick because they make us feel better. That good feeling becomes its own reward: It builds its own momentum. One healthy choice leads to another healthy choice, and another.

It all starts with listening to our bodies. When we tune in to the feedback our bodies give us and tap into that flow, healthy choices stop being a chore and start becoming our default. They become *intuitive*. When we shift away from ultra-processed foods, for example, we might go through a transition period of craving those inflammatory, hyperpalatable, lab-created foods. Once we're over that hump, though, we begin to crave what nourishes us.

THYROID30 acts like a radio dial, helping you tune into how your choices make you feel on a physical, cognitive, and emotional level. We don't *judge* the bad mood, the headache, or the belly bloat: We notice what choices may have contributed to it and if we see a pattern, we adjust accordingly. By listening to the feedback our bodies are constantly giving us about our choices, inputs, and habits, we begin to realize just how much control we have over how we feel, our symptoms, and our vitality—not total control, but a lot of control nonetheless.

This awareness becomes a never-ending power supply for your healing journey.

Building Your "House of Wellness"

You don't need superhuman discipline or perfect compliance to succeed at reclaiming your health. The people who get the most meaningful and sustainable results from THYROID30 are the ones who, quite simply, show up and stick with it, even (and almost always) imperfectly.

What you're building is your personal "House of Wellness," and, as with any house, you need to start with a solid foundation. Your mindset is that foundation. So:

- Meet yourself where you are.

- Know that relapse/failure is part of success.

- Speak kindly to yourself.

- Ditch the diet culture and listen to your body.

- Trust *your* process, and *your* journey, and in doing so, you will build trust in yourself.

Once you experience the empowerment of knowing how to nourish, nurture, and heal yourself—and of feeling better because of it—there's no turning back.

You've already taken a powerful first step in giving yourself this book as a resource. Now, all you really need to do is take the next small step—and keep going.

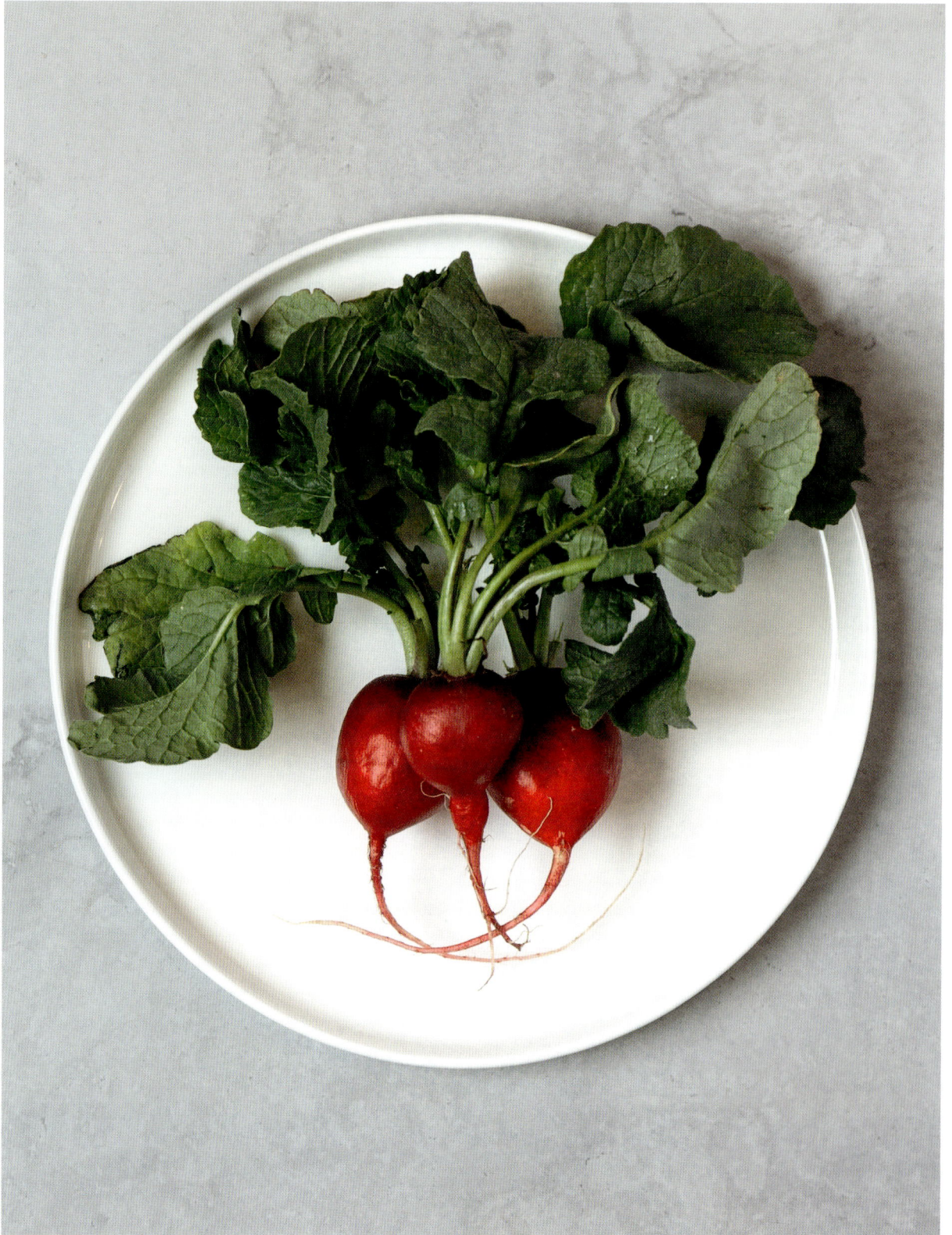

6

Getting Started with THYROID30

It's time to begin your THYROID30 journey! I'm so excited to support you in taking this powerful step toward reclaiming your energy and feeling your best. This isn't just a wellness challenge; it's a whole-health reset and a thirty-day adventure in thriving. You'll learn about thyroid-friendly food and lifestyle choices, gain priceless insights about your body, and get the tools, guidance, and encouragement to make meaningful improvements to your health and vitality. If you're not sure where to start, don't worry. In this chapter, I'll walk you through it all step-by-step so you can get the most out of your experience.

How It Works

THYROID30 follows a flexible thirty-day structure that includes:

- **Days 1 to 7, Prep Week:** This is a gentle on-ramp where you can start preparing your environment, exploring the 8 Daily Rituals, and easing yourself into thyroid-friendly choices. This week is all about setting yourself up for success, so you won't be scoring yourself during it.

- **Days 8 to 28, the 21-Day Challenge:** This is the heart of THYROID30. Each day you'll score yourself based on how many of the 8 Daily Rituals of Thyroid-Healthy Living you complete. These are the habits that can help you feel more energized, resilient, and in control of your health.

- **Days 29 to 30, Reflection and Integration Days:** This is a soft landing. Use these days to reflect on what you've learned, identify what felt most impactful, and celebrate your wins. This is also a chance for you to keep the momentum going by choosing your next steps. Whether you decide to repeat the challenge, shift your focus, or maintain the progress you've made, these final days will help you transition with intention.

To track your progress during the 21-Day Challenge, you'll use a printable score sheet to record your daily points for each of the 8 Rs. The complete score sheet packet also includes a Prep Week checklist, scoring instructions, goal-setting prompts, and reflection questions—everything you need to stay focused and supported from start to finish! You can download it at hypothyroidchef.com/cookbook or by scanning the QR code below.

Scoring

Each of the 8 Daily Rituals is worth 1 point, except for "Refuel" (food and drink), which is worth 3 points. Each time you stray from your designated dietary goals you take away one of your 3 "Refuel" points. This way you have some flexibility built in and don't have to take an all-or-nothing approach to thyroid-healthy food and beverage choices.

THYROID30 SCORE BREAKDOWN:
The 8 Daily Rituals of Thyroid-Healthy Living

1 **REMEMBER:** Did you remember to take your medications and supplements? **(1 point)**

2 **REFUEL:** Did you follow your chosen dietary guidelines? **(Up to 3 points. Remove a point for each dietary slip or deviation.)**

3 **REACTIVATE:** Did you get ten or more minutes of physical activity? **(1 point)**

4 **REPAIR:** Did you do one small thing to nourish your gut health? **(1 point)**

5 **REJUVENATE:** Did you enjoy ten or more minutes of self-care? **(1 point)**

6 **REDUCE:** Did you do one small thing to reduce your toxin exposure? **(1 point)**

7 **RELISH:** Did you celebrate your wins or connect with your support system? **(1 point)**

8 **RECHARGE:** Did you stick to your sleep goals? **(1 point)**

TOTAL: 10 daily points possible

Resources

Throughout THYROID30, you'll have the opportunity to sample the recipes or use the meal plans from this book, which are labeled according to the three dietary levels outlined on page 79 (GF/DF, paleo, and AIP). If you'd like additional support, such as thyroid-friendly workout, meditation, or breathwork videos as well as expert-written guides on topics like toxins or gut health, you can unlock a treasure trove of resources in my online thyroid community, the Thrivers Club.

Getting Ready for Your Wellness Adventure

Follow these steps to get started:

1. Answer the preliminary questions in step 1.

2. Pick your primary goal or focus.

3. Pick your start date, including a Prep Week to prepare for the challenge.

4. Gather your support system.

5. Select your meal plan (or personalized dietary approach).

6. Set your lifestyle goals (for example, hours of sleep, ounces of hydration).

7. Prepare your environment during your Prep Week (Days 1 to 7).

8. Start your 21-Day Challenge (Days 8 to 28)!

Each step is covered in detail. Go through each one and you'll be set up for the ultimate THYROID30!

1. First, Answer These Questions

When you know where you want to go, it's a lot easier to get there. The questions below will help you gain clarity on what you want for your health, why you want it, and what could stand in your way on your journey. Grab your journal or open a fresh document and spend some time answering these questions:

1. What are my greatest current health challenges?

2. If I could wave a magic wand and have the health of my dreams, what would that look like? What would I be doing? Where would I be? Who would I be with?

3. What are three to five steps I could take now to move toward that vision of better health?

4. What could get in my way of achieving this vision of better health?

Answering these questions will help you lay the essential groundwork for a meaningful and effective THYROID30 experience. It will also help you answer one more essential question: **What is your primary goal or focus during this 30-day wellness adventure?**

2. Pick Your Primary Goal or Focus

Picking a primary goal or focus for your THYROID30 will help you pinpoint your priorities. This way, on those days when life gets busy or you just don't have time to practice all 8 Daily Rituals, you'll have a guidepost to help you decide which activities you should devote your time and energy to. To pick your primary goal or focus, review your answers to the preliminary questions in step 1, along with the 8 Daily Rituals. Which area feels most important to your current needs? You might choose to prioritize one or two rituals, or to set a primary goal that's uniquely your own.

Record your primary goal or focus in the designated area of your THYROID30 score sheet. This handy reminder will keep you focused and moving toward the health and vitality of your dreams.

3. Pick a Start Date

Timing is everything. Choosing when to begin your THYROID30 experience is about setting yourself up for success: You're making a thirty-day commitment to yourself, so take into consideration any upcoming holidays, plans, or projects on your calendar. Can you work around them? If so, this is a great way to create realistic expectations for yourself and increase your chances of success.

Would you like to do your THYROID30 with community support? Check the Hypothyroid Chef website to see when the next THYROID30 group wellness adventure is happening inside the Thrivers Club. If you choose this route, this will determine your start date.

Once you've identified a start date that will work for you, add it to your calendar, noting the dates for Prep Week (Days 1 to 7), the 21-Day Challenge (Days 8 to 28), and two Reflection and Integration days (Days 29 to 30).

4. Gather Your Support System

Support makes all the difference. Whether it's a friend, a family member, or an online community, having people to cheer you on and check in with can significantly boost your chances of success.

If you prefer to embark on your THYROID30 journey solo and at your own pace, that's totally fine, but do consider sharing your intention with someone you trust to strengthen your commitment and provide encouragement when you need it most. That said, group support is one of the most effective ways to stay consistent with healthy changes. If you'd like to do THYROID30 alongside a supportive community, we'd love to have you join our next wellness adventure in the Thrivers Club. You can learn more or sign up at hypothyroidchef.com/membership.

5. Select Your Meal Plan

There are three carefully curated meal plans to choose from on your THYROID30 journey, each featuring the recipes in this book. While not required, these thirty-day meal plans are designed to support you throughout your entire THYROID30 experience. You can use them during Prep Week to ease yourself into dietary changes, follow them during the 21-Day Challenge, or continue using them afterward to maintain momentum. Think of them as flexible support tools to guide your journey.

While there is no one-size-fits-all "thyroid diet," these plans represent three levels of thyroid-healthy eating based on commonly recommended dietary templates (GF/DF, paleo, and AIP). Think of these levels as a stair-step approach, where each level becomes progressively more restrictive while also offering greater potential for healing. Remember: Your long-term goal is a healthy gut and a customized dietary approach. To get there, you'll need to go through a process of discovering your unique and personalized dietary needs and sensitivities: in other words, which foods you thrive on and which foods you don't. This typically requires the process of elimination and reintroduction, which we covered in chapter 3. Each of the three dietary levels represents a variation of an elimination diet, designed to help guide that discovery. The three dietary levels, or templates, have two benefits. First, they offer a starting point for beginning that process and can be modified and adapted over time to reflect your bio-individual nutritional needs. Second, they offer us a common language that enables us to communicate with each other about our dietary needs and search for the resources and recipes that fit our chosen approach.

Also, Thyroid Thrivers may use other dietary templates depending on their individual needs, like low-FODMAP or low-histamine diets. While there are too many possibilities to cover in this book, know that you can use the THYROID30 framework to implement the dietary approach that's appropriate for your needs. Always consult with your health care provider before making major food or lifestyle changes.

NOTE: FOLLOWING THE MEAL PLANS IS OPTIONAL! You can choose from the three dietary levels outlined on the next page, each with an accompanying meal plan, or you can customize your eating approach and make your own menus based on your bio-individual needs.

Level 1: Gluten and Dairy-Free (GF/DF)

This level eliminates gluten and dairy, the two most common dietary triggers for thyroid patients: While not all thyroid patients will feel better after eliminating these foods, a majority do report improvements in symptoms.

In addition to eliminating gluten and dairy, this level also excludes:

- Refined sugars
- Ultra-processed foods (UPFs) including industrially refined seed and vegetable oils
- Soy

All of the recipes in this book adhere to these guidelines, enabling you to pick and choose from any of the recipes in this book.

Level 2: Paleo

This level takes a thyroid-friendly paleo approach, which balances nutritional diversity with increased potential for healing by removing common dietary irritants. Contrary to popular belief, paleo is not a meat-centric diet. Paleo meals are created from three primary building blocks: plenty of colorful plant foods, high-quality animal proteins, and healthy fats. It's a diet rich in nutrients that support thyroid function, gut health, hormones, and blood sugar balance.

Paleo is often used therapeutically to help reduce inflammation, particularly for those dealing with autoimmune conditions or metabolic issues.

In Level 2, you'll avoid all the same foods as Level 1 (gluten, dairy, sugar, UPFs, soy) and will also exclude:

- Grains
- Legumes
- White potatoes (optional; sometimes excluded in strict paleo)

Level 3: The Autoimmune Protocol (AIP)

The AIP is an expanded version of the paleo diet and is sometimes referred to as "Autoimmune Paleo." It's specifically designed to reduce inflammation and manage symptoms in those with autoimmune diseases like Hashimoto's or Graves'. This therapeutic elimination diet offers a comprehensive anti-inflammatory reset by focusing on gut healing and eliminating potential trigger foods before systematically reintroducing them.

Completing the entire AIP entails five phases: an initial elimination phase of at least thirty days (sometimes more), which is the most restrictive of the five phases, followed by reintroduction phases one through four.

Moving through all five phases of AIP can take several months. After the initial elimination phase (which will last throughout your THYROID30), the reintroduction phases of AIP walk participants through a systematic process of reincorporating foods one at a time and in a strategic order to identify personal dietary triggers.

It's important to note that the elimination phase of AIP is not intended for long-term use. The ultimate goal is to heal the gut, calm inflammation, and then reintroduce foods, thus restoring food freedom and maintaining nutritional diversity while avoiding known triggers.

Level 3: AIP excludes the same foods as Levels 1 and 2 (gluten, dairy, refined sugar, UPFs, alcohol, grains, and legumes) and additionally eliminates:

- Nightshades (tomatoes, potatoes, eggplant, peppers, and nightshade-based spices)
- Seeds and seed-based spices and oils
- Nuts and nut oils
- Eggs
- Caffeine
- Alcohol

WHICH MEAL PLAN IS RIGHT FOR ME?

Use the criteria here to help you identify which dietary level might be the best starting point for you, given your current needs. If you're working with a functional, holistic, or integrative practitioner, you can use THYROID30 to follow their recommendations or use the criteria to communicate with them about your current needs, readiness, and goals.

Remember: Meet yourself where you are when choosing your dietary level. You can always move up or down the levels as needed.

Consider Level 1 (GF/DF) If:
- You're new to thyroid-friendly eating.
- You've never tried eliminating gluten or dairy before.
- You want a gentle first step that's powerful but sustainable.
- You're not sure if food is affecting your symptoms but want to find out.
- You aren't ready for a bigger commitment.

Consider Level 2 (Paleo) If:
- You've already tried removing gluten and dairy (as well as refined sugar, soy, and UPFs) from your diet and are ready to test your sensitivity to grains and legumes.
- You're managing inflammation or symptoms related to digestion, blood sugar, or hormones.
- You're up for a bigger shift and want a nutrient-dense reset balanced with more food freedom than a full-blown elimination diet.
- You're not in a major autoimmune flare but still want to support healing.

Consider Level 3 (AIP) If:
- You're in an active autoimmune flare or dealing with persistent, hard-to-manage symptoms.
- You're ready for a more intensive thirty-day reset.
- You want to test your sensitivity to as many potential trigger foods as possible.
- You have the time, energy, and resources to cook most of your meals at home and follow a more structured elimination plan.

6. Set Your Lifestyle Goals

You can fill in specific hydration and sleep goals on your THYROID30 score sheet. Define these goals depending on your personalized needs.

For hydration: A standard rule of thumb is to aim for a minimum of eight 8-ounce (240 ml) glasses of water per day, or a total of 64 ounces (1.9 L). If you're very active or live in a hot climate, this may not be sufficient for your hydration needs. Choose a minimum number of ounces that feels realistic and adequate for you based on your current lifestyle.

For sleep: The agreed-upon target range for sleep is seven to nine hours per night. Anything less is considered "short sleep" and is associated with health risks. Anything more is also associated with health risks and could indicate an underlying health issue (like under-treated hypothyroidism). Set a realistic goal when trying to improve your sleep hygiene and sleep quality with THYROID30: For instance, if you're currently sleeping five hours each night, aiming for eight hours might be too much of a leap. You can always push further toward your long-term sleep goal in your next THYROID30.

7. Prep Week: Preparing Your Environment (Days 1 to 7)

It's a lot easier to reach your goals when you've planned and prepared. Prep Week is your dedicated time to do just that, and it's built right into your thirty-day journey for a reason. It gives you space to ease yourself in without overwhelm, set clear intentions and goals, gather supportive resources, and refresh your understanding of why thyroid-friendly food and lifestyle choices matter. Below are some helpful action steps you can choose from to prepare your environment in a way that will support rather than suppress those healthy choices you're trying to make. That said, how far you go with planning and preparing is up to you: This is another opportunity to meet yourself where you are.

Prep Week Checklist:

☐ Mark the dates of your THYROID30 on the calendar.

☐ Learn more about the general guidelines and principles of thyroid-friendly food and lifestyle by reading chapters 1 through 7 of this book.

☐ Declutter your living space to promote focus and mental clarity.

☐ Gather your THYROID30 materials and support resources, including your scorecard, recipes, and meal plans (if using).

☐ Browse this book for recipes that adhere to your current dietary needs.

☐ Do a fridge and pantry sweep and get rid of any expired, unhealthy, or off-plan foods.

☐ Create a simple self-care plan and gather any needed supplies.

☐ Outline and prepare for a movement plan that feels realistic and energizing.

☐ Make any necessary adjustments to your chosen meal plan (if using).

☐ Make a shopping list and stock up on groceries and any supplements you plan to use.

8. Start Your 21-Day Challenge! (Days 8 to 28)

It's go time! If you follow steps 1 through 7 and use Prep Week to ease in, get organized, and build a strong foundation, you're all set for a fantastic wellness adventure. By tracking your daily score throughout the 21-Day Challenge, you'll gain valuable insights into what's going well and the areas in which you might need a little extra attention.

The built-in Reflection and Integration Days (Days 29 to 30) at the end of THYROID30 will give you space to pause, reflect, and lock in your wins, while walking away with a clear plan for your next steps.

Remember, THYROID30 isn't about getting a perfect score; it's about building momentum through small but mighty steps. Show up for yourself each day, relish those wins, and you *will* make progress. That's the magic of THYROID30.

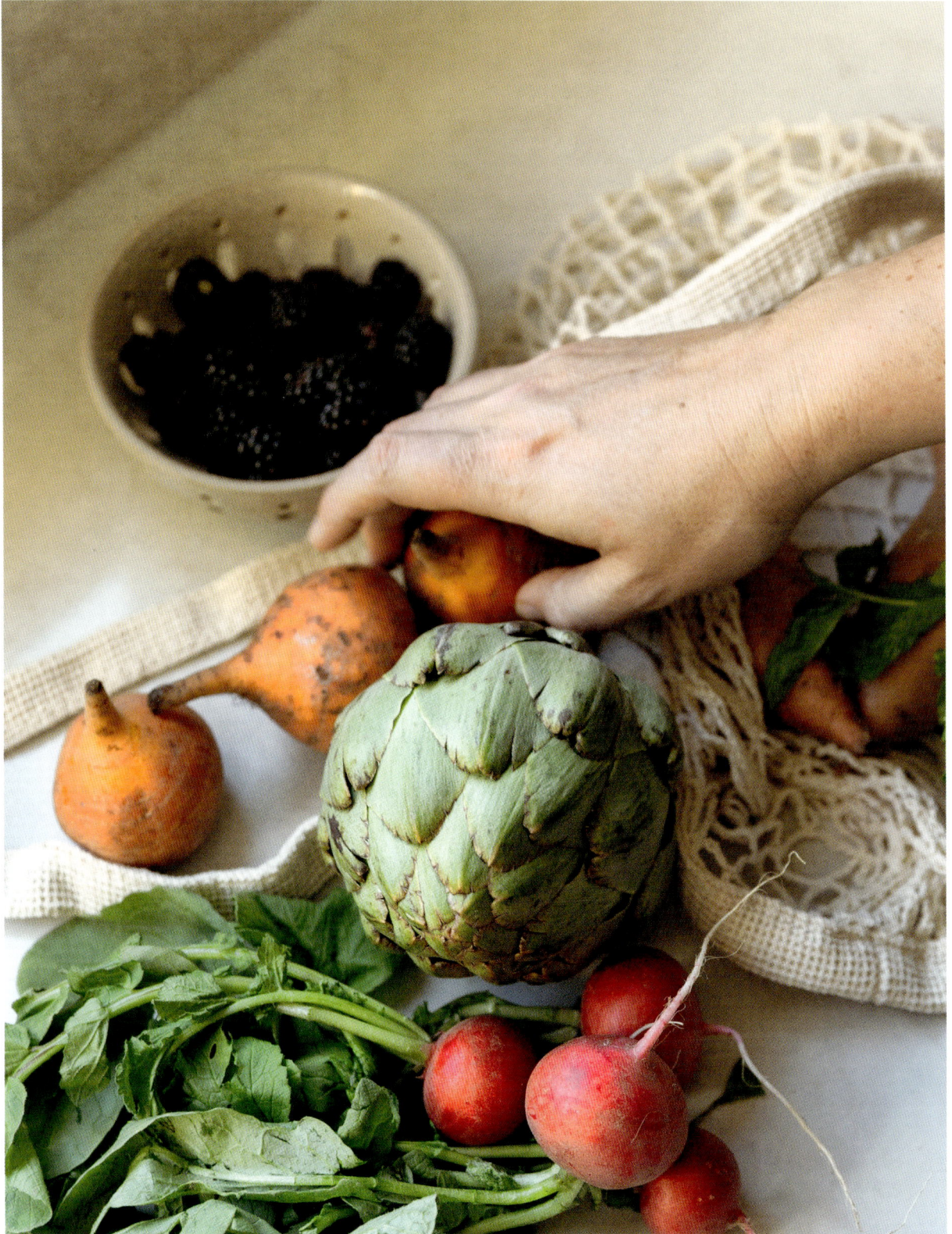

7

What Comes After THYROID30?

As your 30-day THYROID30 adventure comes to a close, you may be wondering: *What's next?* This is a crucial phase, one that determines whether your positive changes become lifelong habits or short-lived experiments. This phase is especially important for those who want to identify their unique dietary needs and sensitivities.

Sticking the Landing of Your THYROID30 with Strategic Reintroductions

If you followed one of the three dietary levels, you now have a valuable opportunity to discover which foods work for you and which don't. This requires gathering meaningful personal data by following the reintroduction process outlined in chapter 3.

The elimination phase helped calm inflammation and reset your system. Now, it's time to systematically reintroduce foods to pinpoint your triggers and tolerances.

Here's a simple framework for successful reintroductions:

1. **Start with the least likely triggers.** The four reintroduction phases of the AIP (see table on the next page) are a helpful guide. These phases begin with the foods you're most likely to tolerate.

2. **Follow the one-food, three-day rule.** Introduce one food at a time, then wait three to five days before introducing another. This helps catch delayed reactions.

3. **Document everything.** Note what you reintroduce, how much you consume, and any physical, mental, or emotional reactions.

4. **Be patient.** Especially for AIP, the full reintroduction process can take weeks. Going slow is worth it: What you learn can guide your choices for years to come.

5. **Create your personal food map.** By the end, you'll have a clear picture of your "yes," "no," and "sometimes" foods—a bio-individual blueprint for sustainable, thyroid-friendly eating.

See chapter 3 for a more detailed guide to elimination and reintroduction.

Beyond Food: Lifestyle Changes You Can Stick With

The lifestyle changes you implemented as part of the 8 Daily Rituals aren't just for your THYROID30 experience: They're tools you can carry with you forever. So, to keep the momentum going:

- **Identify your nonnegotiables.** Which rituals made the biggest difference? Try to prioritize and stick with those, no matter what.

- **Create systems, not just goals.** Systems make follow-through easier. Instead of saying, "I'll exercise three times per week," try, "I'll leave my workout clothes next to the bed and move first thing each morning."

- **Build in regular resets.** Consider doing THYROID30 quarterly or semiannually to realign and refresh your habits.

- **Find your tribe.** Surround yourself with those who support your health journey, whether that's friends, family, or our Thrivers Club community.

- **Celebrate your progress.** Acknowledge your wins, big or small. This reinforces the brain pathways that help make healthy choices feel more automatic.

When to Consider Another Full THYROID30

There's no limit to how many times you can return to THYROID30. In fact, many Thrivers come back to it again and again as life evolves. Consider another round when:

- You're experiencing a symptom or autoimmune flare.

- You've drifted away from your healthy habits and need a reset.

- You're entering a new life phase and want to reconnect with your wellness routine.

- You're aiming for a new goal you didn't focus on last time.

- You're ready to try a different dietary level (for example, moving from Level 1 to Level 2).

Each time you return to THYROID30, you'll gain new insights and deepen your understanding of what your unique body needs to thrive.

THE FOUR REINTRODUCTION PHASES OF THE AUTOIMMUNE PROTOCOL

After the elimination phase of AIP, foods are systematically reintroduced, one at a time, according to the four phases below. These phases are determined by the foods to which you are least likely to react: After working so hard to reduce inflammation and heal your gut, you wouldn't want to blast your body with the most inflammatory foods right away, would you? Better to start with the foods you're most likely to tolerate, says the logic of the four reintroduction phases.

Even if you didn't choose to do the AIP (Level 3), this list can be useful in helping you determine which of your eliminated foods you should reintroduce first.

PHASE 1	PHASE 2	PHASE 3	PHASE 4
Bean sprouts	Alcohol (GF) in small amounts	Bell peppers	Alcohol (GF) in moderate amounts
Cacao	Daily coffee	Chickpeas	Ashwagandha
Chocolate	Egg whites	Eggplant	Beans
Egg yolks	Grass-fed butter	Grass-fed dairy	Chile peppers
Fruit or berry-based spices	Nuts	Lentils	Gluten-free grains
Ghee	Seeds	Paprika	Nightshade spices
Green beans		Peeled potatoes	Peanuts
Macadamia oil		Split peas	Pseudograins
Occasional coffee			Tomatillos
Peas			Tomatoes
Seed-based spices			Unpeeled potatoes
Sesame oil			
Snow peas			
Sugar snap peas			
Walnut oil			

Wrapping It All Up

True health is about honoring your body's needs with curiosity, compassion, and consistency. The skills you've developed over the past thirty days are now yours to keep, ready to support you through whatever comes next.

Whether this is the start of your thyroid-friendly lifestyle or one more step along your healing path, know this: You have everything you need to become your own best health advocate. Your thyroid condition doesn't define you. It can be the catalyst for vibrant well-being and meaningful self-discovery.

Next up: The meal plans and recipes! Let's get cooking. It's time to make your dream of better health a reality, one delicious meal at a time.

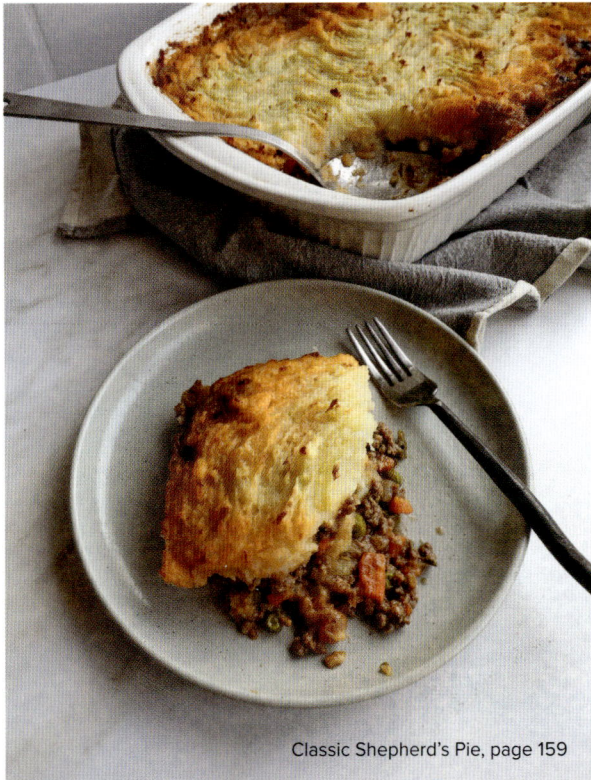
Classic Shepherd's Pie, page 159

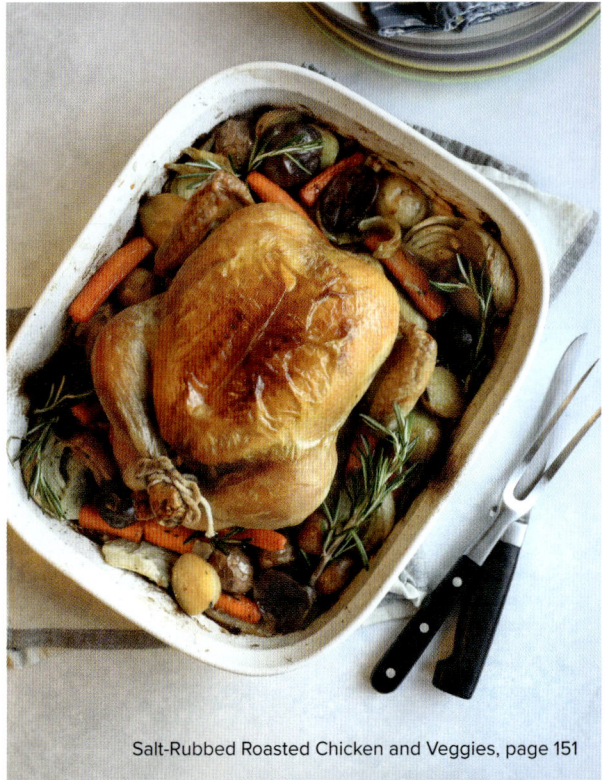
Salt-Rubbed Roasted Chicken and Veggies, page 151

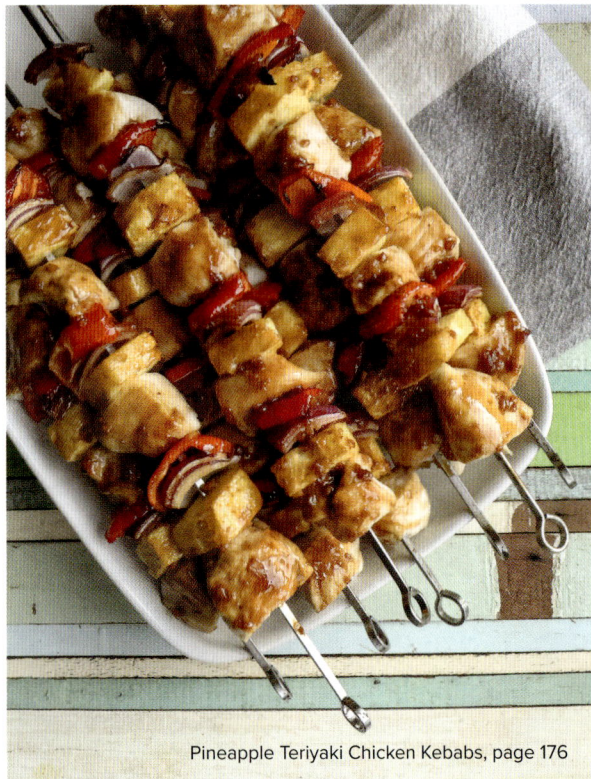
Pineapple Teriyaki Chicken Kebabs, page 176

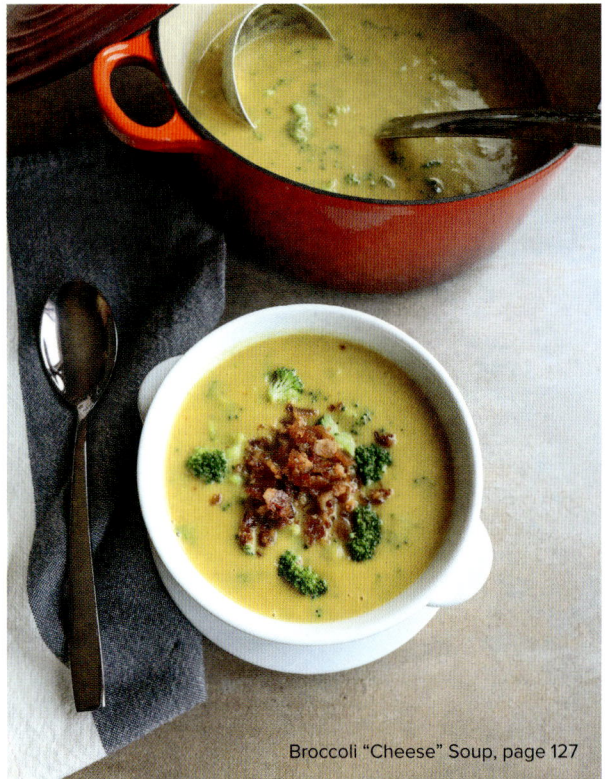
Broccoli "Cheese" Soup, page 127

(8)

The Meal Plans

To help you put what you've learned into practice, I've created three thirty-day meal plans, one for each dietary level in this program:

● ● **Level 1:** GF/DF   ● **Level 2:** Paleo   ● **Level 3:** AIP

Note that the meal plans do not use all of this book's 100 recipes. That's because all of these plans are flexible frameworks, not rigid prescriptions. Feel free to swap meals, adjust for your preferences, and lean on leftovers where it makes sense. Many recipes are batch-cook friendly to simplify your prep and reduce time spent in the kitchen.

How to Use the Meal Plans:

1. **Choose your dietary level.** Pick the plan that best aligns with your needs and goals.

2. **Look for days with recipes highlighted in bold.** These recipes need to be made from scratch.

3. **Look for (L).** These meals use leftovers and don't require cooking.

4. **Review the menus.** Make any changes or substitutions you'd like before shopping or prepping.

5. **Use the five-day block structure.** Each plan is organized in five-day chunks, including breakfast, lunch, and dinner. When planning, shop for the ingredients for the recipes within each five-day block to stay organized and reduce overwhelm.

You'll get the feel for it right away and can easily tweak things to fit your household, doubling recipes, adding snacks or treats, and adjusting portions as needed.

30-DAY GF/DF LEVEL 1 MEAL PLAN

Key: **Bold** = Make from scratch,
(L) = Leftovers/no cooking required

DAY	BREAKFAST	LUNCH	DINNER
1	**Zucchini Basil Frittata** with simple green salad	**Spiced Red Lentil Stew**	**Spice-Rubbed Slammin' Salmon** and **Slow-Roasted Miso Butter Sweet Potatoes**
2	(L) Zucchini Basil Frittata with simple green salad	(L) Spice-Rubbed Slammin' Salmon and Slow-Roasted Miso Butter Sweet Potatoes	(L) Spiced Red Lentil Stew
3	**Sweet and Savory Breakfast Hash**	(L) Zucchini Basil Frittata with simple green salad	**Classic Clean Fajitas**
4	(L) Sweet and Savory Breakfast Hash	(L) Classic Clean Fajitas	**Vietnamese-Style Spring Roll Salad**
5	(L) Sweet and Savory Breakfast Hash	(L) Vietnamese-Style Spring Roll Salad	(L) Classic Clean Fajitas
6	**Banana Buckwheat Waffles**	**Broccoli "Cheese" Soup**	**Coconut-Crusted Mahi-Mahi** with **Mango Slaw** and white rice
7	(L) Banana Buckwheat Waffles	(L) Coconut-Crusted Mahi-Mahi with Mango Slaw and white rice	(L) Broccoli "Cheese" Soup
8	**Everyday Breakfast Salad** with eggs and bacon	(L) Broccoli "Cheese" Soup	**Sausage, Beans, and Greens Pasta**
9	(L) Everyday Breakfast Salad with eggs and bacon	(L) Sausage, Beans, and Greens Pasta	**Savory Korean-Style Chuck Roast** with rice and **Japanese-Style Cucumber Salad**
10	(L) Banana Buckwheat Waffles	(L) Sausage, Beans, and Greens Pasta	(L) Savory Korean-Style Chuck Roast with rice and Japanese-Style Cucumber Salad
11	**Turkey and Sweet Potato Breakfast Tacos**	**Cowboy Caviar Quinoa Salad**	**Smoky Bison Chili**
12	(L) Turkey and Sweet Potato Breakfast Tacos	(L) Smoky Bison Chili	(L) Cowboy Caviar Quinoa Salad
13	**Tropical Delight Chia Pudding**	(L) Cowboy Caviar Quinoa Salad	**Sushi-Style Buddha Bowl**
14	(L) Tropical Delight Chia Pudding	(L) Sushi-Style Buddha Bowl	**Balsamic-Marinated Chicken Breasts** with **Citrus-Glazed Beets** and green salad with Italian dressing
15	(L) Turkey and Sweet Potato Breakfast Tacos	(L) Balsamic-Marinated Chicken Breasts with Citrus-Glazed Beets and green salad with Italian Dressing	(L) Smoky Bison Chili

DAY	BREAKFAST	LUNCH	DINNER
16	**Blueberry Breakfast Salad** with **Zesty Homemade Breakfast Sausage Patties**	**BLAT Wraps**	**Chile Lime Shrimp (or Fish) Tacos**
17	(L) Blueberry Breakfast Salad with Zesty Homemade Breakfast Sausage Patties	(L) Chile Lime Shrimp (or Fish) Tacos	(L) BLAT Wraps
18	**Scrambled Egg Breakfast Tacos with Harissa**	(L) BLAT Wraps	**White Bolognese Sauce** with pasta (GF)
19	(L) Scrambled Egg Breakfast Tacos with Harissa	(L) White Bolognese Sauce with pasta (GF)	**Salt-Rubbed Roasted Chicken and Veggies**
20	(L) Scrambled Egg Breakfast Tacos with Harissa	(L) Salt-Rubbed Roasted Chicken and Veggies	White Bolognese Sauce with pasta (GF)
21	**Everything Seed Loaf with toppings**	**Mediterranean Gundi Bowls**	**Classic Shepherd's Pie**
22	(L) Everything Seed Loaf with toppings	(L) Classic Shepherd's Pie	(L) Mediterranean Gundi Bowls
23	**Energizing Green Goddess Smoothie** (make double for leftovers) with a side of **Zesty Homemade Breakfast Sausage Patties**	(L) Classic Shepherd's Pie	**Thai-Style Chicken (or Shrimp) Red Curry** with white rice
24	(L) Energizing Green Goddess Smoothie with a side of Zesty Homemade Breakfast Sausage Patties	(L) Thai-Style Chicken (or Shrimp) Red Curry with white rice	**Herb-Marinated Pork Tenderloin with Fennel-Olive Sauce** and **Garlicky Sheet Pan Broccoli**
25	(L) Everything Seed Loaf with toppings	(L) Herb-Marinated Pork Tenderloin with Fennel-Olive Sauce and Garlicky Sheet Pan Broccoli	(L) Thai-Style Chicken (or Shrimp) Red Curry with white rice
26	**Samurai Breakfast Bowls with Steel-Cut Oats**	**Super Simple Lemon Chicken Soup**	**Spice-Rubbed Slammin' Salmon** with **Lemony Cauliflower Pasta**
27	(L) Samurai Breakfast Bowls with Steel-Cut Oats	(L) Spice-Rubbed Slammin' Salmon with Lemony Cauliflower Pasta	**Pub Mash with Sausage and Caramelized Onion and Mushroom Gravy** and simple green salad
28	**Carrot Ginger Breakfast Soup**	(L) Pub Mash with Sausage and Caramelized Onion and Mushroom Gravy and simple green salad	(L) Super Simple Lemon Chicken Soup
29	(L) Carrot Ginger Breakfast Soup	(L) Super Simple Lemon Chicken Soup	**Thai Beef Lettuce Wraps** with white rice
30	(L) Carrot Ginger Breakfast Soup	(L) Thai Beef Lettuce Wraps with white rice	(L) Pub Mash with Sausage and Caramelized Onion and Mushroom Gravy and simple green salad

30-DAY PALEO LEVEL 2 MEAL PLAN

Key: **Bold** = Make from scratch,
(L) = Leftovers/no cooking required

DAY	BREAKFAST	LUNCH	DINNER
1	**Scrambled Eggs and Greens** with **Zesty Homemade Breakfast Sausage Patties** (make a triple batch of sausage and freeze 2 pounds [0.9 kg] for upcoming menus)	**Blackened Shrimp Caesar Salad**	**Classic Clean Fajitas**
2	(L) Scrambled Eggs and Greens with Zesty Homemade Breakfast Sausage Patties	(L) Classic Clean Fajitas	(L) Blackened Shrimp Caesar Salad
3	**Almond Berry Sweet Potato Toast**	(L) Classic Clean Fajitas	**Pasta (Cassava) with White Bolognese Sauce**
4	(L) Almond Berry Sweet Potato Toast	(L) Pasta (Cassava) with White Bolognese Sauce	**Crispy Chicken and Veggie Nuggets** with **Oven-Roasted Garlic Fries**
5	(L) Scrambled Eggs and Greens with Zesty Homemade Breakfast Sausage Patties	(L) Crispy Chicken and Veggie Nuggets with Oven-Roasted Garlic Fries	(L) Pasta (Cassava) with White Bolognese Sauce
6	**Sweet and Savory Breakfast Hash**	**Eat the Rainbow Chopped Salad**	**Spice-Rubbed Slammin' Salmon** with **Lemony Cauliflower Pasta**
7	(L) Sweet and Savory Breakfast Hash	(L) Spice-Rubbed Slammin' Salmon with Lemony Cauliflower Pasta	(L) Eat the Rainbow Chopped Salad
8	**Everyday Breakfast Salad** with eggs and bacon	(L) Sweet and Savory Breakfast Hash	**Balsamic-Marinated Chicken Breasts** with **Citrus-Glazed Beets** and green salad with Italian dressing
9	(L) Everyday Breakfast Salad with eggs and bacon	(L) Balsamic-Marinated Chicken Breasts with Citrus-Glazed Beets and green salad with Italian dressing	**Thai Beef Lettuce Wraps** with cauliflower rice
10	(L) Everyday Breakfast Salad with eggs and bacon	(L) Thai Beef Lettuce Wraps with cauliflower rice	(L) Balsamic-Marinated Chicken Breasts with Citrus-Glazed Beets and green salad with Italian dressing
11	**Turkey and Sweet Potato Breakfast Tacos**	**BLAT Wraps**	**Herb-Marinated Pork Tenderloin** with **Garlicky Sheet Pan Broccoli**
12	(L) Turkey and Sweet Potato Breakfast Tacos	(L) BLAT Wraps	(L) Herb-Marinated Pork Tenderloin with Garlicky Sheet Pan Broccoli
13	**Blueberry Breakfast Salad** with **Zesty Homemade Breakfast Sausage Patties**	(L) Turkey and Sweet Potato Breakfast Tacos	**Creamy Ginger Scallion Chicken Soup**
14	(L) Blueberry Breakfast Salad with Zesty Homemade Breakfast Sausage Patties	(L) Creamy Ginger Scallion Chicken Soup	**Crispy "Parmesan" Cabbage and Bratwurst Sheet Pan Meal**
15	(L) Blueberry Breakfast Salad with Zesty Homemade Breakfast Sausage Patties	(L) Crispy "Parmesan" Cabbage and Bratwurst Sheet Pan Meal	(L) Creamy Ginger Scallion Chicken Soup

DAY	BREAKFAST	LUNCH	DINNER
16	**Zucchini Basil Frittata** with simple green salad	**Curried Pumpkin Soup**	**Chile Lime Shrimp (or Fish) Tacos**
17	(L) Zucchini Basil Frittata with simple green salad	(L) Chile Lime Shrimp (or Fish) Tacos	**Salt-Rubbed Roasted Chicken and Veggies**
18	**Everyday Breakfast Salad** with eggs and bacon	(L) Curried Pumpkin Soup	(L) Salt-Rubbed Roasted Chicken and Veggies
19	(L) Curried Pumpkin Soup	(L) Everyday Breakfast Salad with eggs and bacon	**Steak Frites with Homemade Worcestershire Sauce** and **Wilted Greens with Toasted Garlic Chips**
20	(L) Everyday Breakfast Salad with eggs and bacon	(L) Zucchini Basil Frittata with simple green salad	(L) Steak Frites with Homemade Worcestershire Sauce and Wilted Greens with Toasted Garlic Chips
21	**Sweet and Savory Breakfast Hash**	**Broccoli "Cheese" Soup**	**Thai-Style Chicken (or Shrimp) Red Curry** with cauliflower rice
22	(L) Sweet and Savory Breakfast Hash	(L) Thai-Style Chicken (or Shrimp) Red Curry with cauliflower rice	**Mediterranean Gundi Bowls**
23	**Sweet Potato Toast with Sausage Crumbles and Avocado**	(L) Broccoli "Cheese" Soup	(L) Thai-Style Chicken (or Shrimp) Red Curry with cauliflower rice
24	(L) Sweet and Savory Breakfast Hash	(L) Mediterranean Gundi Bowls	**Savory Korean-Style Chuck Roast** with cauliflower rice and **Japanese-Style Cucumber Salad**
25	(L) Sweet Potato Toast with Sausage Crumbles and Avocado	(L) Broccoli "Cheese" Soup	(L) Savory Korean-Style Chuck Roast with cauliflower rice and Japanese-Style Cucumber Salad
26	**Scrambled Egg Breakfast Tacos with Harissa**	**Lamb Burger Salad with Lemon, Garlic, and Dill Aioli**	**Sheet Pan Harissa Chicken with Carrots and Olives**
27	(L) Scrambled Egg Breakfast Tacos with Harissa	(L) Sheet Pan Harissa Chicken with Carrots and Olives	(L) Lamb Burger Salad with Lemon, Garlic, and Dill Aioli
28	**Carrot Ginger Breakfast Soup**	(L) Lamb Burger Salad with Lemon, Garlic, and Dill Aioli	**Veggie-Packed Meatloaf Muffins** and **Sweet Potato Fries with Fry Sauce**
29	(L) Scrambled Egg Breakfast Tacos with Harissa	(L) Carrot Ginger Breakfast Soup	**Seared Chicken Breasts with Mushroom Caper Pan Sauce** and **Roasted Brussels Sprouts with Bacon**
30	(L) Carrot Ginger Breakfast Soup	(L) Seared Chicken Breasts with Mushroom Caper Pan Sauce and Roasted Brussels Sprouts with Bacon	(L) Veggie-Packed Meatloaf Muffins and Sweet Potato Fries with Fry Sauce

30-DAY AIP LEVEL 3 MEAL PLAN

Key: **Bold** = Make from scratch,
(L) = Leftovers/no cooking required

DAY	BREAKFAST	LUNCH	DINNER
1	**Sweet Potato Toast with Sausage Crumbles and Avocado** (make a triple batch of sausage and freeze 2 pounds [0.9 kg] for the next two five-day menus)	**Super Simple Lemon Chicken Soup**	**Coconut-Crusted Mahi-Mahi** with **Mango Slaw** and cauliflower rice
2	(L) Sweet Potato Toast with Sausage Crumbles and Avocado	(L) Coconut-Crusted Mahi-Mahi with Mango Slaw and cauliflower rice	(L) Super Simple Lemon Chicken Soup
3	**Everyday Breakfast Salad** with chicken	(L) Super Simple Lemon Chicken Soup	**Sticky Thai-Style Zingy Wings** with **Rainbow Roasted Root Veggies** and simple green salad
4	(L) Everyday Breakfast Salad with chicken	(L) Sticky Thai-Style Zingy Wings with Rainbow Roasted Root Veggies and simple green salad	**White Bolognese Sauce** with spaghetti squash or cassava pasta
5	(L) Sweet Potato Toast with Sausage Crumbles and Avocado	(L) Everyday Breakfast Salad with Chicken	(L) White Bolognese Sauce with spaghetti squash or cassava pasta
6	**Blueberry Breakfast Salad** with **Homemade Sausage Patties**	**Creamy Ginger Scallion Chicken Soup**	**Savory Korean-Style Chuck Roast** with cauliflower rice and **Japanese-Style Cucumber Salad**
7	(L) Carrot Ginger Breakfast Soup	(L) Savory Korean-Style Chuck Roast with cauliflower rice and Japanese-Style Cucumber Salad	**Butternut, Chard, and Chicken Curry** over cauliflower rice
8	(L) Blueberry Breakfast Salad with Homemade Sausage Patties	(L) Creamy Ginger Scallion Chicken Soup	(L) Butternut, Chard, and Chicken Curry over cauliflower rice
9	(L) Carrot Ginger Breakfast Soup	(L) Butternut, Chard, and Chicken Curry over cauliflower rice	**Steak Frites with Homemade Worcestershire Sauce** and **Roasted Brussels Sprouts with Bacon**
10	(L) Blueberry Breakfast Salad with Homemade Sausage Patties	(L) Steak Frites with Homemade Worcestershire Sauce and Roasted Brussels Sprouts with Bacon	(L) Creamy Ginger Scallion Chicken Soup
11	**Energizing Green Goddess Smoothie** (make double for leftovers) with a side of **Zesty Homemade Breakfast Sausage Patties**	**Golden Leek and Cabbage Soup**	**Herb-Marinated Pork Tenderloin** with **Fennel-Olive Sauce** and **Lemony Cauliflower Pasta (Cassava)**
12	(L) Energizing Green Goddess Smoothie with a side of Zesty Homemade Breakfast Sausage Patties	(L) Golden Leek and Cabbage Soup	(L) Herb-Marinated Pork Tenderloin with Fennel-Olive Sauce and Lemony Cauliflower Pasta (Cassava)
13	**Turkey and Sweet Potato Breakfast Tacos**	**Super Simple Lemon Chicken Soup**	**Veggie-Packed Meatloaf Muffins** with **Velvety Truffle Mashed Cauliflower and Sweet Potatoes**
14	(L) Turkey and Sweet Potato Breakfast Tacos	(L) Super Simple Lemon Chicken Soup	**Balsamic-Marinated Chicken Breasts** with **Citrus-Glazed Beets** and green salad with Italian dressing
15	(L) Turkey and Sweet Potato Breakfast Tacos	(L) Balsamic-Marinated Chicken Breasts with Citrus-Glazed Beets and green salad with Italian dressing	(L) Veggie-Packed Meatloaf Muffins with Velvety Truffle Mashed Cauliflower and Sweet Potatoes

DAY	BREAKFAST	LUNCH	DINNER
16	**Sweet and Savory Breakfast Hash**	**Broccoli "Cheese" Soup**	**Seared Chicken Breasts with Mushroom Caper Pan Sauce** and **French Carrot Salad with Mint**
17	(L) Sweet and Savory Breakfast Hash	(L) Seared Chicken Breasts with Mushroom Caper Pan Sauce and French Carrot Salad with Mint	(L) Broccoli "Cheese" Soup
18	**Everyday Breakfast Salad** with chicken	(L) Sweet and Savory Breakfast Hash	**Steak Frites with Homemade Worcestershire Sauce** and **Wilted Greens with Roasted Garlic Chips**
19	(L) Everyday Breakfast Salad with chicken	(L) Steak Frites with Homemade Worcestershire Sauce and Wilted Greens with Roasted Garlic Chips	**Sticky Thai-Style Zingy Wings** with **Caramelized Cauliflower** and simple green salad
20	(L) Everyday Breakfast Salad with chicken	(L) Sticky Thai-Style Zingy Wings with Caramelized Cauliflower and simple green salad	(L) Seared Chicken Breasts with Mushroom Caper Pan Sauce and French Carrot Salad with Mint
21	**Turkey and Sweet Potato Breakfast Tacos**	Leftovers of choice	**Crispy Chicken and Veggie Nuggets** with **Oven-Roasted Garlic Fries**
22	(L) Turkey and Sweet Potato Breakfast Tacos	(L) Crispy Chicken and Veggie Nuggets with Oven-Roasted Garlic Fries	**Veggie-Packed Meatloaf Muffins** with **Savory Butternut Slices**
23	**Carrot Ginger Breakfast Soup**	(L) Veggie-Packed Meatloaf Muffins with Savory Butternut Slices	**Herb-Marinated Pork Tenderloin** and **Roasted Brussel Sprouts with Bacon**
24	(L) Carrot Ginger Breakfast Soup	(L) Herb-Marinated Pork Tenderloin and Roasted Brussel Sprouts with Bacon	**Savory Korean-Style Chuck Roast** with cauliflower rice and **Japanese-Style Cucumber Salad**
25	(L) Turkey and Sweet Potato Breakfast Tacos	(L) Carrot Ginger Breakfast Soup	(L) Savory Korean-Style Chuck Roast with cauliflower rice and Japanese-Style Cucumber Salad
26	**Blueberry Breakfast Salad** with **Zesty Homemade Breakfast Sausage Patties**	Leftovers of choice	**Coconut-Crusted Mahi-Mahi with Mango Slaw** and cauliflower rice
27	(L) Blueberry Breakfast Salad with Zesty Homemade Breakfast Sausage Patties	(L) Coconut-Crusted Mahi-Mahi with Mango Slaw and cauliflower rice	**White Bolognese Sauce** with zoodles (or cassava pasta)
28	**Sweet Potato Toast with Sausage Crumbles and Avocado**	(L) White Bolognese Sauce with zoodles (or cassava pasta)	**Salt-Rubbed Roasted Chicken and Veggies**
29	(L) Blueberry Breakfast Salad with Zesty Homemade Breakfast Sausage Patties	(L) Salt-Rubbed Roasted Chicken and Veggies	**Super Simple Lemon Chicken Soup** (make broth from roasted chicken bones)
30	(L) Sweet Potato Toast with Sausage Crumbles and Avocado	(L) Super Simple Lemon Chicken Soup (make broth from roasted chicken bones)	(L) White Bolognese Sauce with zoodles (or cassava pasta)

Sweet and Savory
Breakfast Hash,
page 110

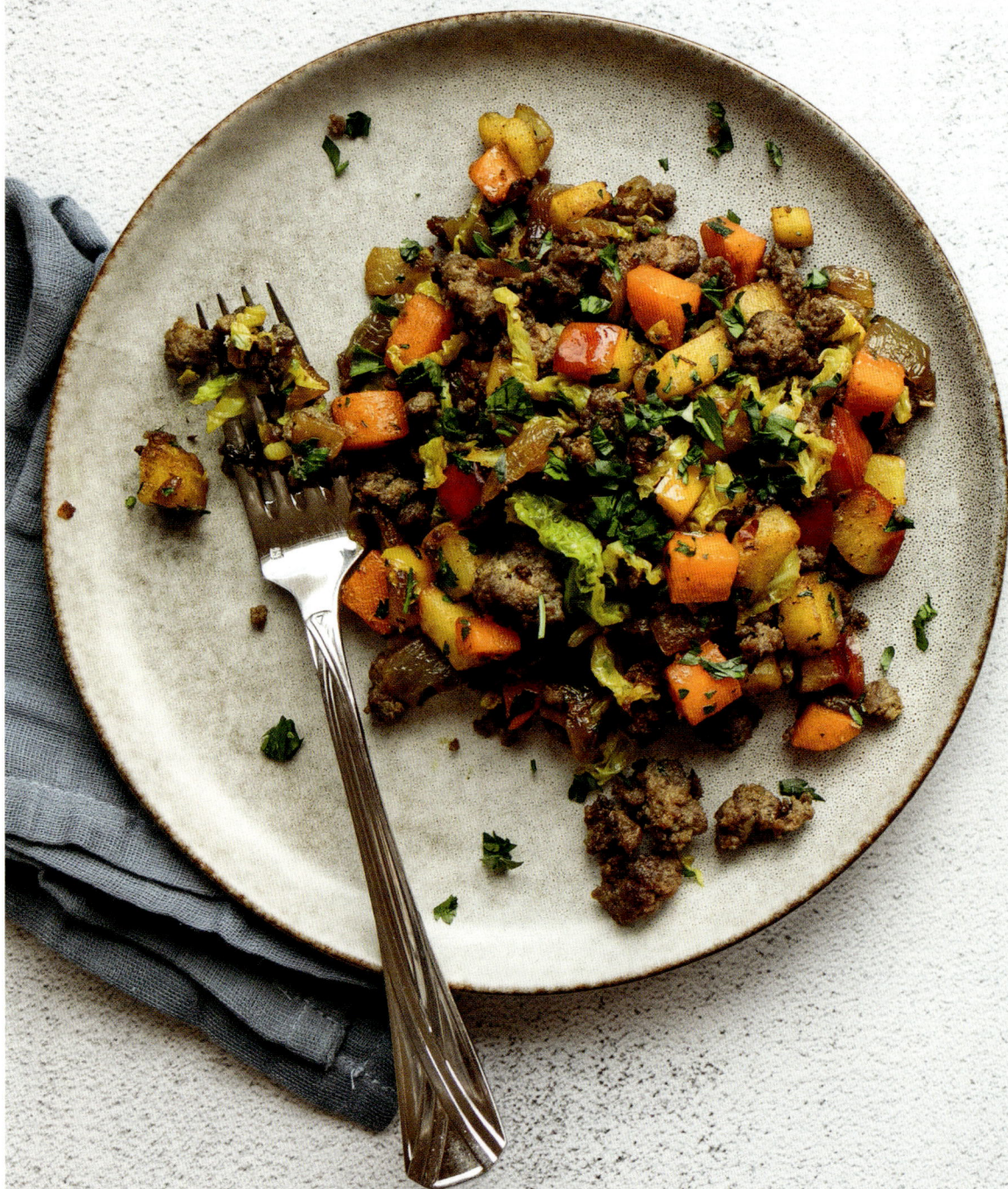

9

Breakfasts

When you're navigating dietary changes like going gluten-free, dairy-free, or even skipping grains and eggs, breakfast can suddenly feel like a bit of a conundrum because so many traditional standbys are, quite literally, off the table.

In this chapter, I invite you to reimagine breakfast through a thyroid-friendly lens—one that supports all-day energy, blood sugar balance, digestion, and nutrient intake. Starting your day with a balanced blend of colorful produce, satiating protein, fiber, and healthy fats creates a foundation for how you feel—not just in the morning, but all day long.

That's because breakfast is more than just a meal. It's a daily opportunity to set the tone for how you're going to nourish your body. By shifting the way we approach it, we can move the needle on everything from our energy levels to our long-term metabolic health. In the pages to come, you'll discover what that can look like, with reinventions of old favorites and creative alternatives that will transform the way you think about your fast-breaking meal.

SCRAMBLED EGGS AND GREENS

This is one of those simple staples you can whip up in ten minutes and use in dozens of different ways. Pair it with fresh fruit and Zesty Homemade Breakfast Sausage Patties (page 107) for a complete breakfast; wrap it in a gluten- or grain-free tortilla with crispy bacon and salsa for a breakfast taco; or pile it onto a piece of gluten-free toast or Sweet Potato Toast (page 102) with Quick and Easy Harissa (page 220). The possibilities are endless!

● **GLUTEN-FREE**　　● **DAIRY-FREE**　　● **PALEO**

DIETARY LEVELS 1, 2

SERVINGS 2
PREP TIME 5 minutes
COOK TIME 5 minutes
TOTAL TIME 10 minutes

4 eggs, lightly beaten

1 tablespoon (15 ml) water

¼ teaspoon herbes de Provence (optional but recommended)

¼ teaspoon fine sea salt

Freshly ground black pepper, to taste

1 tablespoon (15 ml) extra-virgin olive oil

1 small shallot, finely minced (about 2–3 tablespoons [20–30 g])

2 cups (60 g) roughly chopped greens, like baby spinach, Swiss chard, or kale

1. Add the eggs, water, herbes de Provence, salt, and pepper to a small bowl and whisk to combine.

2. Heat the olive oil in a medium skillet over medium heat until shimmering. Add the shallot and cook, stirring, until soft and translucent, about 2 minutes. Add the greens and cook, stirring, until wilted and tender, about 2 to 3 minutes.

3. Pour in the eggs and cook, gently scraping the pan occasionally with a spatula, until scrambled and fully set, about 3 to 4 minutes. Taste and adjust seasoning as desired, and serve with your favorite breakfast additions.

CARROT GINGER BREAKFAST SOUP

Soup for breakfast? Absolutely! Pureed soups are an excellent thyroid-friendly option: gentle on digestion, packed with nutrients, and easy to prepare in advance. This vibrant soup combines sweet carrots, apples, and onions with warming ginger, curry powder or turmeric, and citrus for a flavor-packed, anti-inflammatory, gut-friendly meal. See the note below for an AIP-friendly version.

● GLUTEN-FREE ● DAIRY-FREE ● PALEO ● AIP-FRIENDLY ● VEGAN

DIETARY LEVELS 1, 2, 3

SERVINGS 4
PREP TIME 20 minutes
COOK TIME 30 minutes
TOTAL TIME 50 minutes

3 tablespoons (42 g) grass-fed ghee (sub coconut oil for AIP)

1 sweet onion or yellow onion, roughly chopped

1 large shallot, roughly chopped

3 tablespoons (18 g) finely minced fresh ginger, or to taste, divided

2 cups (260 g) (about 5 medium) roughly chopped carrots

1 medium apple, peeled and roughly chopped

1 teaspoon curry powder (sub turmeric for AIP)

1 teaspoon fine sea salt, plus more to taste

Pinch white pepper, or to taste (omit for AIP)

4 cups (946 ml) Easy Homemade Chicken Bone Broth (page 218), or vegetable broth for a vegan version

⅔ cup (158 ml) freshly squeezed orange juice

1 tablespoon (15 ml) fresh lemon juice (optional)

Finely chopped parsley or green onion (optional)

1. Melt the ghee or coconut oil in a large Dutch oven or soup pot over medium heat. Add the onion and shallot and sauté until softened, about 5 minutes. Add 1 tablespoon (6 g) of the ginger, and the carrots, apple, curry powder or turmeric, sea salt, and white pepper. Cook, stirring occasionally, until carrots have begun to soften, about 5 minutes.

2. Add the broth of choice, bring to a boil, then reduce the heat. Simmer, covered, for 20 minutes or until the carrots are very tender.

3. Remove from the heat and add the orange juice and the remaining 2 tablespoons (12 g) of ginger. Blend until smooth using an immersion blender or upright blender (see note).

4. Taste and adjust seasoning as desired. To brighten the flavors, add a spritz of fresh lemon juice, if desired. Garnish with parsley or green onion, if desired, and enjoy! Store in an airtight container (without garnishes) in the refrigerator for up to 5 days or freeze for up to 2 months.

NOTES

Use caution when blending hot liquids in an upright blender, as steam can build up and pop the top. Prevent this by working in batches, leaving ample headroom. Start at the lowest speed, increasing speed slowly. If possible, hold the top very slightly ajar so that steam can escape.

What is ghee? Ghee is essentially clarified butter that has had all the milk solids removed, making it paleo-friendly. While it is *technically* a dairy product, most people who are intolerant to dairy have no issue with ghee because the lactose, whey, and casein have been removed. However, if you are highly sensitive to dairy and cannot tolerate ghee, you can substitute extra-virgin olive oil.

ZUCCHINI BASIL FRITTATA

Frittatas are a great kitchen-sink meal—the perfect way to use up all those bits and bobs from the produce drawer. But sometimes the simplest flavor combos create something more transcendent. This one starts with sweet, caramelized onion and savory garlic, tossed with tons of fluffy grated zucchini—a nutrient-dense powerhouse of a vegetable if there ever was one—and an herbal hint of fresh basil. The result? A soufflé-like texture that pairs beautifully with the acidity of a fresh tomato topping. For extra flavor, try a light dusting of Brazil Nut "Parmesan" (page 225). Add a simple green salad and you've got a showstopping breakfast plus leftovers for grab-and-go meals throughout the week!

● GLUTEN-FREE   ● DAIRY-FREE   ● PALEO

DIETARY LEVELS 1, 2

SERVINGS 8
PREP TIME 20 minutes
COOK TIME 20 minutes
INACTIVE COOK TIME 20 minutes
TOTAL TIME 1 hour

1½ pounds (680 g) (about 2 medium) zucchini, grated

1 teaspoon fine sea salt, plus more as needed

1 tablespoon (14 g) grass-fed ghee (optional) or (15 ml) extra-virgin olive oil

1 tablespoon (15 ml) extra-virgin olive oil

1 medium sweet onion, diced

Freshly ground black pepper, to taste

2 cloves garlic, minced

½ cup (20 g) loosely packed basil leaves, finely chopped

1 tablespoon (9 g) nutritional yeast (optional, but recommended)

8 organic eggs, lightly beaten

OPTIONAL GARNISHES

1 cup (150 g) cherry tomatoes, sliced or quartered

Fresh basil leaves

Brazil Nut "Parmesan" (page 225)

1. Preheat the oven to 350°F (175°C).

2. Place the zucchini in a colander and sprinkle with the sea salt. Toss to coat and let it sit to drain for about 15 minutes.

3. Heat the ghee, if using, or olive oil, and olive oil (you need a total of 2 tablespoons [30 ml]) in a 10-inch (25.4 cm) oven-safe skillet over medium heat. Add the diced onion and season with salt and pepper to taste. Cook, stirring occasionally, for about 10 minutes or until the onion is golden brown and caramelized. Add the garlic and cook, stirring, until fragrant, about 1 minute more.

4. Squeeze out the excess liquid from the zucchini, then add to the skillet. Cook, stirring, for about 5 minutes or until the zucchini is soft and cooked through. Stir in the basil and nutritional yeast (if using) and stir to combine. Taste the filling before adding the eggs: It should be well seasoned but not overly salty. Adjust the seasoning if necessary.

5. Add the eggs to the skillet and stir to evenly distribute the veggies. Transfer to the center of the oven and bake for about 20 minutes or until eggs are set in the middle. (The frittata may also puff up in the center.)

6. Remove the frittata from the oven and let sit for about 5 minutes before slicing into wedges. Sprinkle with diced tomatoes, fresh basil, or Brazil Nut "Parmesan," if desired, and serve warm or at room temperature.

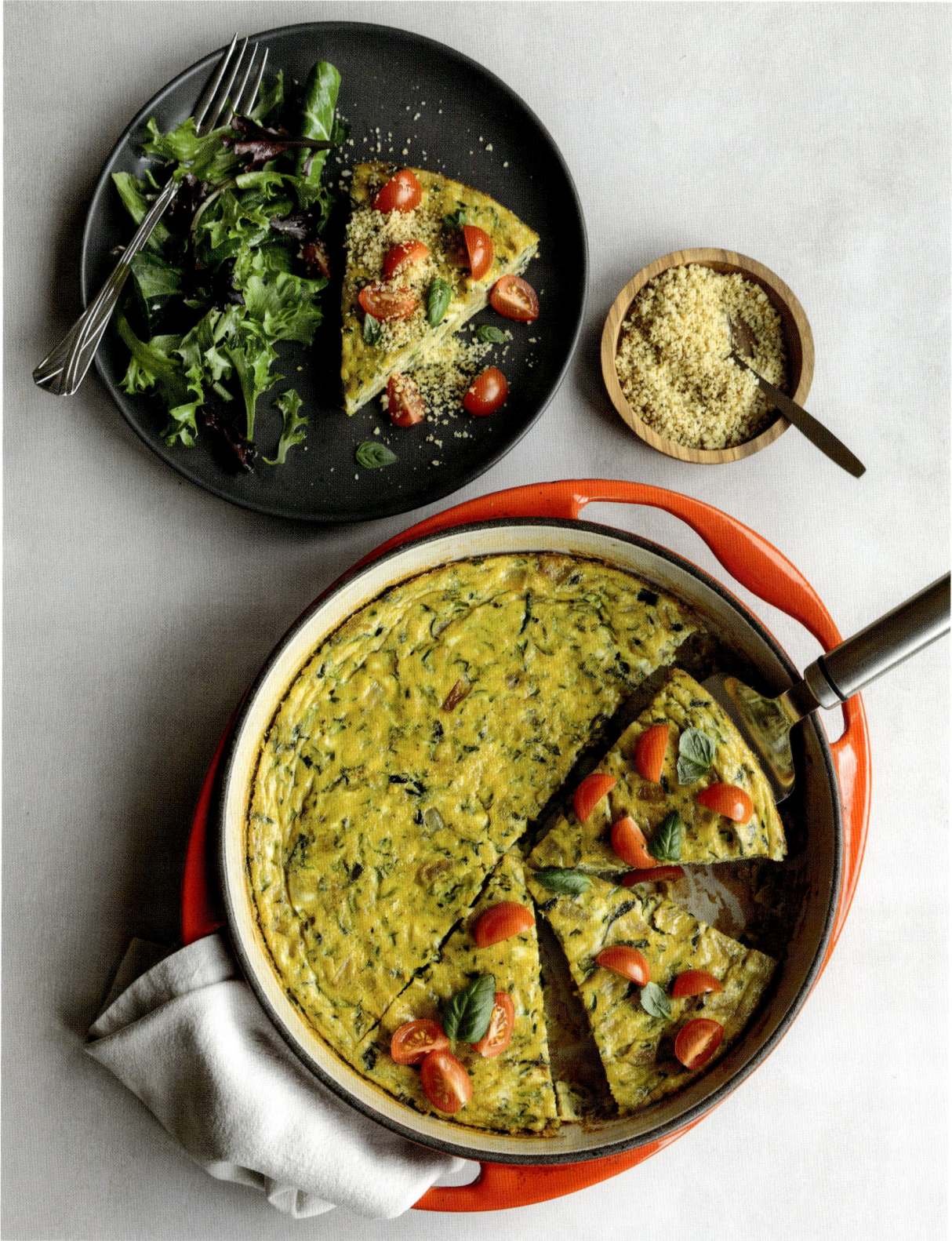

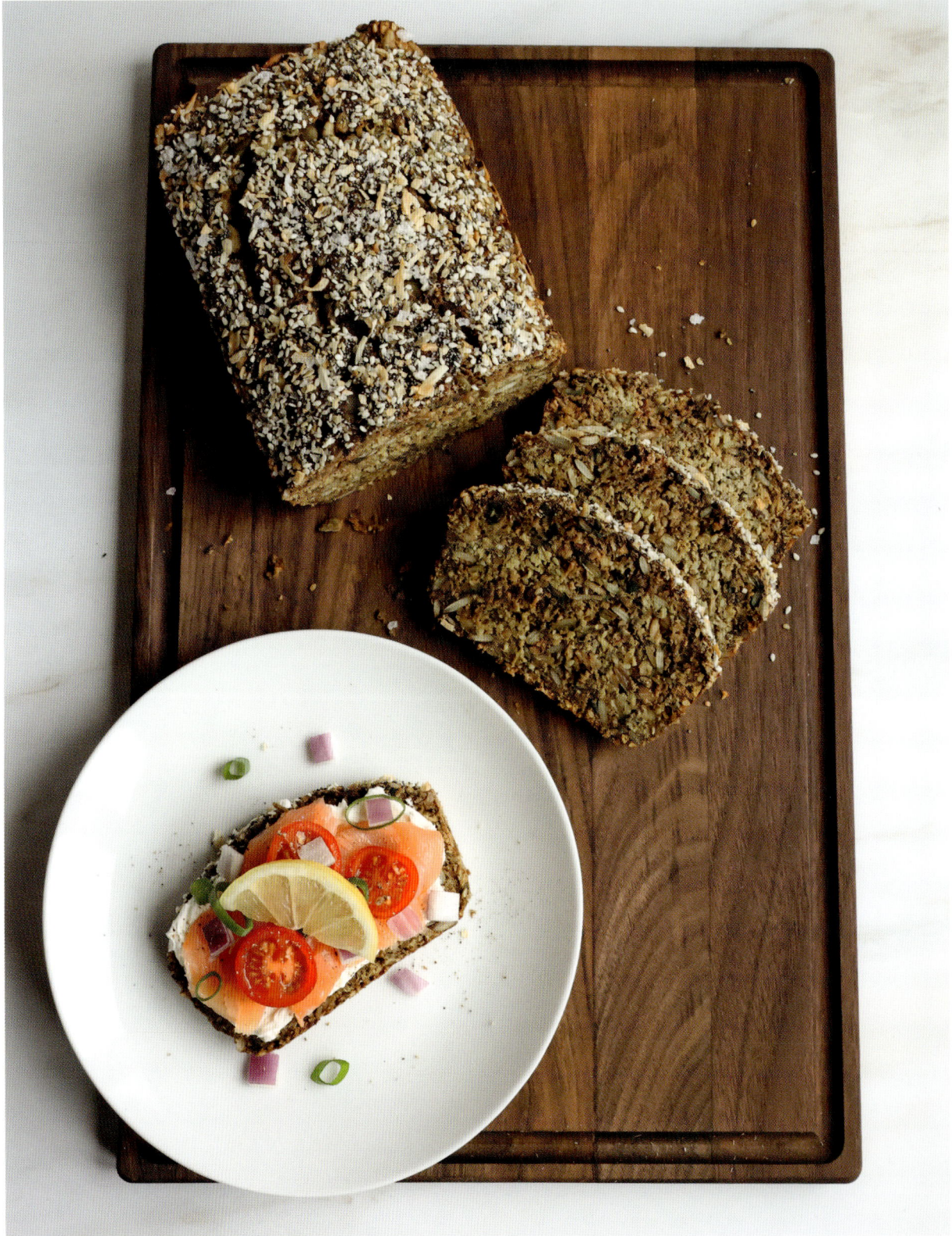

EVERYTHING SEED LOAF

This nutrient-packed loaf takes inspiration from traditional seed breads but features a bold twist—everything-bagel seasoning! Enjoy it toasted and topped with chickpea miso and avocado for a probiotic boost, or go classic everything bagel–style with dairy-free cream cheese and smoked salmon.

● GLUTEN-FREE   ◑ DAIRY-FREE

DIETARY LEVELS 1

SERVINGS 12 slices
PREP TIME 20 minutes + an overnight soak
COOK TIME 1 hour
TOTAL TIME 1 hour 20 minutes + overnight

FOR EVERYTHING-BAGEL SEASONING

2 tablespoons (16 g) sesame seeds

1 tablespoon (11 g) poppy seeds

1 tablespoon (7 g) dried minced onion

1 tablespoon (10 g) dried minced garlic

FOR BREAD

½ cup (75 g) pumpkin seeds

½ cup (75 g) sunflower seeds (see note)

¼ cup (33 g) ground flaxseed

¼ cup (40 g) chia seeds

¼ cup (33 g) sesame seeds

⅓ cup (40 g) buckwheat flour

1½ cups (165 g) certified gluten-free rolled oats

1½ teaspoons fine sea salt

¼ cup (35 g) Everything-Bagel Seasoning, divided

1 tablespoon (20 g) maple syrup

2 tablespoons (30 ml) extra-virgin olive oil

1½ cups (355 ml) water

2 eggs, lightly beaten

1 teaspoon baking soda

1 tablespoon (15 ml) apple cider vinegar

½ teaspoon flaky sea salt, or to taste (optional, for topping)

To Make the Everything-Bagel Seasoning
1. Combine all the ingredients for the Everything-Bagel Seasoning in a small bowl.

To Make the Bread
2. In a medium mixing bowl, combine the seeds, buckwheat flour, oats, fine sea salt, and 3 tablespoons (26 g) of the Everything-Bagel Seasoning. Add the maple syrup, olive oil, and water. Mix until well combined. Cover and refrigerate overnight (or at least 8 hours).

3. Preheat the oven to 325°F (160°C) and line a loaf pan with parchment paper.

4. Mix in the eggs until fully incorporated. Sprinkle the baking soda over the dough, add the vinegar (it will fizz), and mix thoroughly to combine.

5. Transfer the dough to the prepared loaf pan and smooth the top with a rubber spatula. Sprinkle the remaining 1 tablespoon (9 g) of Everything-Bagel Seasoning on top of the dough, along with the flaky sea salt, if using.

6. Bake uncovered for 30 minutes before tenting loosely with foil to protect the seasoning from scorching. Continue baking for 30 to 40 minutes more or until the loaf is golden brown and firm to the touch.

7. Let cool for 30 minutes in the pan, then transfer to a wire rack to cool completely before slicing. Slice, toast, and top as desired. Store in an airtight container at room temperature for up to 4 days, refrigerate for up to 7 days, or freeze for up to 3 months.

NOTES
Sunflower seeds contain a natural compound that reacts with baking soda and heat, sometimes turning them greenish-blue. They're safe to eat, but you can keep them from changing color by toasting them before using.

Soaking the seeds improves texture and digestibility while neutralizing "antinutrients" like phytic acid and making beneficial nutrients more bioavailable.

SWEET POTATO TOAST WITH SAUSAGE CRUMBLES AND AVOCADO

This recipe combines sweet and savory flavors with healthy doses of protein, fat, and complex carbs and is sure to start your day off right. Crispy-edged sweet potato toast provides a sturdy base for creamy avocado and flavorful homemade sausage crumbles, while optional toppings add color, texture, and a customizable twist. This nutrient-dense, meal prep–friendly option is as satisfying as it is simple.

● **GLUTEN-FREE** ● **DAIRY-FREE** ● **PALEO** ● **AIP-FRIENDLY** ● **VEGAN**

DIETARY LEVELS 1, 2, 3

SERVINGS 4
PREP TIME 10 minutes
COOK TIME 15 minutes
TOTAL TIME 25 minutes

1 large sweet potato, trimmed and peeled

1 tablespoon (15 ml) avocado or olive oil

¾ teaspoon fine sea salt, divided

½ teaspoon garlic powder

½ teaspoon smoked paprika (omit or substitute with turmeric for AIP)

½ pound (8 ounces) (227 g) Zesty Homemade Breakfast Sausage Patties, loose (page 107)

2 ripe avocados, mashed

2 teaspoons fresh lemon juice

OPTIONAL TOPPINGS

Sliced radishes

Microgreens

Fresh herbs

Green onions

Scrambled egg (omit for AIP)

1. Preheat the oven to 400°F (200°C). Line a baking sheet with parchment paper.

2. Slice the sweet potato lengthwise into slabs approximately ¼-inch (6 mm) thick.

3. Combine the oil, ½ teaspoon of the sea salt, garlic powder, and smoked paprika or turmeric in a small bowl and stir well. Arrange the sweet potato slices in a single layer on the prepared baking sheet. Brush on both sides with the oil mixture. Transfer to the oven and bake for 12 to 15 minutes, flipping halfway through. The slices are done when they are fork-tender but still firm enough to hold their shape, like toast.

4. Meanwhile, cook the sausage crumbles. Heat a medium skillet over medium heat. Add the loose Zesty Homemade Breakfast Sausage Patties and cook, breaking them up with a spatula, until browned and fully cooked (about 5 to 7 minutes). Set aside.

5. Mash the avocado with the lemon juice and the remaining ¼ teaspoon of sea salt in a small bowl.

6. To assemble, spread the mashed avocado evenly over the roasted sweet potato slices. Top with sausage crumbles. Add any optional toppings for extra flavor and color. Serve warm as a hearty breakfast, snack, or light meal.

NOTE
The sweet potato toasts (without toppings) can be made ahead of time, stored, and reheated. Let cool and store leftovers in an airtight container in the refrigerator for up to 5 days. Reheat slices in a toaster, toaster oven, or oven until warmed through, then add toppings.

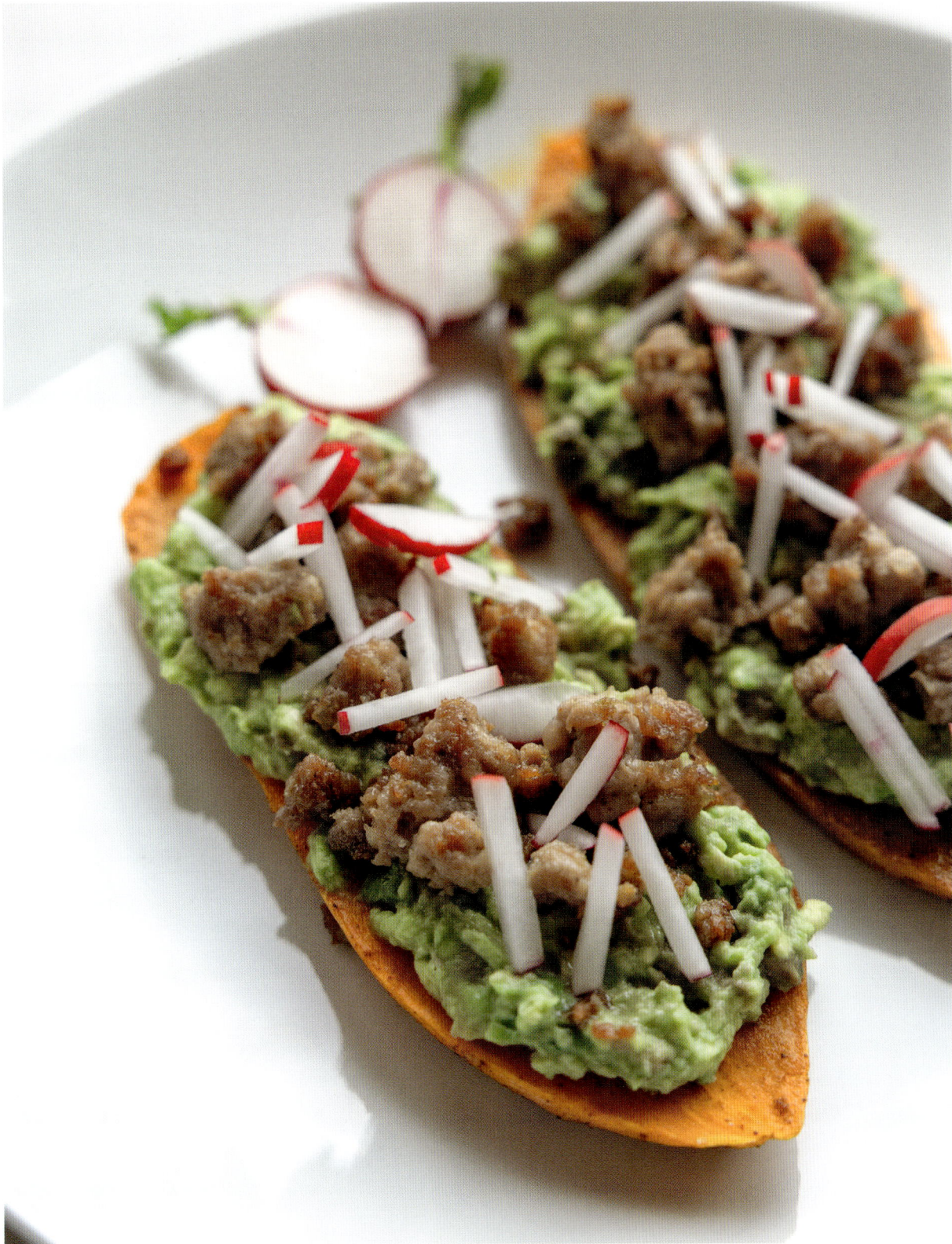

ALMOND BERRY SWEET POTATO TOAST

Sweet potato toast is endlessly versatile, and this version is packed with flavor, texture, and nutrients. It's perfect for meal prep: Just reheat the sweet potato slices in the toaster or air fryer and then add toppings for a quick, satisfying meal, snack, or dessert. Feel free to riff on this combo with different nut butters or your favorite seasonal fruits. But the combination below has it all: creamy almond butter, juicy berries, warm cinnamon, and a satisfying crunch. For a balanced meal, pair it with a protein side.

● GLUTEN-FREE   ● DAIRY-FREE   ● PALEO   ● VEGAN

DIETARY LEVELS 1, 2

SERVINGS 4
PREP TIME 10 minutes
COOK TIME 15 minutes
TOTAL TIME 25 minutes

1 large sweet potato, trimmed and peeled

¾ cup (195 g) unsweetened almond butter

1 tablespoon (20 g) honey or maple syrup (optional)

¼ teaspoon cinnamon

Pinch fine sea salt

1½ cups (225 g) fresh mixed berries, such as blueberries, raspberries, or sliced strawberries

1 tablespoon (7 g) sliced almonds or chopped walnuts (optional)

OPTIONAL TOPPINGS
Hemp nuggets
Toasted coconut flakes
Cacao nibs

1. Preheat the oven to 400°F (200°C). Place a wire rack on a rimmed baking sheet.

2. Slice the sweet potato lengthwise into slabs approximately ¼-inch (6 mm) thick. Arrange in a single layer on the wire rack. Transfer to the oven and bake for 12 to 15 minutes, flipping halfway through. The slices are done when they are fork-tender but still firm enough to hold their shape, like toast. Let cool slightly.

3. Meanwhile, combine the almond butter, maple syrup or honey (if using), cinnamon, and sea salt in a small bowl and mix until smooth. (If the almond butter is too thick, warm it slightly to make it easier to spread.) Taste and adjust seasoning as needed.

4. To assemble, spread a thin layer of almond butter on each sweet potato slice. Top with fresh berries and nuts (if using). For extra texture, sprinkle with optional toppings like hemp seeds, toasted coconut flakes, or cacao nibs. Serve immediately.

NOTE
For meal prep: Let sweet potato toasts cool completely, then store (without toppings) in an airtight container in the fridge for up to 3 days. To reheat, pop the slices into a toaster or air fryer until warm and slightly crisp, then add toppings.

GLUTEN-FREE BANANA BUCKWHEAT WAFFLES

Despite its name, buckwheat has nothing to do with wheat. It's naturally gluten-free and isn't actually a grain at all. Like quinoa, this "pseudograin" is a complete source of plant-based protein and packed with microbiome-supporting prebiotic fiber. It's an excellent alternative flour for those of us who want to avoid inflammatory refined white flour and gluten, and in this recipe, its dark color and earthy flavor are perfectly balanced by the fragrant spices and the sweetness of banana.

● GLUTEN-FREE   ● DAIRY-FREE

DIETARY LEVELS 1

SERVINGS Makes 10–12 waffles (depending on your waffle maker)

PREP TIME 25 minutes

COOK TIME 20 minutes

TOTAL TIME 45 minutes

1 cup (120 g) buckwheat flour

1 cup (92 g) oat flour

1 teaspoon cinnamon

½ teaspoon nutmeg

2 teaspoons baking powder

1½ teaspoons baking soda

½ teaspoon fine sea salt

1 cup (225 g) (about 2 large) mashed banana

2 eggs, lightly beaten

2 tablespoons (40 g) pure maple syrup

1 can (14-ounces [224 g]) light coconut milk

1 teaspoon vanilla extract

½ cup (118 ml) avocado oil

1 tablespoon (15 ml) apple cider vinegar

OPTIONAL GARNISHES

Fresh banana slices

Toasted chopped pecans

More maple syrup

1. Whisk together the buckwheat and oat flours, cinnamon, nutmeg, baking powder, baking soda, and salt in a medium mixing bowl until well combined.

2. Add the mashed banana to another medium mixing bowl. Add the eggs and whisk to combine, followed by the maple syrup, coconut milk, vanilla, avocado oil, and apple cider vinegar. Whisk well to blend.

3. Pour the wet ingredients into the dry ingredients and stir until no lumps remain. Let the batter sit for about 10 minutes to allow the flours to hydrate.

4. Meanwhile, preheat your waffle maker according to the manufacturer's instructions.

5. Ladle batter into your preheated waffle maker, using an amount suited to its size (I used about ⅓ cup [78 ml] per square Belgian waffle). Cook until brown and crisp, then carefully remove from waffle maker. Repeat with the remaining batter.

6. Serve waffles topped with fresh banana slices, toasted chopped pecans, and more maple syrup, if desired, and enjoy! Waffles can be stored in an airtight container in the refrigerator for up to 1 week. To freeze, cool completely on a wire rack to prevent condensation, then transfer to a resealable freezer bag and store for up to 2 months. To reheat, place in toaster until heated through.

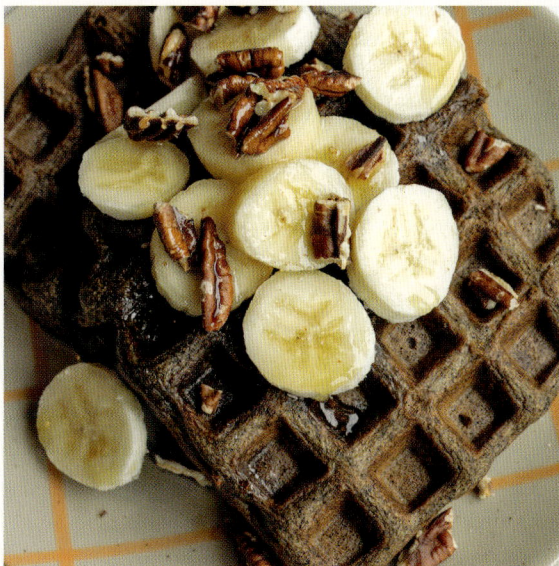

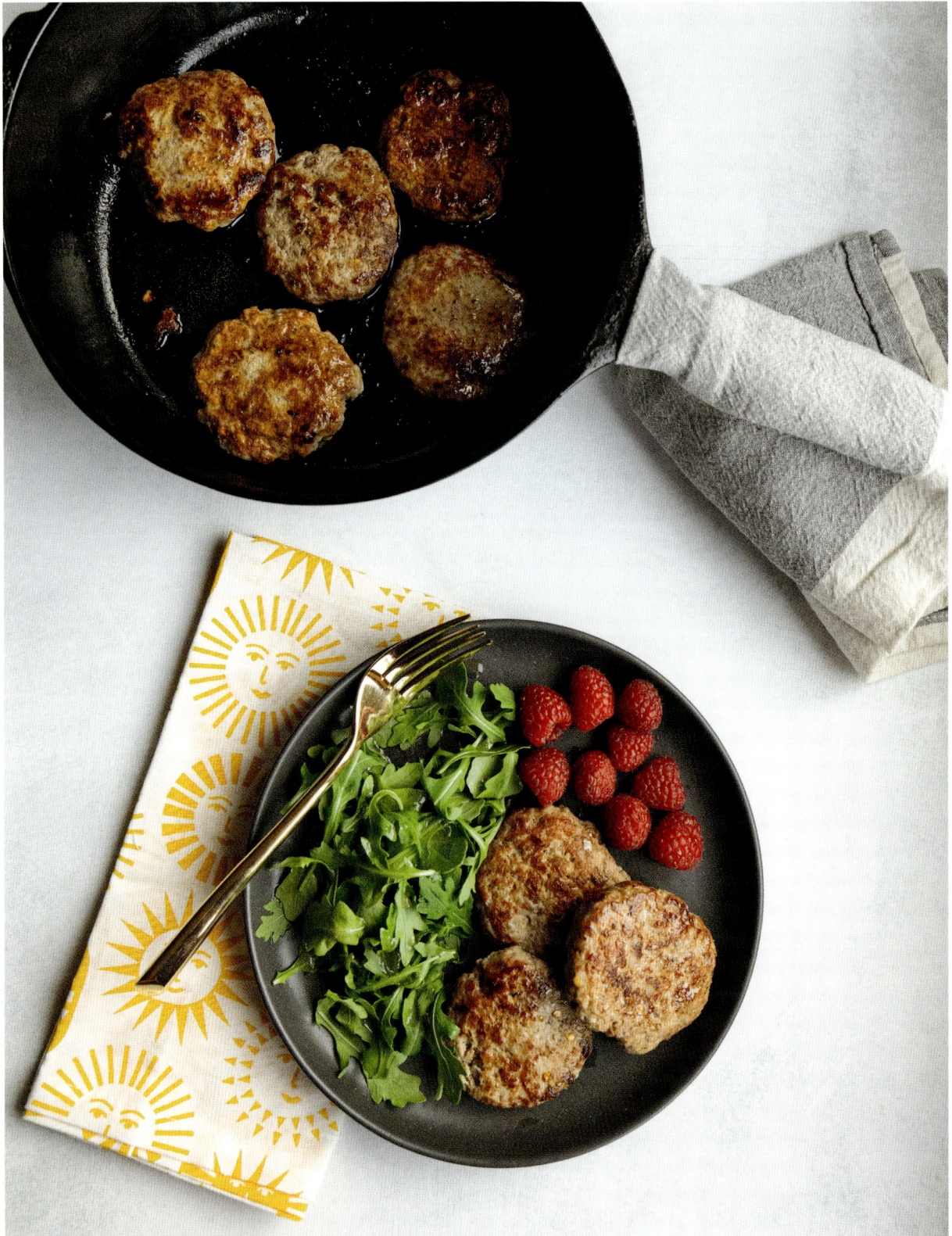

ZESTY HOMEMADE BREAKFAST SAUSAGE PATTIES

This handy meal-prep staple makes for convenient, protein-rich breakfasts and can easily be doubled or tripled, and extras can be frozen. Feel free to get creative with flavoring options like fresh thyme, rosemary, or your favorite spices. A built-in flavor booster here is a splash of apple cider vinegar, which brings the seasonings to life and helps keep the patties moist and juicy. Pair them with fresh or wilted baby greens, eggs (if tolerated), avocado slices, and some fermented sauerkraut (see note on page 119) for a balanced, thyroid-friendly breakfast!

● **GLUTEN-FREE**   ● **DAIRY-FREE**   ● **PALEO**   ● **AIP-FRIENDLY**

DIETARY LEVELS 1, 2, 3

SERVINGS 4
(about 8 small patties)

PREP TIME 10 minutes

COOK TIME 10 minutes

TOTAL TIME 20 minutes

1 pound (454 g) pastured ground turkey or pork

1 tablespoon (15 ml) water

1 teaspoon coconut aminos

1 tablespoon (20 g) pure maple syrup

1 tablespoon (15 ml) apple cider vinegar

½ teaspoon garlic powder

1 teaspoon onion powder

½ teaspoon ground allspice (sub scant ¼ teaspoon each of ground cinnamon, cloves, and ginger for AIP)

1 teaspoon dried rubbed sage

¼ teaspoon red pepper flakes (optional, omit for AIP)

¾ teaspoon fine sea salt

Freshly ground black pepper, to taste (optional, omit for AIP)

1. Combine all the ingredients in a medium mixing bowl and mix with your hands just until blended. Avoid overmixing to keep the sausage tender. For the best flavor, cover and refrigerate overnight to allow the seasonings to meld with the meat: Alternatively, cook immediately.

2. Divide the sausage mixture into 8 equal portions and form into patties about 3 inches (7.6 cm) wide and ⅓-inch (8 mm) thick.

3. Heat a large skillet over medium heat and grease with a little ghee or extra-virgin olive oil. When hot, add the patties, working in batches: Avoid overcrowding the pan. Cook for approximately 3 minutes per side or until cooked through and golden brown in spots. Do not overcook or the sausage will be dry.

4. Enjoy immediately or let cool and store in the fridge or freezer (instructions below) for later use.

NOTES

To freeze prepared patties: Let cool completely, then place in an airtight container, separating layers with parchment paper to prevent sticking. Freeze for up to 3 months.

To reheat frozen patties: Microwave at 50 percent power for 1 to 2 minutes per patty, checking halfway through to avoid overcooking. Alternatively, reheat in a skillet over low heat until warmed through.

To freeze unprepared (loose) sausage: Place 1-pound (454 g) portions in a freezer-safe container, label, date, and thaw when ready to use as desired.

SALMON HASH WITH POACHED EGGS

Crispy, golden potatoes, tender flaked salmon, and a medley of colorful veggies come together in this showstopping hash. A perfectly poached egg on top creates a silky, natural sauce as the warm yolk drizzles over the crispy bits. Enjoy this gluten-free, dairy-free delight as a weekend brunch or satisfying dinner!

● **GLUTEN-FREE**   ● **DAIRY-FREE**

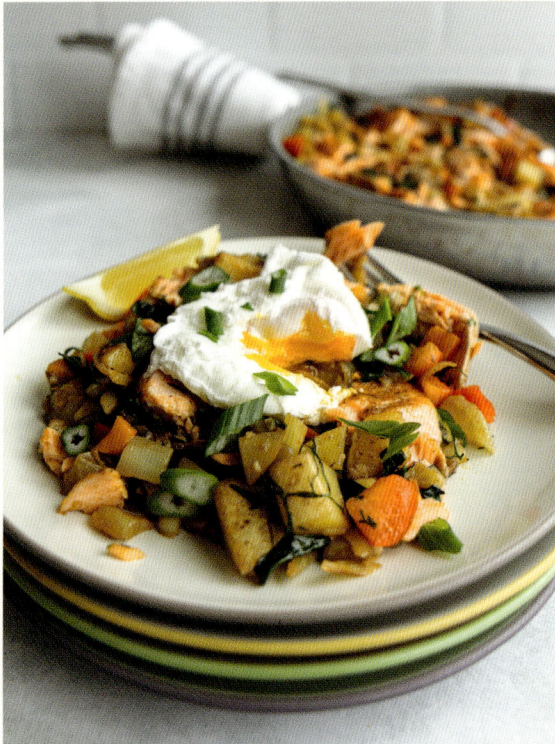

DIETARY LEVELS 1

SERVINGS 4
PREP TIME 30 minutes
COOK TIME 25 minutes
TOTAL TIME 55 minutes

FOR SALMON HASH

1 pound (454 g) wild-caught salmon fillet, skin removed

Fine sea salt, as needed

Freshly ground black pepper, as needed

½ teaspoon ground fennel

½ teaspoon Old Bay Seasoning, divided (see note)

3 tablespoons (45 ml) avocado oil, macadamia oil, grass-fed ghee, or other high-heat-friendly cooking fat, divided, plus more as needed

2 small or 1 large (about ¾ pound) (340 g) Yukon Gold potatoes, cut into ⅓-inch (9 mm) cubes

⅔ cup (107 g) diced sweet onion

1 fennel bulb, diced (reserve 1 tablespoon [3 g] chopped fronds)

4 cloves garlic, minced

1 medium carrot, peeled and finely diced

1 medium red bell pepper, seeded and diced

½ teaspoon ground cumin

½ teaspoon ground coriander

2 cups (60 g) baby spinach, roughly chopped

Juice of ¼–½ lemon

FOR POACHED EGGS AND GARNISH

4 eggs

1 tablespoon (15 ml) white wine vinegar

1 tablespoon (3 g) chopped chives or 2 green onions

4 lemon wedges

Gluten-free hot sauce, to serve (optional)

To Make the Salmon Hash

1. Season the salmon on both sides with the sea salt, pepper, ground fennel, and ¼ teaspoon of the crab seasoning.

2. Heat a large, heavy-bottomed or nonstick skillet over medium-high heat. Add 1 tablespoon (15 ml) of the oil. When the oil is hot and shimmery, place the salmon in the skillet. It should sizzle. Cook for about 4 minutes on each side until brown and crispy and just barely cooked through (do not overcook). Remove from skillet and set aside. If salmon has rendered a lot of fat or juice, discard it and wipe the pan lightly with a paper towel.

3. Meanwhile, parcook the potato. Toss the potato cubes with the 1 tablespoon (15 ml) of the oil in a microwave-safe bowl and season generously with sea salt and pepper. Mix to combine. Microwave for 4 minutes on full power. Set aside until ready to add to the hash.

4. Cook the vegetables. Return the skillet to medium-high heat and add the remaining 1 tablespoon (15 ml) of oil. When hot, add the diced onion and fennel bulb. They should sizzle. Cook, stirring occasionally, until soft and beginning to brown, 3 to 5 minutes. Add the garlic, season with salt and pepper, and cook 2 minutes more.

5. Add the parcooked potatoes and diced carrots to the skillet. Continue cooking, occasionally scraping the brown bits from the bottom of the skillet. Reduce the heat if the bottom of your skillet is becoming too dark (black, not brown). If necessary, deglaze the skillet with 1–2 tablespoons (15–30 ml) of water, scraping up the brown bits. Let the liquid evaporate, and continue browning. Sauté until everything is beginning to brown and crisp, about 7 to 10 minutes, adding more oil if needed to prevent sticking.

6. Add the bell pepper, cumin, coriander, and the remaining ¼ teaspoon of crab seasoning. Season with salt and pepper to taste and continue to cook, stirring occasionally, about 3 minutes more. When everything is tender and nicely browned, reduce heat to medium-low and stir in the chopped fennel fronds and baby spinach to wilt. Taste and adjust seasoning as needed with more salt, pepper, or spices.

7. Combine all ingredients. Roughly chop the salmon into large chunks with the edge of your spatula, removing any bones. Add the salmon to the skillet, spritz everything with the lemon juice, and toss very gently to combine, being careful not to break up the salmon too much.

To Make the Poached Eggs and Garnish

8. Poach the eggs while the hash is cooking. Fill a high-sided skillet with 2–3 inches (5–8 cm) of water. Bring to a boil, then reduce heat to a simmer. Add the vinegar to help the egg whites coagulate faster and maintain their shape. Crack 1 egg at a time into a small dish; this makes it easier to slide them into the water. When you're ready to add the egg, stir the water in the pan in a circle to create a vortex, and pour the cracked egg into the center of the swirl. The spinning water will help neatly wrap the white around the egg. Once firm enough to move, you can scoot the egg to the edge of the pan and repeat the process to add another egg, keeping track of which went in first.

   Poach eggs for 4 to 7 minutes each, depending on your desired degree of doneness. Firm whites with a runny yolk is recommended. Either let the poached eggs rest on a paper towel–lined plate to absorb excess water or, if the hash is ready, place a poached egg atop each serving.

9. Garnish hash with chives or green onion and lemon wedges. Serve with your favorite hot sauce, if desired, and enjoy!

NOTE
Old Bay Seasoning doesn't have artificial colors, flavors, preservatives, or anticaking agents like some other seasoning products.

SWEET AND SAVORY BREAKFAST HASH

This breakfast hash has it all—color, flavor, texture, and spice! And few breakfast options provide a more balanced and energizing way to start the day. Note that this calls for a batch of the loose Zesty Homemade Breakfast Sausage Patties (page 107): You can substitute plain ground pork, turkey, beef, lamb, bison, or chicken, but if you do, jazz up your meat with a little salt and whatever spices suit your dietary needs to provide extra flavor. The secret to a great hash lies in caramelization at every stage of cooking. To achieve this, you'll need plenty of fat, heat, and patience. Resist the urge to stir too often: Let the ingredients sit undisturbed in the skillet to develop those golden, crispy edges. Adjust the heat as needed to avoid overbrowning, and enjoy the mouthwatering results!

● GLUTEN-FREE ◍ DAIRY-FREE ● PALEO ● AIP-FRIENDLY

DIETARY LEVELS 1, 2, 3

SERVINGS 4
PREP TIME 20 minutes
COOK TIME 25 minutes
TOTAL TIME 45 minutes

1 pound (454 g) Zesty Homemade Breakfast Sausage Patties (page 107), loose

1 medium red onion, diced

2 medium carrots, peeled and diced

1 large or 2 small parsnips, peeled and diced

¼ teaspoon ground cinnamon

¼ teaspoon ground ginger

¼ teaspoon ground turmeric

Fine sea salt, to taste

Freshly ground black pepper, to taste (omit for AIP)

2 cups (180 g) finely chopped green cabbage

1 medium tart apple, diced (peeled, if preferred)

1 tablespoon (15 ml) coconut aminos

¼ cup (15 g) chopped fresh parsley

1. Brown the breakfast sausage in a large skillet over medium-high heat, breaking it up with a spatula. Cook until well-browned and crisp in spots, about 5 to 7 minutes. Remove the sausage from the skillet with a slotted spoon, leaving 2–3 tablespoons (30–44 ml) of the rendered fat in the pan. Discard any extra fat or save for another use.

2. Add the onion and cook, stirring, until nicely browned in spots, about 5 minutes.

3. Add the carrots, parsnips, cinnamon, ginger, and turmeric. Season with salt and pepper to taste, and cook, stirring, until veggies are brown in spots and beginning to soften, about 5 to 7 minutes.

4. Add the cabbage, apple, and coconut aminos, and cook for 5 to 7 minutes more until the cabbage is tender and the apple is softened. Add the parsley and cooked sausage to the skillet and stir to combine. Season to taste with salt and pepper, and enjoy!

NOTE

Serving suggestion: Serve alongside a scoop of fermented sauerkraut (see note on page 119) for added probiotics and flavor, a few slices of ripe avocado for color and richness, or a poached egg for added protein (omit egg for AIP).

SCRAMBLED EGG BREAKFAST TACOS WITH HARISSA

These vegetarian breakfast tacos are so simple and tasty. Starting the eggs off with a bit of golden-brown onion is a great way to add lots of flavor (and nutrients) in very little time. (For meal prep, feel free to cook all the eggs and store them in the fridge for heat-and-eat leftovers.) Harissa makes the tacos extra special, but you can substitute a quality store-bought salsa for convenience. Pair these tacos with your favorite side, like roasted sweet potatoes, fresh berries, or pineapple.

● GLUTEN-FREE　　● DAIRY-FREE　　● PALEO

DIETARY LEVELS 1, 2

SERVINGS 4
PREP TIME 20 minutes
COOK TIME 10 minutes
TOTAL TIME 30 minutes

8 eggs

1 tablespoon (14 g) ghee, (15 ml) extra-virgin olive oil, or (15 ml) avocado oil

½ onion, diced

½ teaspoon fine sea salt

Freshly ground black pepper, to taste

2 cups (60 g) baby spinach, arugula, or greens of your choice, roughly chopped

8 small gluten-free or grain-free tortillas (see note on page 113)

1 batch Quick and Easy Harissa (page 220) or store-bought

1 large ripe avocado, sliced

1. Crack the eggs into a small bowl and whisk with a fork until blended.

2. Heat the ghee or oil over medium heat in a medium skillet. Add the onion, salt, and pepper, and cook, stirring occasionally, until softened and golden brown in spots. Add the greens and cook, stirring, until wilted, about 1 minute. Add the eggs and cook, stirring occasionally with a spatula, until eggs are scrambled and fully cooked.

3. To serve, heat the tortillas according to package instructions. (See the note on page 113 to help you decide what type of tortilla is right for your dietary needs.) Smear each tortilla generously with Quick and Easy Harissa, then top with scrambled eggs and avocado slices. Enjoy!

TURKEY AND SWEET POTATO BREAKFAST TACOS

These satisfying AIP-friendly breakfast tacos are such a flavorful way to start the day. The combination of savory ground turkey, sweet potato, and warming spices like cinnamon and mace makes for a delicious, well-balanced filling. A bright, herby lime and cilantro sauce adds a refreshing contrast to the creamy avocado. A few slivers of citrusy quick-pickled red onion add extra zing, making every bite feel balanced and satisfying. See notes on the opposite page regarding store-bought tortilla options, or substitute a lettuce wrap.

● GLUTEN-FREE   ● DAIRY-FREE   ● PALEO   ● AIP-FRIENDLY

DIETARY LEVELS 1, 2, 3

SERVINGS 4 (about 8 tacos)
PREP TIME 20 minutes
COOK TIME 30 minutes
TOTAL TIME 50 minutes

FOR QUICK-PICKLED RED ONIONS

2 tablespoons (30 ml) freshly squeezed lime juice (about 1 large lime)

¼ teaspoon fine sea salt

⅛ teaspoon ground mace (optional)

1 teaspoon honey

½ red onion, thinly sliced

FOR LIME CILANTRO GREEN SAUCE

1 cup (16 g) fresh cilantro leaves

1 green onion, roughly chopped

2 tablespoons (30 ml) freshly squeezed lime juice (about 1 large lime)

2 tablespoons (30 ml) avocado oil

¼ teaspoon fine sea salt, or more to taste

1 tablespoon (15 ml) water, if needed

FOR TURKEY AND SWEET POTATO FILLING

2 tablespoons (30 ml) avocado oil

1 tablespoon (10 g) minced garlic, about 3 cloves

1 pound (454 g) ground turkey

2 cups (260 g) grated sweet potato

¾ teaspoon fine sea salt

½ teaspoon ground cinnamon

¼ teaspoon ground mace

¼ teaspoon dried Mexican or regular oregano

Freshly ground black pepper to taste (omit for AIP)

2 tablespoons (30 ml) water

FOR ASSEMBLY

8 gluten-free or grain-free tortillas (see note)

1 ripe avocado, sliced

OPTIONAL GARNISHES

Extra cilantro

Microgreens

To Make the Quick-Pickled Red Onions

1. Combine the lime juice, salt, mace (if using), and honey in a small bowl or jar. Stir well to blend. Add the sliced red onion and toss to combine. Let marinate at room temperature for 15 to 20 minutes, stirring occasionally, while you prepare the remaining ingredients. (Store leftovers in the refrigerator for up to 1 week.)

To Make the Lime Cilantro Green Sauce

2. Add the cilantro, green onion, lime juice, avocado oil, and sea salt to a small blender or food processor and blend until smooth. If needed, add up to a tablespoon (15 ml) of water to reach a pourable consistency.

To Make the Turkey and Sweet Potato Filling

3. Heat a large, lidded skillet or Dutch oven over medium heat. Add the oil, then the garlic, and cook, stirring until fragrant, 1 to 2 minutes. Add the ground turkey, breaking it up with a spatula. Cook until no longer pink (about 5 minutes). Stir in the grated sweet potato, salt, cinnamon, mace, oregano, and pepper, if using.

   Add the water, cover, and let cook for 5 to 10 minutes, stirring occasionally, until the sweet potato is soft and lightly caramelized. If needed, uncover for the last 2 minutes to evaporate excess liquid.

To Assemble

4. Heat the tortillas according to package instructions until soft and pliable. Spoon the Turkey and Sweet Potato Filling onto warm tortillas. Top with sliced avocado, a drizzle of Lime Cilantro Green Sauce, and a few slivers of pickled onion. Garnish with fresh cilantro or microgreens, if using.

   Store leftover pickled onions, sauce, and filling separately in airtight containers in the refrigerator for up to 3 days.

NOTE

We're lucky to have so many options for gluten-free tortillas these days. You can use classic corn tortillas for a gluten- and dairy-free option, but be sure to check the label carefully to avoid hidden wheat. For a grain-free option, try chickpea flour tortillas. Paleo options include almond, coconut, or cassava flour tortillas. AIP options include cassava or coconut-based options. Read labels carefully to avoid unwanted ingredients.

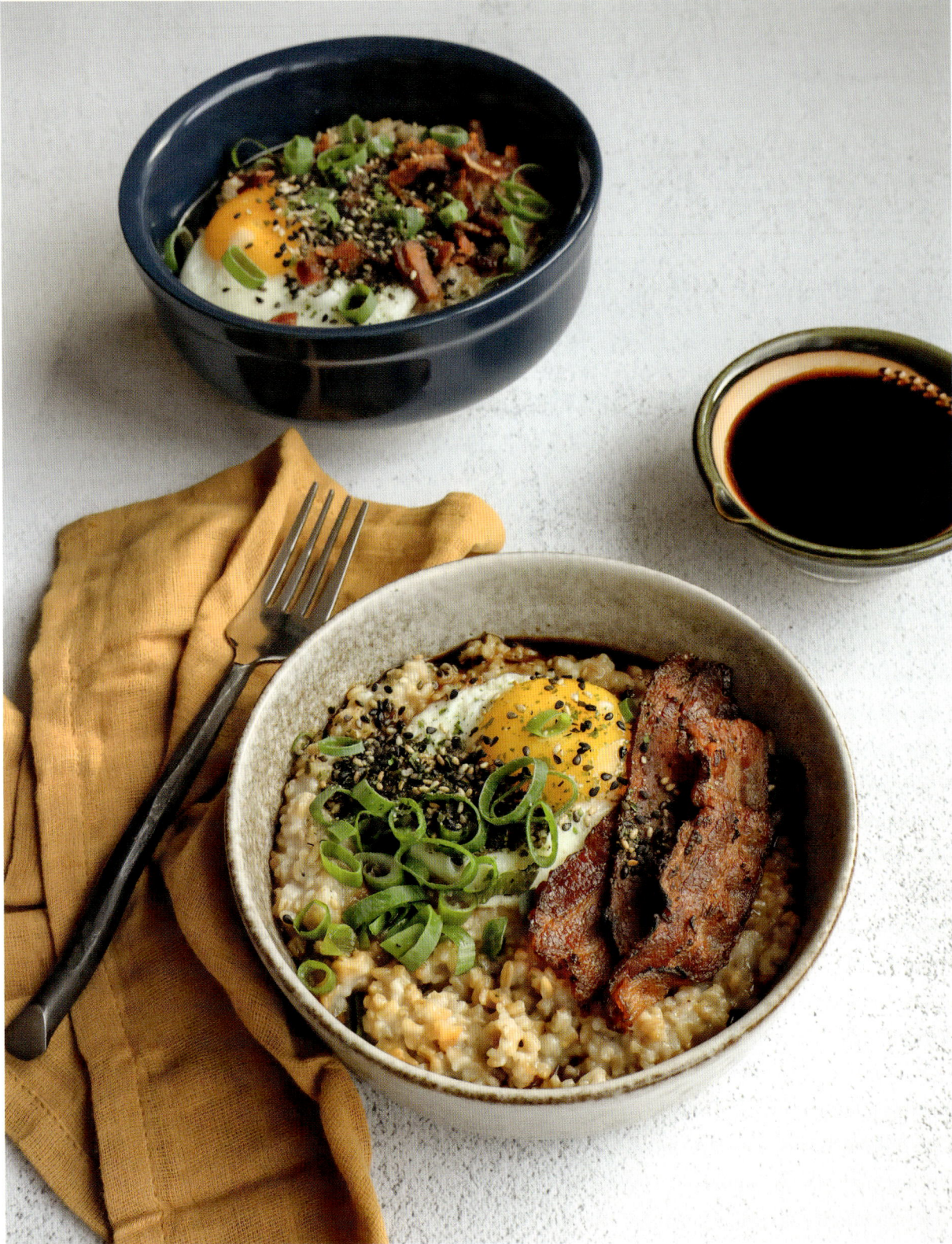

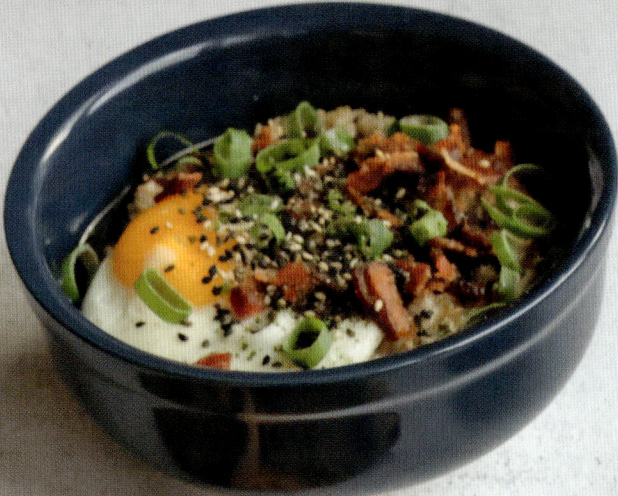

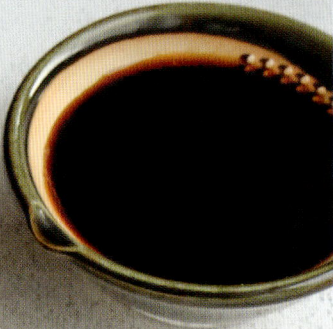

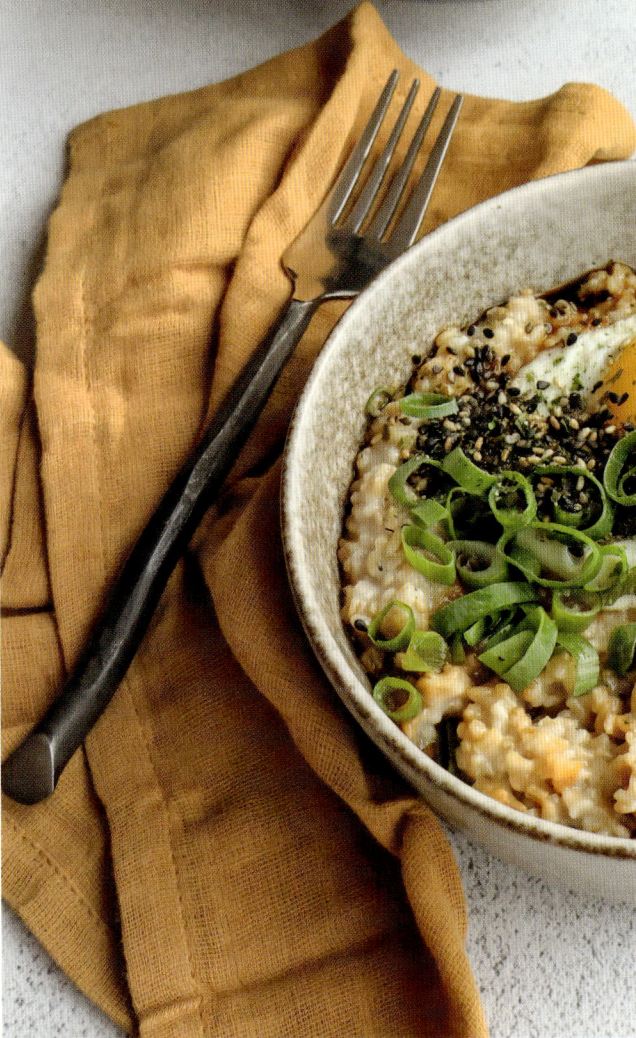

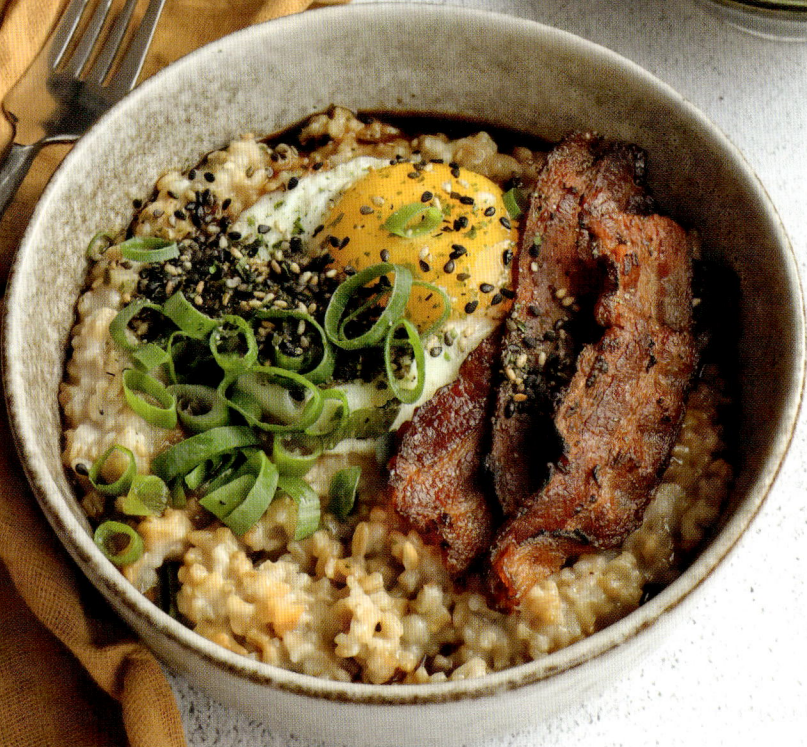

SAMURAI BREAKFAST BOWLS WITH STEEL-CUT OATS

If you've only ever had oatmeal topped with fruit and brown sugar—a surefire way to spike your blood sugar—this recipe will be a game-changer. These savory oatmeal bowls are a power breakfast created by my husband, Noah, for ski days and adventure fuel, and they supply steady energy that'll keep you full and focused for hours. Complex carbs in the form of slow-burning steel-cut oats are balanced out by protein-rich eggs and bacon, then topped with scallions, furikake (a Japanese sesame-seaweed seasoning), and coconut aminos for a deeply satisfying umami kick. Steel-cut oats differ from rolled oats in that they aren't rolled, making them chewier and more toothsome. They also require a bit more cooking time to soften. We'll toast them first here for extra flavor.

● **GLUTEN-FREE** ● **DAIRY-FREE**

DIETARY LEVELS 1

SERVINGS 2–3
PREP TIME 10 minutes
COOK TIME 30 minutes
TOTAL TIME 40 minutes

1 cup (90 g) certified gluten-free steel-cut oats

1 tablespoon (14 g) ghee

3 cups (710 ml) water

¼ teaspoon fine sea salt

4 ounces (113 g) compliant bacon (see note)

3 eggs

1–2 green onions, thinly sliced

OPTIONAL TOPPINGS

Furikake

Crumbled seaweed sheets

Dulse flakes (a seaweed with a mild, baconlike flavor)

2–3 tablespoons (30–44 ml) coconut aminos, to taste

1. Combine the oats and ghee in a medium saucepan over medium heat and cook, stirring occasionally, until oats are golden and fragrant, about 5 to 7 minutes.

2. Remove the saucepan from the heat and add the water (use care to avoid sputtering and steam if your pan is still hot), then return to the heat, stir in the salt, and bring to a boil. Reduce the heat, cover, and simmer for 20 minutes, stirring occasionally. Remove the oatmeal from the heat and let sit for 10 minutes, stirring occasionally, until excess water is absorbed.

3. Meanwhile, cook the bacon to your desired crispness, and fry, poach, or hard-boil the eggs.

4. Spoon the oatmeal into bowls and top each with bacon, eggs, green onions, and optional toppings (if using). Enjoy!

NOTES
Squeeze in extra veggies by topping with wilted greens, or add sliced avocado for a creamy contrast to those umami flavors.

For paleo compliance, select a nitrate-free, sugar-free bacon. For AIP compliance, be sure to use brands that do not contain added sugar, nightshade spices, or preservatives. See THYROID30 Support and Resources on page 246 for suggestions.

EVERYDAY BREAKFAST SALAD

Tender greens, freshly grated beets and carrots, pumpkin seeds, protein-packed poached eggs, bacon, and a delicate vinaigrette—I love this salad and could eat it every day, hence the name! Prep all the ingredients on the weekend and you can build your salad in minutes come weekday mornings. Makes a wonderful lunch too.

● **GLUTEN-FREE**　　● **DAIRY-FREE**　　● **PALEO**　　● **AIP-FRIENDLY**

DIETARY LEVELS 1, 2, 3

SERVINGS 4
PREP TIME 15 minutes
COOK TIME 15 minutes
TOTAL TIME 30 minutes

4–8 eggs (1–2 per serving) (sub 2 cups [280 g] shredded chicken for AIP)

8 slices compliant bacon, cooked and crumbled

5 ounces (142 g) favorite baby greens, washed and ready to eat

1 medium red beet, peeled and grated

1 large carrot, peeled and grated

⅓ cup (47 g) raw pumpkin seeds (sub diced avocado for AIP)

Freshly ground black pepper, to taste (omit for AIP)

Nigella Seed Vinaigrette (page 224) (sub olive oil and lemon juice for AIP)

1. Fill a large saucepan halfway with water and bring to a boil. If including eggs, gently add the eggs (still in their shells) and cook at a medium boil for 7 to 8 minutes for jammy eggs and 10 minutes for a dry yolk. When done, immediately rinse the eggs under cold water and let them sit for a few minutes until cool enough to handle.

2. Meanwhile, cook and crumble the bacon.

3. Build your salads by topping a generous handful of greens with the grated veggies, pumpkin seeds or diced avocado, cooked egg or chicken, and bacon. Top each with freshly ground black pepper and a light drizzle of Nigella Seed Vinaigrette.

NOTE
Store any leftover ingredients separately for ready-to-build breakfasts. Store leftover hard-boiled eggs in the fridge in a sealed container (to contain odor) for up to 1 week.

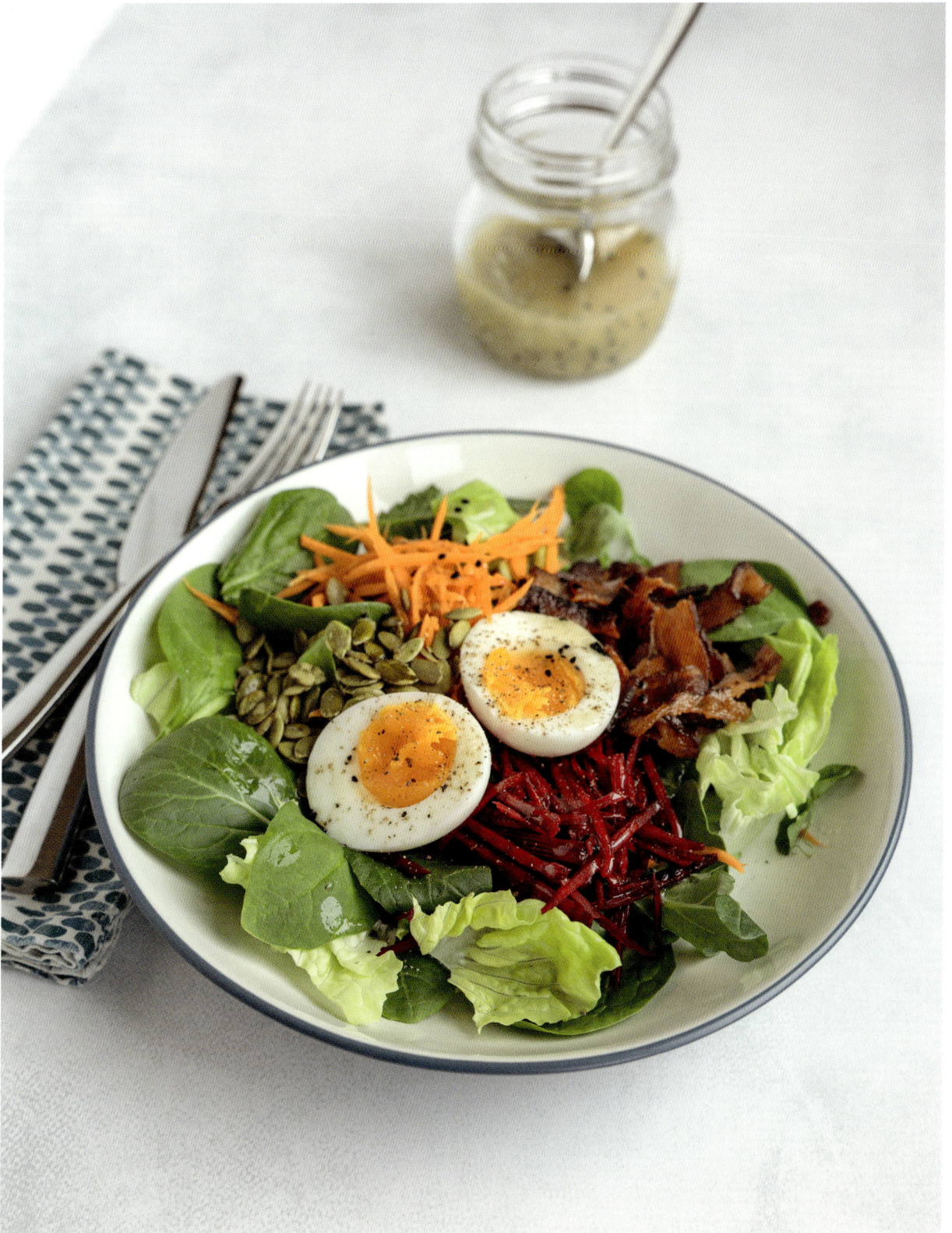

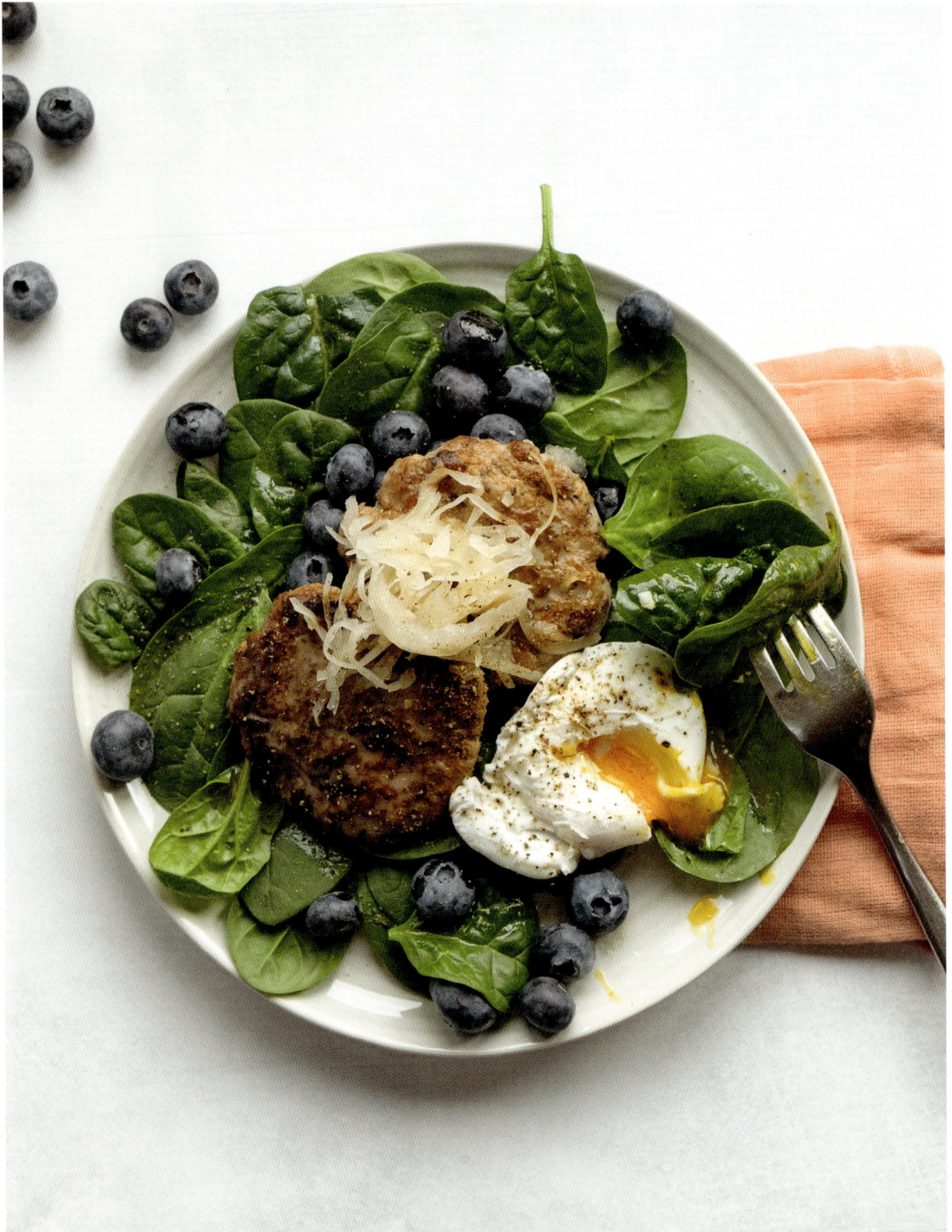

BLUEBERRY BREAKFAST SALAD
WITH HOMEMADE SAUSAGE PATTIES

This fresh, flavorful breakfast salad brings together an unexpected combination of sweet, savory, and tangy flavors. Juicy blueberries and fermented sauerkraut create a surprisingly delightful contrast to the savory homemade sausage patties. With ample protein, fiber, healthy fat, and phytonutrients, this meal is a complete power breakfast. Top with an egg for even more protein, if you like, and drizzle with one of the paleo- or AIP-friendly dressings noted below.

● GLUTEN-FREE   ● DAIRY-FREE   ● PALEO   ● AIP-FRIENDLY

DIETARY LEVELS 1, 2, 3

SERVINGS 4

PREP TIME 10 minutes (plus extra to prepare sausage and dressing, if necessary)

TOTAL TIME 10 minutes

5 ounces (141 g) baby spinach

1 cup (145 g) fresh blueberries

1 batch Zesty Homemade Breakfast Sausage Patties (page 107), prepared

1 cup (142 g) fermented sauerkraut (see note)

4 poached, fried, or hard-boiled eggs (optional, omit for AIP)

Nigella Seed Vinaigrette (page 224, see note)

To make each salad, arrange about 2 cups (35 g) of spinach on a plate and sprinkle with ¼ cup (36 g) blueberries. Top with 2 sausage patties and a scoop (about ¼ cup [36 g]) of fermented sauerkraut. Add an egg if desired (omit for AIP) and drizzle with your vinaigrette of choice. Serve immediately.

NOTES
Replace the Nigella Seed Vinaigrette with AIP-Friendly Italian Dressing (page 130) for AIP or simply drizzle with extra-virgin olive oil and spritz with lemon juice (paleo- and AIP-friendly).

Not all sauerkraut is created equal. Look for raw sauerkraut labeled "lacto-fermented," "raw," "unpasteurized," or "with live cultures" in your supermarket's refrigerated section. Avoid shelf-stable or vinegar-based varieties if you want the gut-friendly benefits of traditional fermentation methods.

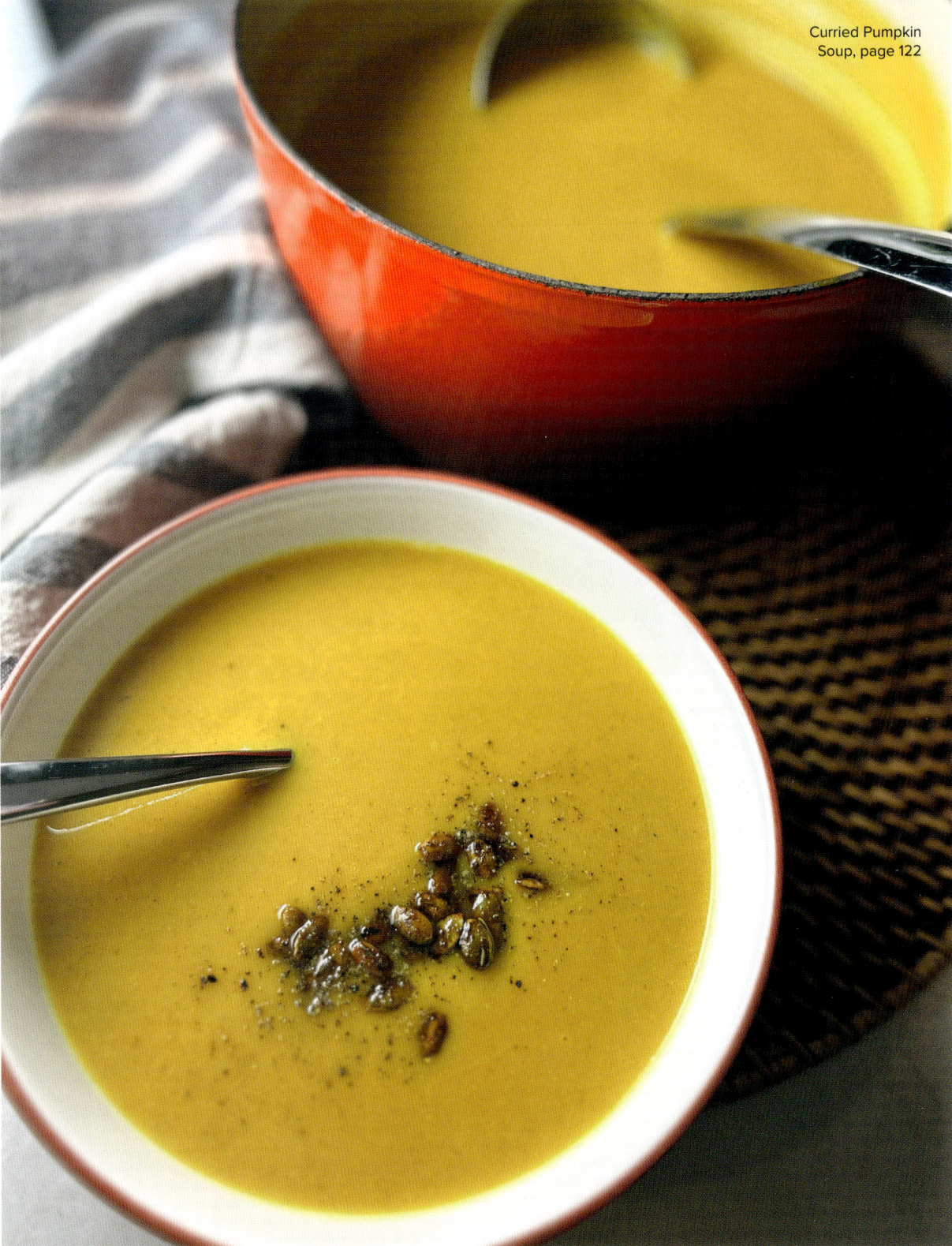

Curried Pumpkin
Soup, page 122

10

Soups

Something magical happens when you combine wholesome ingredients (and a dash of love) in a pot, elevating them into something greater than the sum of their parts. Soups are incredibly healing, enabling us to load up on energizing veggies, gut-soothing broths, and quality protein, all in one comforting bowl. When gut health is compromised, they're gentle and easy to digest. For those with dietary restrictions, soups can even double as a convenient and nourishing breakfast option. Many of the recipes in this chapter also freeze beautifully (because they don't contain dairy or noodles), so you'll always have thyroid-friendly heat-and-eat meals at the ready.

Great soups start with great stock. If possible, use bone broth for the best-tasting and most healing soups. If it's homemade, even better! You'll find my recipe for Easy Homemade Bone Broth (using bones of your choice) in the Snacks and Staples chapter (page 218). That said, store-bought bone broth can be a real time-saver. Even regular boxed broth works in a pinch—just with less collagen and minerals. If you're using a store-bought version, read the label carefully to ensure it aligns with your dietary needs. To keep it thyroid-friendly, avoid bouillon cubes and flavoring packets, which often contain inflammatory additives and, sometimes, gluten.

CURRIED PUMPKIN SOUP

This vibrant creation is visually stunning—its bright orange hue is the perfect backdrop for toppings like pumpkin seeds, cilantro, and green onions—and it's packed with nutrients. The best thing about pureed soups like this, though, is that they are easy to make, freezer-friendly, and portable. If you're looking for a grab-and-go meal, this warming recipe is the perfect fit.

● GLUTEN-FREE ● DAIRY-FREE ● PALEO ● AIP-FRIENDLY ● VEGAN

DIETARY LEVELS 1, 2, 3

SERVINGS 4–6
PREP TIME 10 minutes
COOK TIME 30 minutes
TOTAL TIME 40 minutes

2 tablespoons (28 g) organic, unrefined coconut oil

1 cup (160 g) diced shallots (about 4 medium)

2 cloves garlic, chopped

1 tablespoon (6 g) chopped fresh ginger

1 tablespoon (6g) curry powder (see note for an AIP-friendly option)

¼ teaspoon cinnamon

3 cups (710 ml) Easy Homemade Chicken Bone Broth (page 218) (sub vegetable broth for vegan)

1 cup (224 g) coconut milk

3 cups (735 g, or two 14-ounce cans) pumpkin puree

1 tablespoon (20 g) maple syrup

Fine sea salt, to taste

Freshly ground black pepper, to taste (omit for AIP)

Pinch cayenne pepper, to taste (omit for AIP)

OPTIONAL GARNISHES

Pumpkin seeds or pumpkin seed oil (omit for AIP)

Coconut milk

Fried sage leaves, cilantro, or green onion

1. Heat the coconut oil in a medium pot over medium-high heat. Add the shallot and sauté until soft and translucent, about 4 minutes.

2. Add the garlic and ginger and cook for 1 to 2 minutes or until fragrant. Stir in the spices (according to your dietary preference) and sizzle with the shallot for 1 minute to help the flavors bloom.

3. Next, add the broth, coconut milk, and pumpkin puree. Stir, scraping up any spices stuck to the bottom of the pan. Add the maple syrup and season with salt, pepper, and cayenne.

4. Bring to a boil, reduce the heat to low, cover, and let simmer for about 20 minutes. Remove from the heat and allow to cool slightly, then puree the soup in batches in an upright blender or with a handheld immersion blender until velvety smooth (see note below).

5. Taste and adjust seasoning and garnish as desired. Store in the fridge for 4 to 5 days, or freeze for 2 to 3 months.

NOTES

Use caution when pureeing hot or warm soup in a blender to avoid steam pressure buildup and—literally—a hot mess! Fill the blender only halfway. Start blending at the lowest speed and work your way up, holding the lid slightly ajar to allow steam to escape.

For an AIP-friendly curry powder alternative, substitute with 1 teaspoon ground turmeric powder, ¼ teaspoon ground clove, and ¼ teaspoon ground mace.

SMOKY BISON CHILI

Almost everyone loves chili, which makes it a great gluten-free and dairy-free meal that can be made ahead and served casually from the stovetop or crockpot. It's also perfect for entertaining, because everyone can customize their bowl with colorful toppings. Cheese and sour cream are solid choices for your dairy-loving guests, but it's fun to go outside the box with gluten-free and dairy-free toppings like roasted sweet potatoes, diced red onion, creamy avocado, and crushed plantain or tortilla chips. This recipe doubles easily and freezes well, making it perfect for those nights when you want a homemade meal without the effort. Bison's naturally rich, slightly sweet flavor pairs beautifully with the smoky, earthy depth of chili spices. It's always my first choice here, but if you can't find it, grass-finished beef makes a perfect substitute.

● **GLUTEN-FREE**   ● **DAIRY-FREE**

DIETARY LEVELS 1

SERVINGS 6
PREP TIME 20 minutes
COOK TIME 45 minutes
TOTAL TIME 1 hour, 5 minutes

5 ounces (142 g) compliant bacon, roughly chopped

1 medium yellow onion, peeled and diced

4 cloves garlic, minced

1 pound (454 g) ground bison or grass-finished beef

1 tablespoon (9 g) coconut sugar

1 tablespoon (16 g) tomato paste

2 tablespoons (30 ml) Homemade Worcestershire Sauce (page 222)

1 teaspoon ground cumin

1 teaspoon ground coriander

1 teaspoon smoked paprika

2 teaspoons cacao powder (optional, but recommended)

1 tablespoon (8 g) + 2 teaspoons chile powder

⅛–¼ teaspoon chipotle powder, to taste

1 (28-ounce [899 g]) can crushed tomatoes

1 cup (267 ml) beef broth

2 teaspoons apple cider vinegar or red wine vinegar

1 (4-ounce [113 g]) can diced mild green chiles

1 (14-ounce [400 g]) can black beans, rinsed and drained

1 (14-ounce [400 g]) can pinto beans, rinsed and drained

1½–2 teaspoons fine sea salt, or to taste

OPTIONAL TOPPINGS
Fresh cilantro

Diced red onion

Roasted sweet potatoes

Diced avocado

Crushed plantain or tortilla chips

1. Brown the bacon in a large soup pot over medium heat, stirring occasionally, until just beginning to crisp. Using a slotted spoon, transfer the bacon to a paper towel–lined plate, leaving the rendered fat in the pot.

2. Add the diced onion to the pot and cook, stirring occasionally, until soft and translucent, about 5 minutes. Add the garlic and cook 1 minute more. Add the bison (or beef), and cook, breaking it up with a spatula, until no longer pink.

3. Add the coconut sugar, tomato paste, Worcestershire sauce, cumin, coriander, smoked paprika, cacao (if using), chile powder, and chipotle powder, and stir to combine.

4. Pour in the crushed tomatoes, beef broth, vinegar, chiles, and beans. Return the crisped bacon to the pot. Season with salt and stir well. Bring to a boil, reduce the heat, cover, and let simmer over medium-low heat for about 30 minutes, allowing the flavors to meld.

5. Taste and adjust salt, spice, or acidity as needed. Serve with your toppings of choice, and enjoy!

SUPER SIMPLE LEMON CHICKEN SOUP

This gut-soothing comfort food is as nourishing as it is versatile. Packed with thyroid-supportive ingredients like bone broth to promote gut and immune health, parsley for a dose of antioxidants, and lemon juice to aid digestion, it's the perfect recipe when you need something simple and restorative. It's easy to tweak to make paleo, AIP, and grain-free versions, too, without sacrificing flavor.

● GLUTEN-FREE ● DAIRY-FREE ● PALEO ● AIP-FRIENDLY

DIETARY LEVELS 1, 2, 3

SERVINGS 6
PREP TIME 20 minutes
COOK TIME 40 minutes
TOTAL TIME 1 hour

1–2 tablespoons (14–28 g) ghee (sub extra-virgin olive oil for AIP)

1 large leek, white and light green parts only, finely chopped (see note)

4 celery ribs, finely chopped

2 cloves garlic, finely minced

8 cups (1.9 L) Easy Homemade Chicken Bone Broth (page 218) or store-bought

⅛ teaspoon white pepper (omit for AIP)

1 pound (454 g) boneless skinless chicken breasts

⅔ cup (107 g) white basmati rice, rinsed (sub 10-ounce [132 g] bag cauliflower rice for paleo or AIP)

2 tablespoons (8 g) finely chopped parsley

Fine sea salt, to taste

Freshly ground black pepper, to taste (omit for AIP)

2–3 tablespoons (30–44 ml) fresh lemon juice (about 1 medium lemon)

1. Combine the ghee or oil with the leek and celery in a large Dutch oven over medium heat. Cook, stirring occasionally, until the vegetables are tender, about 5 to 7 minutes. Add the garlic and cook for 1 to 2 minutes more or until fragrant.

2. Add the broth, white pepper, and chicken breasts to the pot and bring to a simmer. Reduce the heat and cook for 10 to 15 minutes or until the chicken breast is cooked through and registers 165°F (74°C) in the thickest part of the breast. Remove chicken from broth and set aside on a plate to cool.

3. Add the rice to the pot and stir. Bring to a simmer, cover, and cook for 20 to 25 minutes or until the rice is soft and tender. (Don't overcook unless you want the soup to have a porridgelike consistency.) If you're making a paleo, AIP, or grain-free version, add the cauliflower rice to the pot, bring to a simmer, cover, and cook until soft and tender, about 10 minutes.

4. While the rice or cauliflower rice is cooking, shred the chicken into bite-size pieces with 2 forks. After the rice is tender, return the chicken to the pot and add the parsley. Season to taste with salt and pepper. Add the lemon juice to taste, starting with about 2 tablespoons (30 ml) of the juice and adding more if needed. Serve hot and enjoy!

NOTE
Rinse and reserve the leek tops for the Easy Homemade Bone Broth on page 218.

CREAMY GINGER SCALLION CHICKEN SOUP

This quick and easy soup combines comforting creamy coconut milk with lively Southeast Asian flavors for a nutrient-dense and deeply flavorful bowl of goodness. Try to use an additive-free brand of fish sauce, such as Red Boat.

● **GLUTEN-FREE**　◍ **DAIRY-FREE**　● **PALEO**　● **AIP-FRIENDLY**

DIETARY LEVELS 1, 2, 3

SERVINGS 4–6
PREP TIME 20 minutes
COOK TIME 20 minutes
TOTAL TIME 40 minutes

1 tablespoon (15 ml) avocado oil or (14 g) unrefined coconut oil

1 large shallot, diced (about ½ cup [80 g])

2 tablespoons (12 g) finely chopped fresh ginger

1 tablespoon (10 g) finely chopped garlic (2–3 cloves)

3 green onions, white and green parts separated, thinly sliced

1 pound (454 g) ground chicken or turkey

1 tablespoon (9 g) coconut sugar

4 cups (946 ml) Easy Homemade Chicken Bone Broth (page 218) or store-bought

1 (14-ounce [392 g]) can full-fat coconut milk

3 tablespoons (45 ml) AIP-compliant fish sauce

1 bunch Lacinato kale, stems removed and roughly chopped (about 4 cups [268 g])

½ cup (8 g) finely chopped fresh cilantro

2 tablespoons (30 ml) freshly squeezed lime juice

Fine sea salt, to taste

Sambal oelek or sriracha, to taste (optional, omit for AIP)

1. Add the oil to a large soup pot over medium-high heat. Add the shallot and cook, stirring, until softened, about 3 minutes. Add the ginger and garlic, and cook, stirring until fragrant, about 2 minutes more.

2. Add the sliced white parts of the green onions to the pot along with the ground chicken or turkey and cook, breaking up the meat with a spatula, until cooked through.

3. Stir in the coconut sugar, broth, coconut milk, and fish sauce, and bring to a simmer. Cook for 5 to 10 minutes to allow flavors to meld. Add the kale and cook for 5 minutes more until tender.

4. Remove from the heat and stir in the cilantro and lime juice. Taste and adjust seasoning as desired.

5. Ladle soup into bowls and garnish with the sliced green onion tops. For extra heat, add a spoonful of sambal oelek or sriracha (omit for AIP).

GOLDEN LEEK AND CABBAGE SOUP

Light, velvety, and deeply nourishing, this golden-hued soup blends sautéed leeks, cabbage, and cauliflower with anti-inflammatory spices for a subtly sweet, gently spiced meal that's freezer-friendly and perfect for all dietary levels. To make a vegan version, just substitute vegetable broth for the bone broth.

⬤ **GLUTEN-FREE**   ◍ **DAIRY-FREE**   ⬤ **PALEO**   ⬤ **AIP-FRIENDLY**   ⬤ **VEGAN**

DIETARY LEVELS 1, 2, 3

SERVINGS 4–6
PREP TIME 15 minutes
COOK TIME 40 minutes
TOTAL TIME 55 minutes

2 tablespoons (30 ml) extra-virgin olive oil, plus more as needed

2 medium leeks, white and light green parts only, thinly sliced

1½–2 teaspoons fine sea salt, or to taste, divided

3 cloves garlic, minced

2 cups (180 g) thinly sliced green cabbage

3 cups (300 g) cauliflower florets

6 cups (1.4 L) Easy Homemade Chicken Bone Broth (page 218) or compliant store-bought broth (sub vegetable broth for vegan)

½ teaspoon ground turmeric

1 tablespoon (30 ml) fresh lemon juice

1. Heat the olive oil in a large soup pot or Dutch oven over medium heat. Add the sliced leeks and a pinch of salt. Sauté, stirring occasionally, for 7 to 10 minutes or until soft and lightly browned.

2. Add the garlic, cabbage, and cauliflower. Sauté for 3 to 5 minutes, stirring occasionally, until the vegetables begin to soften.

3. Add the broth, turmeric, and the remaining 1½ teaspoons of salt. Bring to a gentle boil, then reduce the heat to low. Cover and simmer for 25 to 30 minutes or until the vegetables are very tender.

4. Remove from the heat and use an immersion blender to blend the soup until smooth, or allow to cool slightly and blend in batches in a high-speed blender (see note on page 97).

5. Return the soup to low heat and stir in the lemon juice. Taste and adjust seasoning as needed.

6. Ladle the soup into bowls and drizzle with olive oil, if desired. Store leftovers in an airtight container in the refrigerator for up to 5 days, or freeze for up to 3 months.

BROCCOLI "CHEESE" SOUP

This creamy, comforting Broccoli "Cheese" Soup is so much like the real thing! With the savory richness of nutritional yeast and crispy bacon crumbles for topping, you won't believe this is completely dairy-free. If you're following the AIP meal plan, see the note on page 115 on choosing AIP-friendly bacon.

GLUTEN-FREE **DAIRY-FREE** **PALEO** **AIP-FRIENDLY**

DIETARY LEVELS 1, 2, 3

SERVINGS 4
PREP TIME 20 minutes
COOK TIME 40 minutes
TOTAL TIME 1 hour

6 ounces (170 g) compliant bacon, roughly chopped

1 small onion, peeled and diced

2 cloves garlic, minced

1–2 tablespoons (15–30 ml) water, if needed

2 large carrots, peeled and chopped

1 medium zucchini, peeled and chopped

2 celery stalks, chopped

2 tablespoons (14 g) cassava flour

4 cups (946 ml) Easy Homemade Chicken Bone Broth (page 218) or store-bought

1–1½ teaspoons sea salt, or to taste

Freshly ground black pepper, to taste (omit for AIP)

4 cups (284 g) finely chopped broccoli florets

¼ cup (36 g) + 1 tablespoon (9 g) nutritional yeast

½ cup (112 g) full-fat coconut milk

1–2 teaspoons (15–30 ml) fresh lemon juice

1. Place a large pot or Dutch oven over medium heat. Add the bacon and cook, stirring until crispy and browned, about 7 to 10 minutes. Remove the bacon with a slotted spoon and set it aside to drain on a paper towel–lined plate. Leave about 2–3 tablespoons (30–44 ml) of bacon fat in the pot, draining any excess.

2. Add the onion and garlic to the pot, and cook, stirring, until onions are soft and translucent. (If needed, you can also add 1–2 tablespoons (15–30 ml) of water to the pot to deglaze, scraping up any brown crust left over from frying the bacon.) Add the carrots, zucchini, and celery and sauté over medium heat for 5 to 7 minutes, stirring occasionally, until the vegetables have begun to soften.

3. Sprinkle the cassava flour over the vegetables and stir constantly for about 1 minute to evenly coat. Slowly pour in the broth, stirring constantly to prevent lumps from forming as the broth thickens.

4. Stir in the salt and pepper. Bring the mixture to a gentle boil, then reduce the heat and let simmer for about 15 minutes or until the vegetables are very soft.

5. Meanwhile, lightly steam the broccoli in a saucepan fitted with a steamer basket until tender but still vibrant green. Remove from the heat and set aside.

6. Stir in the nutritional yeast and coconut milk, mixing well to incorporate. Using an immersion or upright blender, carefully blend the soup mixture until velvety smooth (see note on page 97). If using an upright blender, return the blended soup to the pot and place over medium heat. Stir in the steamed broccoli florets and let the soup simmer for an additional 3 minutes.

7. Add the lemon juice, then taste and adjust seasoning as needed. Ladle soup into bowls, garnish with crispy bacon crumbles, and enjoy!

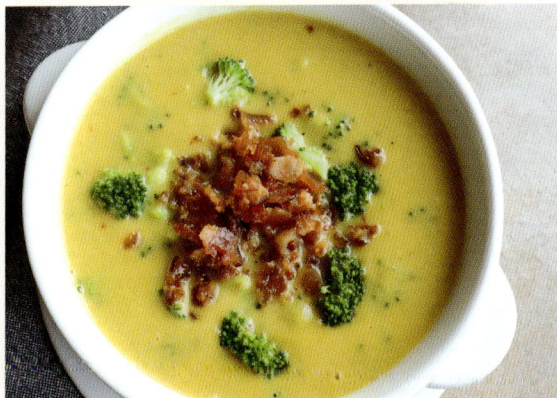

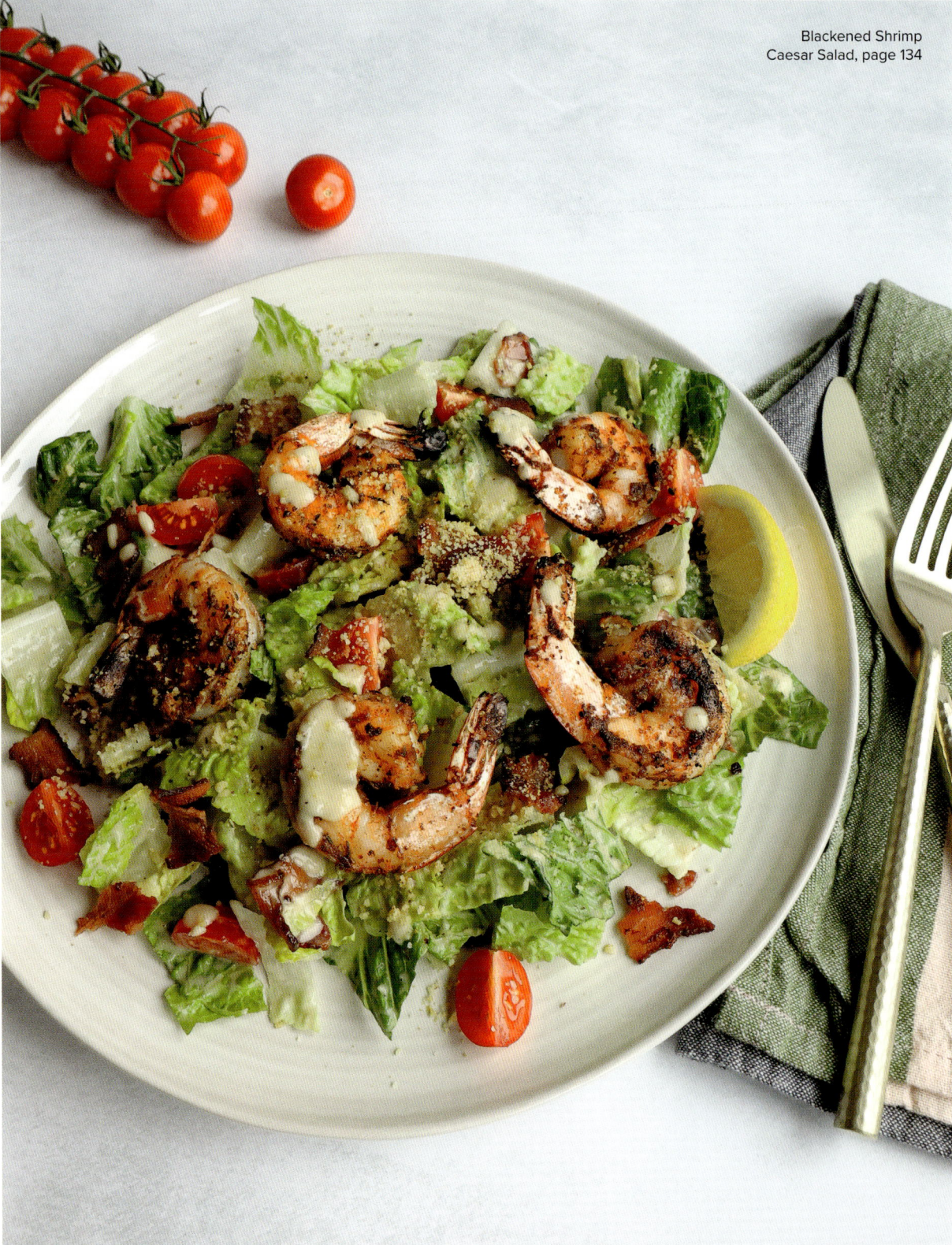

Blackened Shrimp
Caesar Salad, page 134

11

Salads

When it comes to nutrient density, it's hard to beat a really good salad. They brilliantly layer color, fiber, and hydration onto your plate (over 20 percent of our daily water intake comes from our food!). When they're thoughtfully crafted, salads can deliver an energizing mix of leafy greens, colorful veggies, quality proteins, healthy fats, and crunchy textures, all in a single, vibrant meal.

In this chapter, you'll find a collection of flavor-forward recipes that make eating the rainbow easy, delicious, and satisfying. From hearty main-course salads to fresh and festive sides, you'll find options to suit any mood, season, or occasion.

These recipes aren't just good for you: They're satisfying, crave-worthy, and full of life. Feel free to mix, match, and adapt ingredients based on what's in season and your personal needs. A well-made salad isn't just a plate-filler; it's a celebration of what your body can do with the right support.

EAT THE RAINBOW CHOPPED SALAD

This colorful, crunchy chopped salad is a vibrant blend of flavor, fiber, and phytonutrients. Chickpeas contribute plant-based protein and texture; sunflower or pumpkin seeds add extra crunch; and a zesty homemade Italian dressing brings everything together with bold, herby flavor. This recipe makes a big batch—perfect for parties, potlucks, or a week of meal prep—but you can also halve it, if that suits your needs. Serve it alongside the Balsamic-Marinated Chicken Breasts (page 160), Steak Frites (page 175), or Spice-Rubbed Slammin' Salmon (page 161) for a satisfying and colorful meal.

● GLUTEN-FREE   ● DAIRY-FREE

DIETARY LEVELS 1

SERVINGS 8 as a side dish
PREP TIME 25 minutes
TOTAL TIME 25 minutes

FOR ITALIAN DRESSING

1 tablespoon (6 g) Italian Dressing Mix (page 223), dry

1 tablespoon (15 ml) water

2 tablespoons (30 ml) red wine vinegar

1 tablespoon (11 g) Dijon mustard

⅓ cup (79 ml) extra-virgin olive oil

FOR SALAD

4 cups (220 g) chopped romaine or iceberg lettuce

1 cup (150 g) cherry tomatoes, halved or quartered

1 cup (110 g) grated carrot

1 cup (150 g) diced yellow bell pepper

1½ cups (429 g) cooked chickpeas (or one 15-ounce can), rinsed and drained

1 cup (135 g) diced English cucumber

½ cup (50 g) pitted Kalamata olives, halved or sliced

¼ cup (15 g) chopped fresh parsley

Fine sea salt, to taste

Freshly ground black pepper, to taste

¼ cup (34 g) pickled banana peppers (look for sugar-free and sulfite-free brands, like Jeff's Garden Sunshine Mix)

2–3 ounces (57–85 g) chopped uncured salami or pepperoni (look for nitrate- and sugar-free brands like Applegate Naturals Uncured Genoa Salami)

¼ cup (35 g) sunflower or pumpkin seeds

To Make the Italian Dressing

1. Combine all the ingredients for the dressing in an 8-ounce (237 ml) jar with a tight-fitting lid. Shake vigorously to combine. For best results, let sit for at least 15 minutes to allow the flavors to meld.

To Make the Salad

2. Combine all salad ingredients in a large mixing bowl. Add about ½ cup (118 ml) of the prepared dressing and toss well. Taste and add more dressing if desired. Season with sea salt and freshly ground pepper to taste, and serve.

NOTE

For meal prep, store the salad and dressing separately. The undressed salad components can be stored in the fridge for up to 3 days. Extra dressing can be stored in a sealed jar in the fridge for up to 2 weeks; just shake well before using.

BEET SALAD WITH CHICKEN AND MAPLE MUSTARD VINAIGRETTE

If you're still warming up to beets, this salad might just change your mind. Beets are rich in antioxidants, fiber, and essential nutrients like folate and potassium. They also support liver function and promote detoxification thanks to compounds like betalains, which help reduce oxidative stress and aid the body's natural cleansing processes, so they're a great addition to a thyroid-friendly eating approach. You're going to love this dressing too. While it pairs beautifully with just about any salad, it's especially well-suited to the earthy sweetness of beets and the crunch of toasted pecans or walnuts. Cooked chicken makes this a complete meal. Any kind will do, so feel free to use up those leftovers, but the Balsamic-Marinated Chicken Breasts (page 160) are a natural dance partner for these flavors.

● **GLUTEN-FREE** ● **DAIRY-FREE** ● **PALEO**

DIETARY LEVELS 1, 2

SERVINGS 4
PREP TIME 20 minutes
COOK TIME 1 hour
TOTAL TIME 1 hour, 45 minutes (including cooling time for the beets)

FOR BEETS

2 medium red or golden beets, washed, ends trimmed

2 teaspoons extra-virgin olive oil or avocado oil

Fine sea salt, to taste

Freshly ground black pepper, to taste

2–3 tablespoons (30–44 ml) water

FOR VINAIGRETTE

2 tablespoons (22 g) Dijon mustard

1 tablespoon (20 g) maple syrup

1 tablespoon (15 ml) + 1 teaspoon coconut aminos

1 tablespoon (15 ml) + 1 teaspoon balsamic vinegar

2 tablespoons (20 g) finely minced shallot

Fine sea salt

Freshly ground black pepper, to taste

½ cup (118 ml) walnut, avocado, or extra-virgin olive oil

FOR ASSEMBLY

5 ounces (142 g) mixed baby greens

2 cups (280 g) sliced, diced, or shredded cooked chicken

¾ cup (90 g) toasted chopped pecans or walnuts

To Make the Beets

1. Preheat the oven to 400°F (200°C). Place the beets in a medium baking dish and coat with the oil and seasoning. Make sure the beets aren't touching so air can circulate around them. Add the water (this will help steam the beets), then cover the dish with a tight-fitting oven-safe lid or foil. Place in the center of oven and roast for 45 to 60 minutes, depending on the size of the beets. They are done when they can be easily pierced with a paring knife.

2. Remove the beets from the oven and let rest until cool enough to handle. Rub the skins off with your hands or a paper towel (they should rub off easily). Slice, dice, or wedge the beets as desired.

To Make the Vinaigrette

3. While the beets are roasting, prepare the vinaigrette. Combine all the ingredients except the oil in a small mixing bowl or 2-cup (473 ml) glass measuring cup. Whisk with a fork to combine, taste for seasoning, and adjust as needed. Slowly drizzle in the oil, whisking constantly to blend. Taste and adjust seasonings again as desired.

To Assemble

4. Toss the greens with a light coating of the dressing and arrange them on serving plates. Top with roasted beets, cooked chicken, and toasted pecans or walnuts, and enjoy!

VIETNAMESE-STYLE SPRING ROLL SALAD

This one's a fun, fresh, deconstructed take on Vietnamese spring rolls, featuring marinated shrimp, crisp vegetables, and a bright nuoc cham–inspired dressing. If you want to take the extra step, you could wrap the salad mixture in rice paper for a handheld experience, but this laid-back approach comes together quickly with less fuss. If shrimp isn't an option, cooked and shredded chicken makes a fine substitute.

● **GLUTEN-FREE**　　● **DAIRY-FREE**

DIETARY LEVELS 1

SERVINGS 4
PREP TIME 25 minutes
COOK TIME 5 minutes
TOTAL TIME 30 minutes

FOR DRESSING AND MARINADE

¼ cup (59 ml) compliant fish sauce

¼ cup (59 ml) water

1 teaspoon sambal oelek (or 1 finely minced bird's eye chile)

2 tablespoons (30 ml) fresh lime juice

1 tablespoon (15 ml) rice vinegar

1 tablespoon (9 g) coconut sugar

1-inch (2.5 cm) piece fresh ginger, peeled and grated

1 large clove garlic, finely minced

1 green onion, finely chopped

FOR SALAD

1 pound (454 g) shrimp, peeled and deveined

8 ounces (227 g) thin rice vermicelli noodles

2 cups (180 g) shredded green regular or napa cabbage

1 medium carrot, grated

½ English cucumber, sliced into half-moons

1½ cups (75 g) mung bean sprouts (optional)

½ cup (48 g) fresh mint leaves, roughly chopped

½ cup (20 g) fresh basil leaves, roughly chopped

½ cup (8 g) fresh cilantro leaves, roughly chopped

½ cup (75 g) dry-roasted peanuts or macadamia nuts, roughly chopped

1 small fresh Thai or Fresno red chile, thinly sliced (optional)

Lime wedges (optional)

To Make the Dressing and Marinade

1. Combine the dressing and marinade ingredients in a small mixing bowl and whisk to blend until sugar is dissolved.

To Make the Salad

2. Place the shrimp in a separate bowl, toss with 2 tablespoons (30 ml) of the dressing, and marinate while you prepare the salad ingredients.

3. Cook the rice vermicelli according to package instructions until just al dente. Drain and rinse under cold water to prevent sticking. Set aside.

4. Drain and discard the marinade from the shrimp. Heat a medium skillet over medium heat. Add the shrimp and cook, stirring, just until pink and opaque, 2 to 3 minutes. Remove from the heat and set aside. Alternatively, you can skewer and grill the shrimp over a medium flame.

5. Arrange the salad ingredients on a large, rimmed serving platter or shallow bowl, starting with the cabbage, then the rice vermicelli, followed by veggies, shrimp, herbs, peanuts, and finally the sliced chile. Drizzle with the remaining dressing and toss gently just before serving. Garnish with fresh lime wedges, if desired.

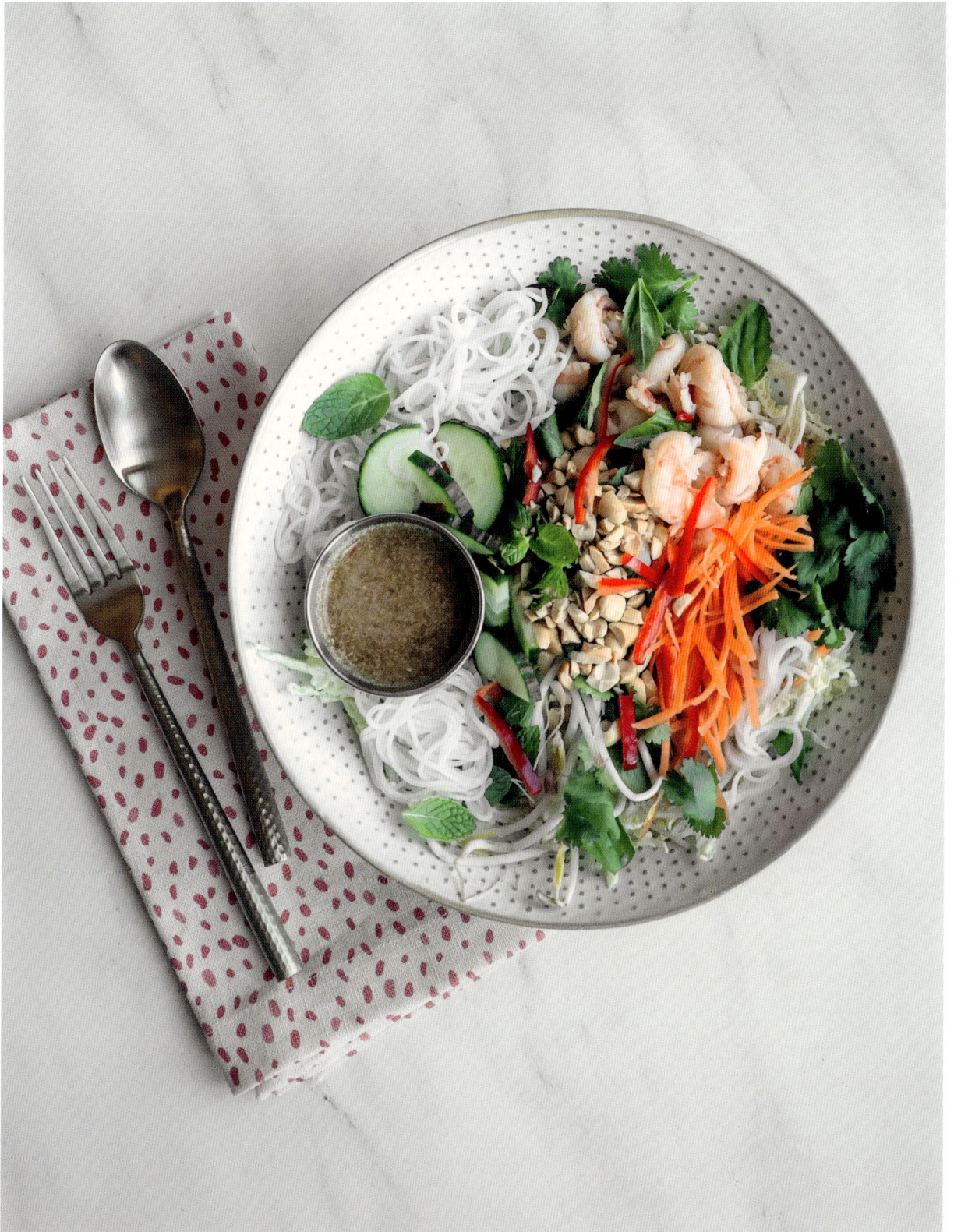

BLACKENED SHRIMP CAESAR SALAD

This flavorful twist on a classic features spice-rubbed blackened shrimp, crispy bacon bits, and juicy tomatoes for a wedge-meets-Caesar vibe—no croutons needed! A bold, dairy-free Caesar dressing ties it all together for a showstopping, grill-friendly meal. (The nutritional yeast in the dressing is optional, but I recommend using it for its Parmesan-esque flavor.)

● **GLUTEN-FREE**　　● **DAIRY-FREE**　　● **PALEO**

DIETARY LEVELS 1, 2

SERVINGS 4 as an entree
PREP TIME 30 minutes
COOK TIME 10 minutes
TOTAL TIME 40 minutes

FOR CAESAR DRESSING

1 large clove garlic, minced

¼ teaspoon fine sea salt

2 tablespoons (30 ml) fresh lemon juice

2 teaspoons minced anchovy (4–5 fillets)

Freshly ground black pepper, to taste

¼ cup (59 ml) + 1 tablespoon (15 ml) extra-virgin olive oil

¼ cup (60 g) paleo or Whole30-compliant mayonnaise

1 teaspoon nutritional yeast (optional)

FOR BLACKENED SHRIMP

½ teaspoon smoked paprika

½ teaspoon sweet paprika

½ teaspoon ground coriander

½ teaspoon garlic powder

½ teaspoon onion powder

¼ teaspoon dried oregano

¼ teaspoon dried thyme

¼ teaspoon dried basil

½ teaspoon fine sea salt

¼ teaspoon black pepper

⅛–¼ teaspoon cayenne pepper, or to taste

1 pound (454 g) large shrimp, peeled and deveined

2 tablespoons (30 ml) avocado oil

FOR ASSEMBLY

2–3 romaine hearts, washed and chopped

4–6 slices cooked compliant bacon, chopped or torn into pieces

1 cup (180 g) diced cherry tomatoes

OPTIONAL GARNISH

Brazil Nut "Parmesan" (page 225)

Fresh lemon wedges

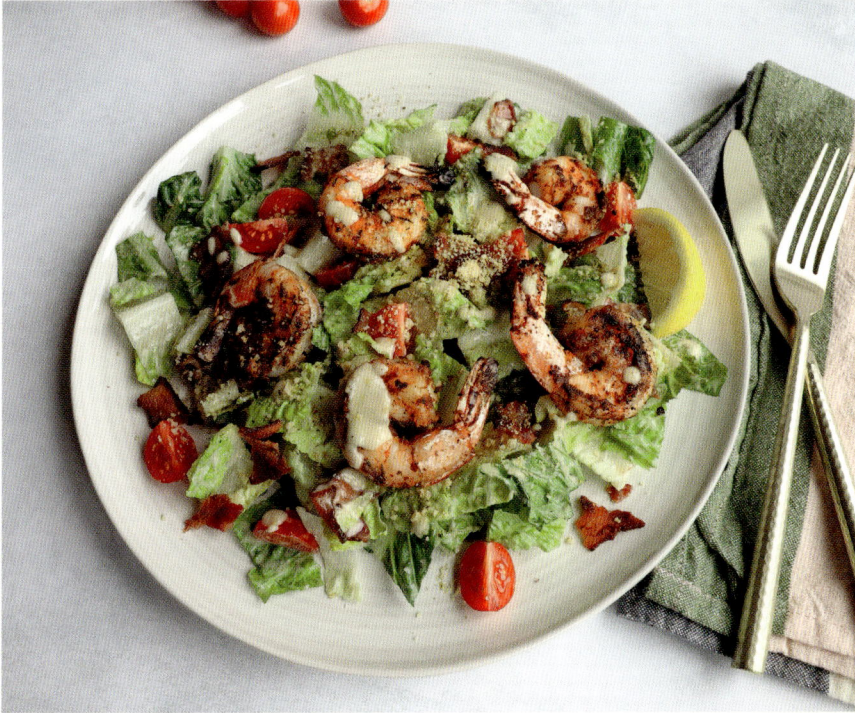

To Make the Caesar Dressing:

1. Whisk together the garlic, salt, lemon juice, anchovy, and pepper, if using, in a small bowl. Slowly whisk in the olive oil, followed by the mayo and nutritional yeast (if using). Adjust seasoning to taste. Alternatively, add all dressing ingredients to a small food processor and blend until smooth. The recipe yields about ¾ cup (177 ml).

To Make the Blackened Shrimp:

2. Preheat the grill to medium-high. Combine the spices and seasonings in a medium bowl and whisk to blend. Pat the shrimp dry with paper towels and toss with the seasoning mixture. Thread onto skewers and brush with oil. Grill over a medium-high flame for 2 to 3 minutes per side or until pink and cooked through.

   Alternatively, cook the shrimp on the stovetop. Heat a large cast-iron skillet over medium-high heat for about 2 minutes. Add the shrimp in a single layer and cook for 2 to 3 minutes per side or until pink and cooked through. Remove from the heat and set aside.

To Assemble:

3. Toss the romaine with the Caesar dressing. Divide among serving plates and top with blackened shrimp, bacon, and tomatoes. Sprinkle with Brazil Nut "Parmesan" and serve with fresh lemon wedges, if desired.

NOTE

To avoid ultra-processed ingredients, look for mayo labeled "Paleo" or "Whole30 approved." See brand suggestions in THYROID30 Support and Resources on page 246.

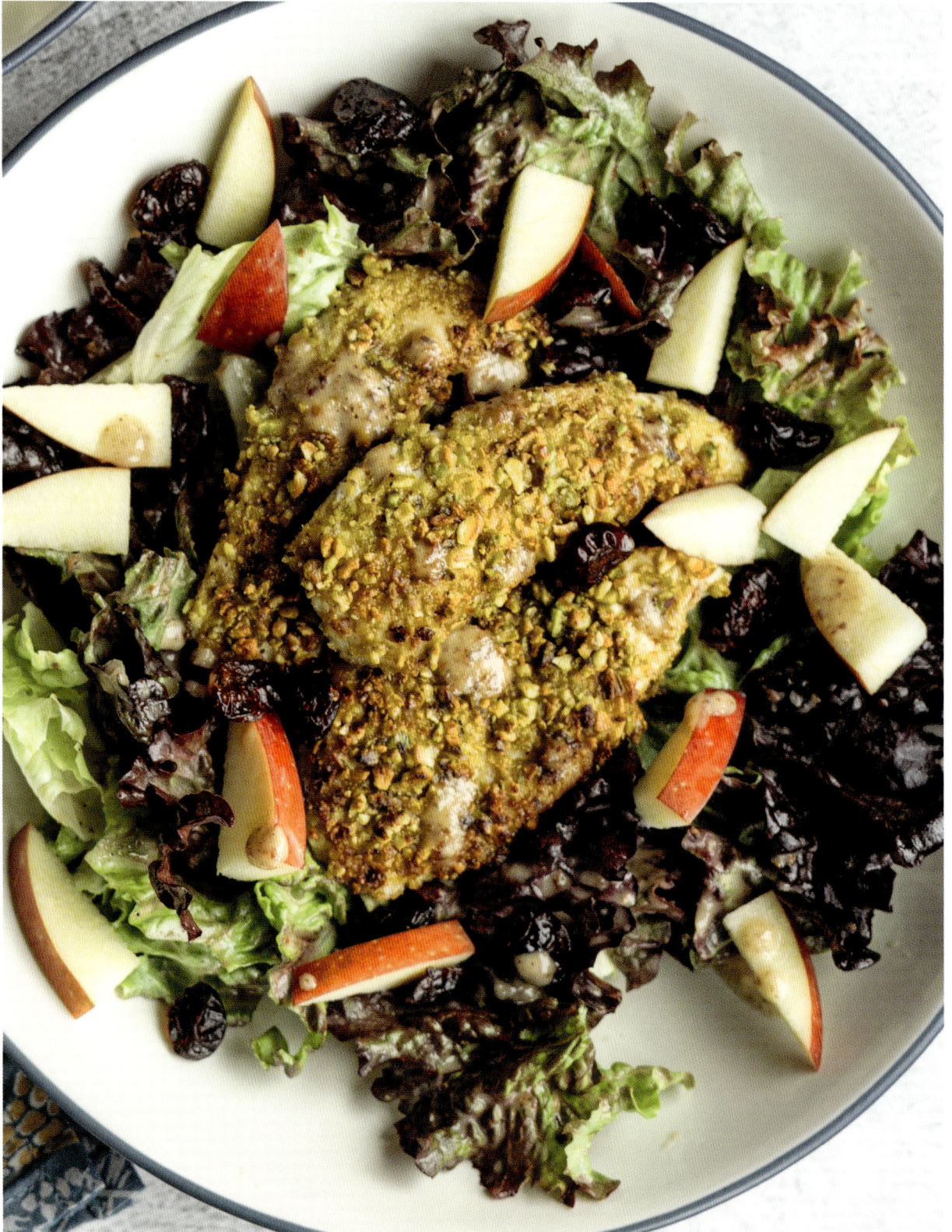

PISTACHIO-CRUSTED CHICKEN SALAD
WITH RAISIN VINAIGRETTE

With its balance of buttery pistachios, tender chicken, and a sweet-yet-tangy dressing, this salad is a real symphony of flavors. If you're not a fan of raisins, don't let their presence here put you off. They don't take center stage: We're mainly using them for their natural sweetness in this elegant vinaigrette.

● **GLUTEN-FREE**   ◐ **DAIRY-FREE**   ● **PALEO**

DIETARY LEVELS 1, 2

SERVINGS 4
PREP TIME 25 minutes
COOK TIME 20 minutes
TOTAL TIME 45 minutes

FOR RAISIN VINAIGRETTE

2 heaping tablespoons (18 g) raisins, preferably golden

Boiling water

1½ tablespoons (15 g) minced shallot

¼ cup (59 ml) avocado oil

2 tablespoons (30 ml) champagne vinegar or white wine vinegar

2 teaspoons Dijon mustard

⅛ teaspoon ground cardamom

¼ teaspoon fine sea salt

Freshly ground black pepper, to taste

FOR CHICKEN

1 cup (123 g) shelled pistachios, preferably unsalted

1 pound chicken breast tenders (or boneless, skinless breasts cut into strips)

Fine sea salt

Freshly ground black pepper, to taste

1 tablespoon (15 ml) avocado or extra-virgin olive oil

FOR ASSEMBLY

1 large head red leaf lettuce, chopped

1 small, tart apple, diced

⅓ cup (40 g) dried cranberries, cherries, or raisins

To Make the Raisin Vinaigrette

1. Place the raisins in a small mug and fill halfway with boiling water. Let the raisins soak for at least 3 minutes or until soft. Measure out 2 tablespoons (18 g) of the raisin soaking liquid and add to a small food processor or blender. Drain and discard the rest of the soaking liquid. Add the raisins to the food processor along with the remaining ingredients. Pulse until the dressing is smooth and creamy. Taste and adjust seasoning as needed, and set aside.

To Make the Chicken

2. Preheat the oven to 350°F (177°C) and line a rimmed baking sheet with parchment paper.

3. Grind the pistachios in a small food processor or coffee grinder, pulsing just until a coarse meal is formed. Place in a wide, shallow dish such as a pie dish.

4. Season the chicken with salt and pepper (use more if using unsalted pistachios and less if using salted pistachios). Roll the chicken tenders (or strips) in the ground pistachios, pressing firmly to adhere. Place on the prepared baking sheet.

5. Brush the chicken lightly with the oil and transfer to the oven. Cook 15 to 18 minutes or until chicken is cooked through and registers 165°F (74°C) internally. Remove from oven and let the chicken rest while you build the salads.

To Assemble

6. Toss the lettuce with a light coating of the dressing and divide among plates or serving bowls. Top each with diced apple and dried fruit. Place 2 or 3 pieces of chicken atop each salad, drizzle with any remaining dressing, and serve immediately.

WARM CHICKEN AND LENTIL SALAD WITH CELERY ROOT, WILTED GREENS, AND RED WINE VINAIGRETTE

This hearty dish offers a combination of plant- and animal-based protein: French green (Puy) or black beluga lentils add a deliciously nutty texture, while shredded chicken makes it extra filling. There's plenty of fiber, too, thanks to roasted celery root (or celeriac) and greens, and when everything's bound together with a simple red wine vinaigrette, this salad is truly irresistible. (It's a good idea to presoak your lentils before cooking: See the note on page 184.)

● **GLUTEN-FREE**   ● **DAIRY-FREE**

DIETARY LEVELS 1

SERVINGS 6
PREP TIME 20 minutes
COOK TIME 30 minutes
TOTAL TIME 50 minutes

FOR LENTILS

1¼ cups (240 g) dried French green (Puy) or black beluga lentils

2 cups (473 ml) Easy Homemade Chicken Bone Broth (page 218) or store-bought

1 cup (267 ml) water

½ teaspoon dried tarragon

½ teaspoon dried thyme

1 garlic clove, finely minced

1 bay leaf

FOR ROASTED CELERY ROOT

1 celery root (about 1½ pounds [180 g]), peeled and cut into ⅓-inch (9 mm) cubes

1 tablespoon (15 ml) extra-virgin olive oil

½ teaspoon fine sea salt

¼ teaspoon freshly ground black pepper

FOR RED WINE VINAIGRETTE

¼ cup (59 ml) red wine vinegar

1 garlic clove, finely minced

½ teaspoon Italian herb blend

2 teaspoons Dijon mustard

½ teaspoon fine sea salt

Freshly ground black pepper, to taste

⅔ cup (158 ml) extra-virgin olive oil

FOR ASSEMBLY

4 cups (560 g) shredded chicken

5 ounces (141 g) hearty baby greens or spinach, roughly chopped

Fine sea salt

Freshly cracked pepper, to taste

Chopped pecans, walnuts, or hazelnuts (optional)

To Make the Lentils

1. Combine all the ingredients for the lentils in a medium saucepan. Bring to a boil, then reduce the heat, cover, and simmer for about 25 minutes or until lentils are tender but still hold their shape. Drain any excess liquid, discard the bay leaf, cover to keep warm, and set aside.

To Make the Roasted Celery Root

2. Preheat the oven to 400°F (200°C) and line a baking sheet with parchment paper. Toss the celery root with the oil and seasoning in a bowl until evenly coated. Spread in a single layer on the baking sheet and roast for 25 minutes, flipping halfway through, until golden brown and fork-tender. Remove from oven and set aside.

To Make the Red Wine Vinaigrette

3. Whisk together all the ingredients except the olive oil in a small bowl. Slowly drizzle in the oil, whisking constantly to blend. Taste and adjust seasoning as needed and set aside.

To Assemble

4. If using cold chicken, warm it briefly in a skillet over low heat, or heat through in the microwave. Combine the warm lentils with the vinaigrette in a large mixing bowl. Toss in the celery root, shredded chicken, and greens, and toss to combine. The greens will wilt slightly from the residual heat. Taste and adjust seasoning with salt and pepper as desired. Top with chopped nuts, if desired, and enjoy! Store leftovers in the fridge for 2 to 3 days.

COWBOY CAVIAR QUINOA SALAD

This recipe brings the bold, zesty flavors of cowboy caviar into a colorful, fiber-rich quinoa salad. Loaded with protein, healthy fats, and fresh summer produce, it makes a satisfying side dish or light main course, and is perfect for make-ahead meal prep. Serve with grilled chicken or fish, or enjoy it on its own for a plant-based meal.

● GLUTEN-FREE   ● DAIRY-FREE   ● VEGAN

DIETARY LEVELS 1

SERVINGS 4–6
PREP TIME 20 minutes
COOK TIME 15 minutes
TOTAL TIME 35 minutes

FOR QUINOA

1¾ cups (414 ml) water

1 cup (173 g) quinoa, rinsed

FOR VINAIGRETTE

¼ cup (59 ml) fresh lime juice (about 2 limes), plus more as needed

1 tablespoon (15 ml) red wine vinegar

1 large clove garlic, minced

1 teaspoon ground cumin

½ teaspoon ground coriander

½ teaspoon chile powder

⅛ teaspoon chipotle powder or cayenne, or to taste

2 teaspoons maple syrup

1 teaspoon fine sea salt, plus more to taste

Freshly ground black pepper, to taste

½ cup (118 ml) extra-virgin olive oil

FOR ASSEMBLY

½ cup (80 g) diced red onion

1 cup (180 g) cherry tomatoes, halved

1 cup (150 g) diced orange bell pepper

1 cup (150 g) fresh or frozen, thawed corn

1 cup (256 g) cooked black beans, rinsed and drained

1 jalapeño pepper, seeded and finely chopped

½ cup (8 g) chopped fresh cilantro

To Make the Quinoa

1. Bring the water to a boil in a medium saucepan. Stir in the quinoa, then cover and reduce the heat to low. Simmer for 12 to 15 minutes or until the liquid is absorbed. Remove from the heat and let sit, covered, for about 5 minutes. Fluff with a fork and spread on a large plate or baking sheet to cool.

To Make the Vinaigrette

2. Combine all the ingredients in a jar with a tight-fitting lid. Close tightly and shake vigorously to combine.

To Assemble

3. Cover the diced red onion with cold water. Soak for 10 minutes, then drain.

4. Combine the cooled quinoa, red onion, cherry tomatoes, bell pepper, corn, black beans, jalapeño, and cilantro in a large mixing bowl. Drizzle the vinaigrette over the salad and toss gently to coat. Taste and adjust seasoning as needed. For best flavor, cover and refrigerate for at least 30 minutes before serving to allow the flavors to meld. Serve chilled or at room temperature.

5. Store leftovers in an airtight container in the fridge for up to 3 days. Give the salad a good stir before serving, as the vinaigrette may settle at the bottom. If needed, refresh with an extra squeeze of lime juice before serving.

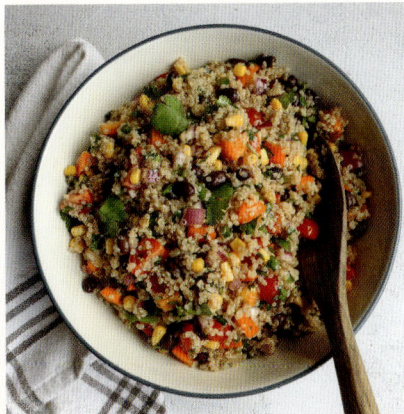

LAMB BURGER SALAD WITH LEMON, GARLIC, AND DILL AIOLI

This satisfying salad is full of Mediterranean flair. It pairs juicy, spiced lamb burgers with a bright, creamy, lemon, garlic, and dill aioli for a mouthwatering flavor combo that's rich, zesty, and herbaceous. Served over crisp greens with fresh toppings, it's a fun twist on burger night.

● **GLUTEN-FREE**   ● **DAIRY-FREE**   ● **PALEO**

DIETARY LEVELS 1, 2

SERVINGS 4
PREP TIME 20 minutes
COOK TIME 15 minutes
TOTAL TIME 35 minutes

FOR BURGERS

¼ cup (40 g) chopped shallot

1 teaspoon ghee or extra-virgin olive oil

1 pound (454 g) ground lamb

2 teaspoons maple syrup

½ teaspoon fine sea salt

¼ teaspoon garlic powder

⅛ teaspoon smoked paprika

1–2 teaspoons Homemade Worcestershire Sauce (page 222)

Freshly ground black pepper, to taste

FOR LEMON, GARLIC, AND DILL AIOLI

2 cloves garlic, minced

2 tablespoons (30 ml) olive oil

Sea salt, to taste

Zest and juice of ½ lemon

1 tablespoon (4 g) minced fresh dill

1 tablespoon (11 g) Dijon mustard

½ cup (115 g) paleo or Whole30-compliant mayonnaise

FOR ASSEMBLY

5 ounces (142 g) tender baby greens of choice

1 cup (180 g) cherry tomatoes, halved

OPTIONAL TOPPINGS

Cucumber

Olives

Pickled beets

Shredded carrot

Dill pickles

To Make the Burgers

1. Sauté the shallot with the ghee or oil in a small skillet over medium-high heat. Season to taste and cook, stirring, until golden brown. Set aside to cool slightly.

2. Combine the ground lamb with the shallot mixture and remaining burger ingredients in a medium mixing bowl. Mix just until combined. Form into 4 patties, then cook over a medium-flame grill for 3 to 4 minutes per side. To cook on the stovetop, sear in a heavy-bottomed skillet over medium-high heat for 3 to 4 minutes per side.

To Make the Lemon, Garlic, and Dill Aioli

3. Combine the garlic and oil in the shallow pan and sauté over medium heat for 3 minutes or until the garlic is fragrant and lightly toasted. Transfer to a small mixing bowl and combine with the remaining ingredients. Taste and adjust seasonings.

To Assemble

4. Divide the greens between 4 bowls. Top each with a burger and sprinkle with cherry tomatoes and other optional salad toppings. Drizzle with the aioli and serve.

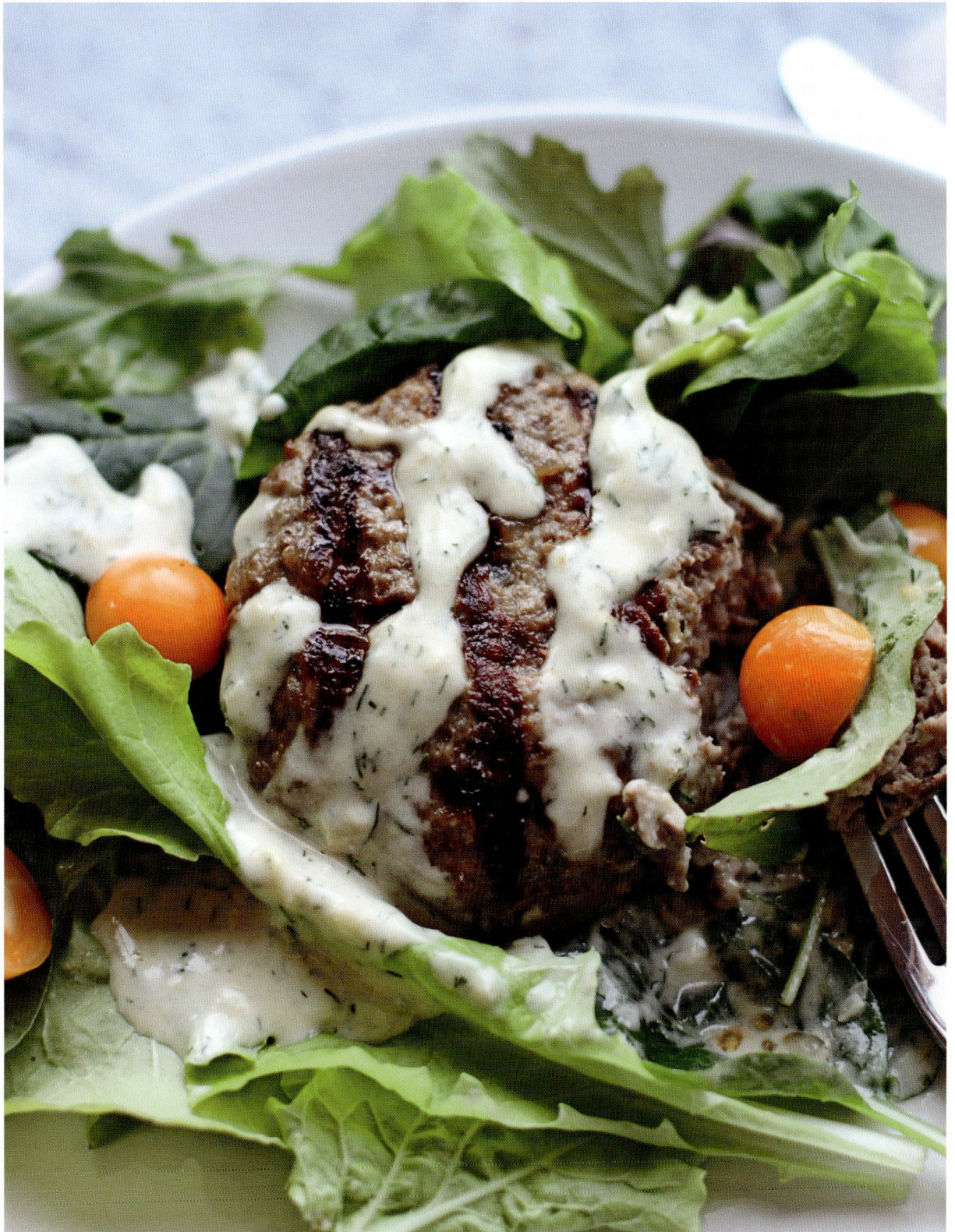

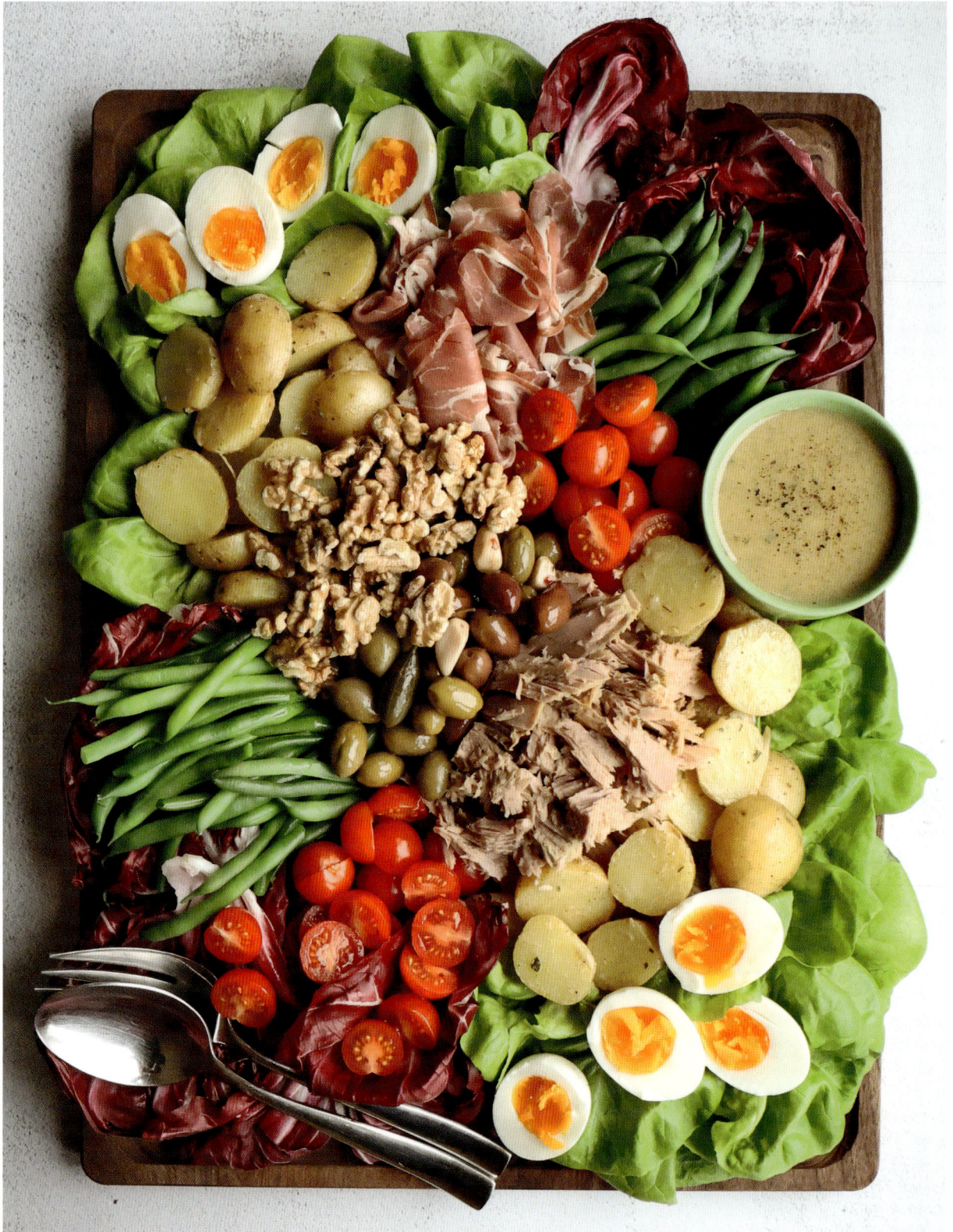

THRIVE BOARD: NIÇOISE EDITION

If you love to graze and nibble, you'll adore this stunning, celebration-worthy platter. Inspired by the classic Niçoise salad, it features a kaleidoscope of flavors and textures: tuna packed in olive oil, prosciutto, boiled eggs, crisp green beans, briny olives, and a mustardy vinaigrette that starts with my Italian Dressing Mix (page 223). It's perfect for a break from the ordinary. That said, this party-sized platter can easily be halved for more casual at-home dining. For meal prep, store components separately so you can build salads or lettuce wraps on demand.

● GLUTEN-FREE ● DAIRY-FREE

DIETARY LEVELS 1

SERVINGS 10
PREP TIME 40 minutes
COOK TIME 20 minutes
TOTAL TIME 1 hour

FOR DRESSING

2 tablespoons (12 g) Italian Dressing Mix (page 223) or store-bought

1 teaspoon dried tarragon

2 tablespoons (30 ml) water

¼ cup (59 ml) champagne vinegar or white wine vinegar

¼ cup (44 g) Dijon mustard

⅔ cup (158 ml) walnut, macadamia, avocado, or extra-virgin olive oil

FOR COOKED INGREDIENTS

4 eggs

1½ pounds (680 g) baby potatoes

Fine sea salt, to taste

12 ounces (340 g) green beans or asparagus

FOR ASSEMBLY

1 small head radicchio, leaves separated

1 small head butter lettuce, leaves separated

1 pint (284 g) cherry tomatoes, halved

1 cup (100 g) mixed olives (Castelvetrano, Kalamata, or your favorite blend), pitted

1 cup (120 g) toasted walnuts

2 (5-ounce [142 g]) jars tuna packed in olive oil, drained and flaked

4 ounces (113 g) prosciutto

OPTIONAL TOPPINGS

Sliced radishes

Artichoke hearts

To Make the Dressing

1. Combine the Italian Dressing Mix with the tarragon, water, vinegar, and Dijon mustard in a 2-cup (473 ml) glass measuring cup. Whisk vigorously with a fork to combine. Slowly drizzle in the oil in a steady stream, whisking constantly with a fork to emulsify. Alternatively, combine all ingredients in a jar with a tight-fitting lid and shake vigorously to combine.

To Make the Cooked Ingredients

2. Bring a medium pot of water to a gentle boil. Carefully lower the eggs (in their shells) into the water and cook for 7 to 8 minutes for jammy yolks or 10 minutes for firm yolks. Immediately rinse the eggs under cold water and let them sit for a few minutes until cool enough to handle, then peel. Slice in half and set aside.

3. Place the potatoes in a large saucepan and cover with water by 1–2 inches (2.5–5.1 cm). Boil until fork-tender, about 10 to 12 minutes. Drain and let cool slightly before slicing in half. In a large bowl, toss the potatoes with a bit of the dressing and a sprinkle of sea salt while still warm.

4. Refill the same pot halfway with water, add a hefty pinch of salt, and bring to a boil. Blanch the green beans or asparagus for 2 to 3 minutes until crisp-tender. Briefly transfer to an ice bath to preserve color, then drain and set aside.

To Assemble

5. Arrange the radicchio and butter lettuce leaves at the ends of a serving platter, cutting board, or baking sheet. Arrange the cherry tomatoes, baby potatoes, green beans or asparagus, olives, and walnuts around the board in distinct clusters. Finish with the tuna, folded slices of prosciutto, and eggs in separate sections.

6. Place the jar of prepared dressing on the board with a spoon for easy drizzling. Add tongs or serving spoons so guests can build their own salads or lettuce wraps, and enjoy!

JAPANESE-STYLE CUCUMBER SALAD

This salad was inspired by my son, James. Cucumber salad is his specialty, and we request it often in our house. The dressing makes a small batch. It might not look like enough, but don't worry; it is. You'll let the cucumbers marinate in the dressing for 10 to 15 minutes for maximum flavor, and as they marinate, they'll release some of their own liquid. This will dilute the dressing slightly, so the final amount will be just right.

● **GLUTEN-FREE**　● **DAIRY-FREE**　● **PALEO**　● **AIP-FRIENDLY**

DIETARY LEVELS 1, 2, 3

SERVINGS 4
PREP TIME 15 minutes
TOTAL TIME 15 minutes

2 English cucumbers, thinly sliced

1 small garlic clove, minced

1 teaspoon finely grated or minced ginger

1 green onion, green parts only, finely minced

1 tablespoon (15 ml) coconut aminos

1 tablespoon (15 ml) avocado oil

1 tablespoon (15 ml) seasoned rice vinegar (sub apple cider vinegar for paleo and AIP)

1 teaspoon honey

½ teaspoon fine sea salt, plus more to taste

Pinch white pepper (omit for AIP)

1. Place the sliced cucumbers in a medium mixing bowl.

2. In a separate small bowl, combine the remaining ingredients for the dressing and whisk vigorously to combine. Taste and adjust seasonings, if needed, and pour dressing over cucumbers.

3. Toss to combine. If possible, let sit for 10 minutes before serving to allow the flavors to meld. This salad is best enjoyed fresh, but you can store in the fridge in an airtight container for up to 24 hours.

SERVING SUGGESTION
Serve atop rice bowls with grilled fish or your favorite protein and some starchy, complex carb–rich plants like the Rainbow Roasted Root Veggies (page 204) for a quick and easy weeknight meal. This salad also pairs beautifully with the Khao Man Gai–Inspired Chicken and Rice (page 166).

FRENCH CARROT SALAD WITH MINT

Carrot salad set the internet on fire as a hormone-balancing side dish. While some claims may have been overhyped, raw carrots do contain unique fibers that can help transport excess estrogen out of the body while also promoting a healthy microbiome. More than anything, though, this salad is cheerful, refreshing, and versatile. Mint, one of the most underused culinary herbs, adds a lively counterpoint to more pedestrian parsley for a flavor combination that feels both elegant and unexpected.

● **GLUTEN-FREE**   ● **DAIRY-FREE**   ● **PALEO**   ● **AIP-FRIENDLY**   ● **VEGAN**

DIETARY LEVELS 1, 2, 3

SERVINGS 4

PREP TIME 10 minutes

TOTAL TIME 10 minutes

1 pound (454 g) carrots (about 5 medium), peeled and grated or cut into matchsticks

1 tablespoon (4 g) finely chopped parsley

1 tablespoon (6 g) finely chopped mint

1 tablespoon (15 ml) champagne vinegar (sub apple cider vinegar for AIP)

½ teaspoon ground coriander (sub with 1 tablespoon [1 g] chopped cilantro leaves for AIP)

¼ teaspoon fine sea salt, or more to taste

Freshly ground black pepper, to taste (omit for AIP)

2 tablespoons (30 ml) extra-virgin olive oil

1 lemon wedge

1. Combine the carrots, parsley, mint, vinegar, coriander, salt, and pepper. Drizzle with the olive oil and toss well to coat. Let the salad sit for 5 to 10 minutes to allow the flavors to blossom.

2. Just before serving, spritz with a lemon wedge, toss once more, and adjust seasoning if needed. Serve immediately. Store leftovers in an airtight container in the fridge for 2 to 3 days.

SERVING SUGGESTION

For a complete meal, serve this alongside Seared Chicken Breasts with Mushroom Caper Pan Sauce (page 170), Steak Frites (page 175) or Artichoke Chicken and Rice Bake (page 165).

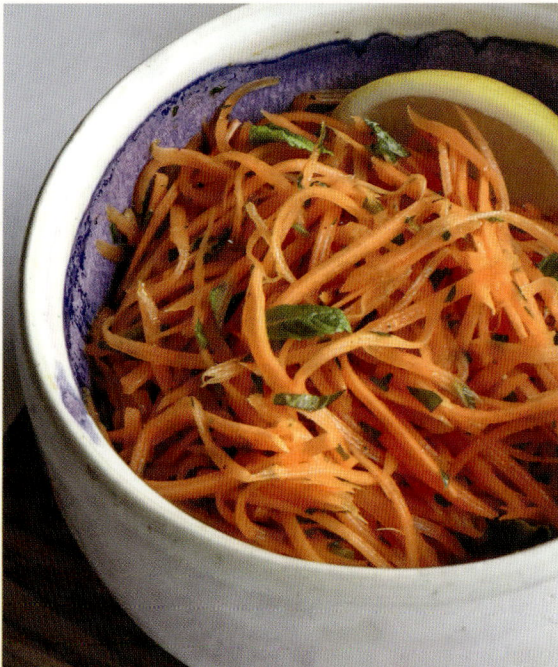

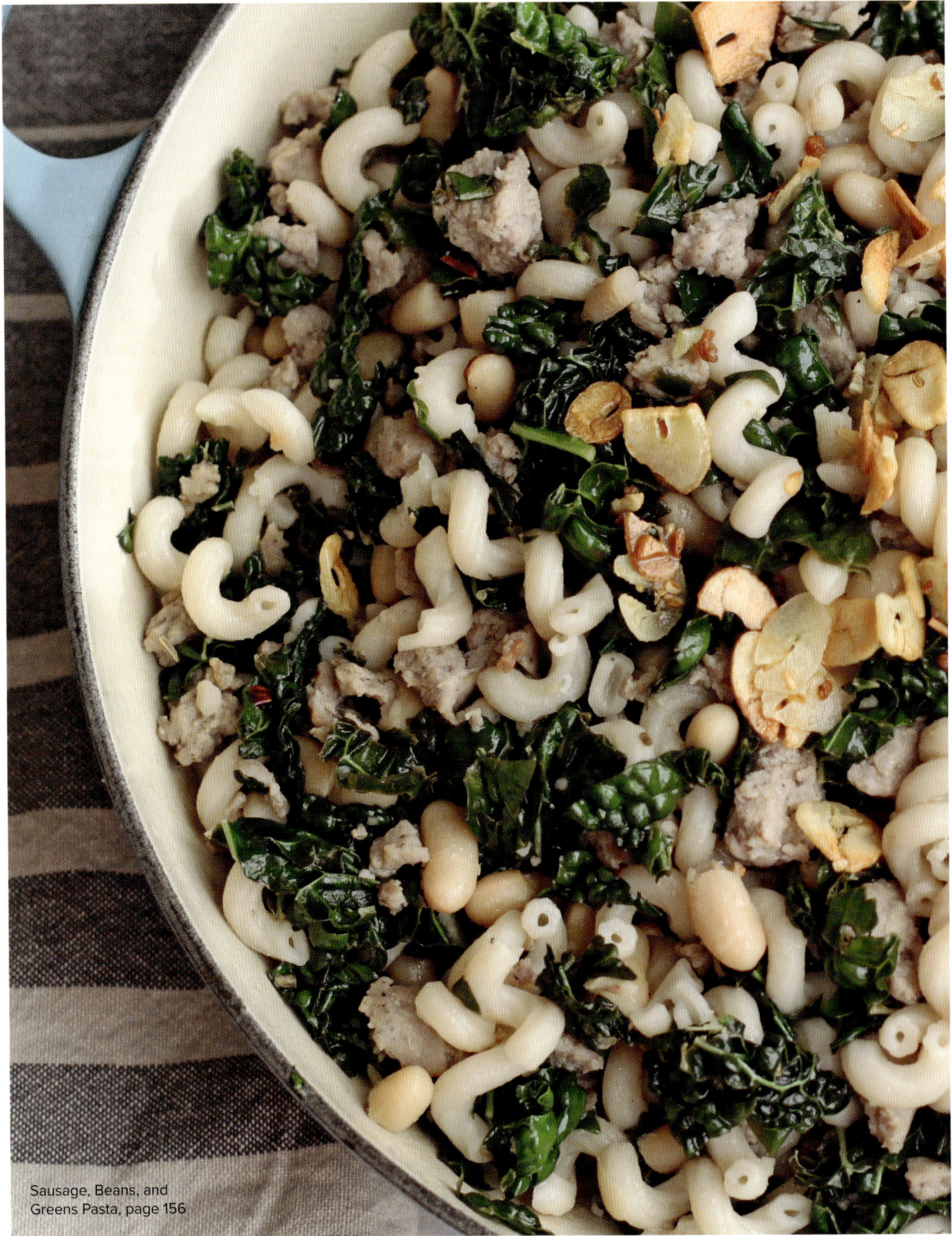

Sausage, Beans, and
Greens Pasta, page 156

12

Mains

Dinner can feel like the biggest hurdle of the day, especially when your energy's flagging and you don't have a plan. This chapter is here to change that. It's all about helping you get dinner on the table with ease and confidence, even on your most depleted days.

Inside, you'll find anti-inflammatory recipes that everyone at the table will love, designed with meal prep, freezer-friendliness, and leftovers in mind to make your tomorrows easier (and more delicious).

These beloved dishes from my own family table have passed the husband test, the kid test (okay, for the most part!), and the test of time. More than that, they're designed to support your healing, not just through nutrient density and blood sugar balance but also by showing you that thyroid-friendly and autoimmune-friendly food doesn't have to be dreary or difficult. Whether it's a sheet pan meal that saves you time and cuts down on dishes, a cozy one-pot wonder, or a flavorful protein to pair with your favorite simple sides, these recipes are built for both real healing and real life.

COCONUT-CRUSTED MAHI-MAHI WITH MANGO SLAW

The tropical sweetness of mango and coconut plus the mild, flaky texture of mahi-mahi—or your favorite flaky white fish—equals a delicious, AIP-friendly meal (see the note on the opposite page). The fish is dredged in a coconut-and-plantain-based coating for a delicious, crunchy crust you're going to love. The recipe makes plenty of coating, so if you'd like to cut the fish into smaller pieces for maximum crust, by all means do! Don't like mango, or don't have a ripe one handy? Feel free to replace it with 1½ cups (248 g) diced fresh pineapple.

● **GLUTEN-FREE**   ● **DAIRY-FREE**   ● **PALEO**   ● **AIP-FRIENDLY**

DIETARY LEVELS 1, 2, 3

SERVINGS 4
PREP TIME 25 minutes
COOK TIME 10 minutes
TOTAL TIME 35 minutes

FOR SLAW

4 cups (360 g) shredded green or red cabbage

1 red bell pepper, cut into strips (sub ½ cup [55 g] shredded carrot for AIP)

1 ripe mango, cut into strips

2 green onions, thinly sliced

¼ cup (4 g) fresh cilantro, roughly chopped

2 tablespoons (30 ml) lime juice

1 tablespoon (20 g) + 1 teaspoon honey

1 tablespoon (15 ml) avocado oil

½ teaspoon Korean gochugaru or Aleppo chile flakes (omit for AIP)

Pinch fine sea salt

Pinch white pepper (omit for AIP)

FOR FISH

4 (6-ounce) mahi-mahi, halibut, or cod fillets

1 cup (150 g) plantain chips (AIP-compliant), ground to a fine crumb texture (about ½ cup ground)

1 cup (80 g) shredded unsweetened coconut

1 teaspoon fine sea salt

½ teaspoon garlic powder

½ teaspoon ground ginger

¼ cup (28 g) tapioca starch or arrowroot starch

⅓ cup (74 g) full-fat, unsweetened coconut milk

1 tablespoon (15 ml) water

½ cup (109 g) unrefined coconut oil (or enough for shallow frying)

OPTIONAL GARNISHES

Flaky sea salt

Fresh cilantro

Lime wedges

To Make the Slaw

1. Combine the cabbage, bell pepper, mango, green onions, and cilantro in a large bowl. Whisk together the lime juice, honey, oil, chile flakes, sea salt, and white pepper in a separate small bowl. Set aside while you prepare the fish.

To Make the Fish

2. Pat the fish fillets dry with a paper towel. Combine the ground plantain chips, coconut, sea salt, garlic powder, and ground ginger in a shallow bowl. Mix with a fork.

3. Whisk together the tapioca starch, coconut milk, and water in a separate small bowl to create a slurry. The consistency should be like a thin pancake batter; add more water if needed. Stir well until no lumps remain.

4. Dip a piece of mahi-mahi into the slurry, shaking off the excess before dredging in the coconut-plantain mixture. Press gently to adhere and ensure an even coating. Set aside on a plate and repeat with the remaining fillets.

5. Heat the coconut oil in a medium skillet over medium heat. The oil should be hot but not smoking. Test by adding a piece of shredded coconut: If it sizzles immediately, the oil is ready. Carefully place the coated fillets into the hot oil. Fry for 3 to 4 minutes per side or until the crust is golden brown and the fish flakes easily with a fork. Adjust the heat as needed; you want it hot enough to crisp the crust without scorching. Transfer the cooked fillets to a paper towel–lined plate to absorb excess oil and sprinkle lightly with flaky sea salt if desired.

6. Pour the dressing over the slaw and toss to combine. Adjust seasoning to taste. Serve the mahi-mahi atop the mango slaw, garnishing with additional cilantro and lime wedges if desired.

NOTE

For an AIP-friendly version of the slaw, replace the red bell pepper with shredded carrot and omit the chile flakes and white pepper.

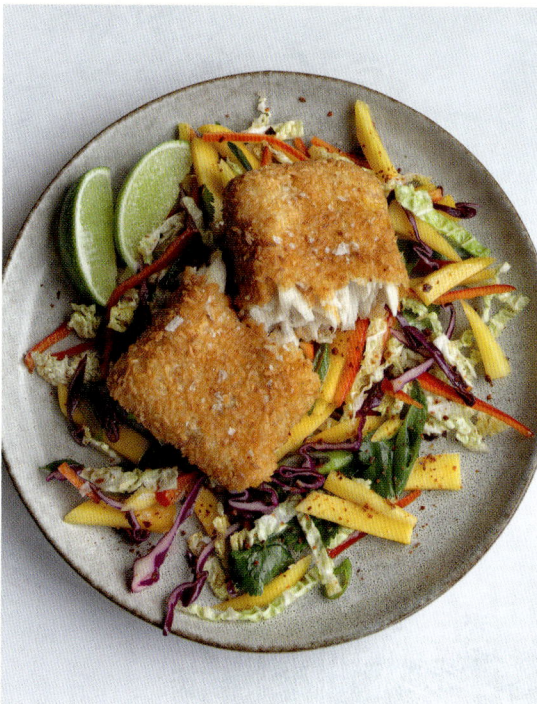

PUB MASH WITH SAUSAGE AND CARAMELIZED ONION AND MUSHROOM GRAVY

Inspired by bangers and mash, this hearty, protein-rich dish features homemade brat-style sausage over dairy-free mashed potatoes with a rich onion-mushroom gravy. A side of sweet peas completes this comforting, family-friendly meal.

● GLUTEN-FREE   ● DAIRY-FREE

DIETARY LEVELS 1

SERVINGS 6
PREP TIME 20 minutes
COOK TIME 40 minutes
TOTAL TIME 1 hour

FOR SAUSAGE

2 pounds (907 g) ground pork (or a mixture of pork and veal)

1¾ teaspoons fine sea salt

Scant ½ teaspoon white pepper

½ teaspoon ground nutmeg

¼ teaspoon ground ginger

¼ teaspoon ground mace (or extra nutmeg)

½ teaspoon dried marjoram

1 teaspoon dried rubbed sage

½ teaspoon onion powder

½ teaspoon garlic powder

2 tablespoons (30 ml) sparkling or filtered water for moisture

FOR MASHED POTATOES

3 pounds (1.4 kg) (about 6 medium) russet potatoes

1 cup (237 ml) warmed Easy Homemade Chicken Bone Broth (page 218) or store-bought

¼ cup (60 g) paleo or Whole30-compliant mayonnaise

1½ teaspoons fine sea salt

¼ teaspoon garlic powder

⅛ teaspoon white pepper (optional)

2 tablespoons (28 g) ghee or (30 ml) extra-virgin olive oil

FOR GRAVY

1½ tablespoons (21 g) ghee or (22 ml) avocado oil

1 medium sweet onion, julienned

4 ounces (113 g) cremini mushrooms, sliced

Fine sea salt, to taste

White pepper, to taste

2 heaping tablespoons (14 g) cassava flour

¼ cup (59 ml) dry white wine

2 cups (473 ml) Easy Homemade Beef Bone Broth [page 218] or store-bought

FOR SERVING

1 (10-ounce [283 g]) bag frozen peas

To Make the Sausage

1. Preheat the oven to 375°F (190°C). Combine ingredients in a medium mixing bowl. Form the mixture into 12 patties about ½-inch (1.3 cm) thick. Place on a parchment paper–lined baking sheet and set aside while you prepare the potatoes.

To Make the Mashed Potatoes

2. Peel the potatoes and cut into 1-inch (2.5 cm) cubes. Place in a medium pot and cover with cool water by at least 1 inch (2.5 cm). Bring to a boil, reduce the heat, and simmer for 20 minutes or until potatoes can easily be pierced with a fork. Drain potatoes, return to pot, and mash with broth and remaining ingredients until smooth. Season to taste and keep warm over very low heat.

To Cook the Sausage

3. Place patties in preheated oven and bake for 15 minutes until firm and cooked through.

To Make the Gravy

4. In a large saucepan over medium-high heat, cook the onion and mushrooms in ghee or oil with salt until browned. Stir in cassava flour to coat, then add wine, stirring to avoid lumps. Gradually add broth, stirring constantly. Bring to a boil and cook until thickened.

To Serve

5. Prepare the peas according to package instructions. Top a scoop of mashed potatoes with sausage patties and gravy and serve with peas.

SALT-RUBBED ROASTED CHICKEN AND VEGGIES

This one-dish dinner is a marriage between two iconic roast chicken recipes from two of my culinary heroes. First, the late and beloved Chef Judy Rodgers of Zuni Café introduced the world to the magic of a presalted bird. Trust me, the preplanning on that part is worth it—you'll know when you bite into that crispy skin and flavorful-to-the-bone meat. Second, Ina Garten has made all of us better home cooks, and her Perfect Roast Chicken is aptly named. Merging these two great techniques in a paleo- and AIP-friendly rendition yields incredible results.

● **GLUTEN-FREE**   ● **DAIRY-FREE**   ● **PALEO**   ● **AIP-FRIENDLY**

DIETARY LEVELS 1, 2, 3

SERVINGS 6

PREP TIME 20 minutes, plus 3 days for presalting

COOK TIME 1–1½ hours

TOTAL TIME 2 hours, 50 minutes, plus 3-day presalt

4–5 pound (1.8–2.3 kg) pasture-raised roasting chicken

4 teaspoons (24 g) fine sea salt, plus more to taste

3–4 medium carrots, peeled and cut into 2-inch (5 cm) pieces

1 pound (454 g) fingerling or baby potatoes, halved or quartered (sub diced celery root for paleo or AIP)

1 fennel bulb, cut into ½-inch (1.3 cm) wedges

3 medium shallots, quartered lengthwise

2 tablespoons (30 ml) extra-virgin olive oil

Freshly ground black pepper, to taste (omit for AIP)

½ bunch fresh thyme or rosemary, divided

½ cup (118 ml) white wine (sub Easy Homemade Bone Broth [page 218] or store-bought chicken broth for AIP)

1 small lemon, preferably Meyer, cut into wedges

4 cloves garlic, smashed

1. First, presalt the chicken. Measure the salt based on the weight of the chicken (¾ teaspoon [5 g] per pound). Rinse the chicken and pat dry thoroughly with paper towels. Rub the salt evenly all over the chicken and in its cavity. Place the chicken breast-side down in a baking dish or a Dutch oven. Cover tightly and refrigerate for 3 days (not 2, not 4!), flipping the bird over on day 2.

2. Preheat the oven to 425°F (218°C). Combine the carrots, potatoes (or celery root), fennel, and shallots in a 9 x 13-inch (22.9 x 33 cm) baking dish. Drizzle with olive oil, season with salt and pepper to taste, and throw in a few pinches of the fresh thyme or rosemary. Toss to coat and pour the white wine or chicken broth into the baking dish.

3. Place the chicken atop the vegetables. Tuck the wing tips behind the bird to prevent scorching. Stuff the cavity with lemon wedges, fresh herb sprigs, and smashed garlic cloves. Cross the legs and tie them together with kitchen twine.

4. Roast on the center rack for 1 to 1½ hours or until the skin is golden brown and crisp and the thickest part of the breast registers 165°F (74°C). Remove from the oven and let rest, uncovered, for about 15 minutes before carving the chicken into serving-sized pieces. Serve atop the roasted vegetables and drizzle with the succulent pan juices.

SERVING SUGGESTION
Pair this with a simple arugula salad. Lightly drizzle baby arugula with extra-virgin olive oil, a spritz of lemon juice or balsamic vinegar, and a pinch of salt and pepper (omit pepper for AIP). Toss to coat. Serve alongside or beneath the roasted chicken and veggies for a bright and lovely counterpoint to the chicken's richness.

MEDITERRANEAN GUNDI BOWLS

Growing up, my Grandma Louise used to make us a dinner she called "Salmagundi," which was really just her way of cleaning out the fridge and feeding me and my four siblings an assorted mash-up of the contents. The name alone is forever etched into our family lore. As it turns out, *salmagundi* is a real dish dating back to seventeenth-century England. Traditionally a hodgepodge of meats, eggs, lettuces, and pickled things, it loosely translates to "a little bit of everything." This updated Gundi Bowl is a little sexier than Grandma's Salmagundi, but still honors that spirit and adds a Mediterranean twist.

● **GLUTEN-FREE**　　● **DAIRY-FREE**　　● **PALEO**

DIETARY LEVELS 1, 2

SERVINGS 4
PREP TIME 30 minutes
COOK TIME 10 minutes
TOTAL TIME 40 minutes

FOR LEMON TAHINI DRIZZLE

½ cup (120 g) tahini

¼ cup (59 ml) fresh lemon juice

2 small cloves garlic, grated or minced

2 tablespoons (30 ml) olive oil

1 teaspoon sea salt

1 teaspoon sumac, plus extra for garnish

¼ cup (60 ml) plus 2 tablespoons (30 ml) cold water, divided, plus more as needed

FOR BOILED EGGS

4 eggs

FOR SPICED MEAT

2 teaspoons olive oil

1 pound (454 g) grass-fed ground beef or lamb

1 teaspoon ground cumin

1 teaspoon ground coriander

½ teaspoon smoked paprika

½ teaspoon ground cinnamon

1 teaspoon sea salt

¼ teaspoon freshly ground black pepper

2 cloves garlic, minced

Juice of 1 lemon

FOR ASSEMBLY

4 ounces (113 g) salad greens (spring mix, butter lettuce, romaine, or iceberg lettuce)

½ Persian cucumber, thinly sliced

1½ cups (270 g) cherry tomatoes, halved

1 cup (135 g) your favorite fermented pickles (see THYROID30 Support and Resources on page 246 for suggested brands)

¼ cup (30) toasted walnuts or pistachios, roughly chopped

¼ cup (24 g) chopped fresh mint

4 lemon wedges (optional)

To Make the Lemon Tahini Drizzle

1. Whisk together all ingredients except the water; the mixture will be very thick. Add ¼ cup (60 ml) cold water, whisking to combine. If needed, add up to 2 tablespoons (30 ml) more water until a smooth and pourable consistency is reached. Set aside.

To Make the Boiled Eggs

2. Bring a medium pot of water to a gentle boil. Carefully lower the eggs into the water and cook for 7 to 8 minutes for soft-boiled, jammy yolks, or 10 minutes for dry yolks. Rinse immediately under cold water and let them sit until cool enough to handle. Peel, slice in half, and set aside.

To Make the Spiced Meat

3. Heat the olive oil in a large skillet over medium heat. Add the ground meat, breaking it up with a spatula. Stir in the spices and seasoning. Cook for about 7 minutes, stirring occasionally, until browned and cooked through. Add the garlic and cook for 30 seconds more, stirring until fragrant. Squeeze in lemon juice, stir, and remove from the heat.

To Assemble

4. Divide the greens between 4 serving bowls. Add the cucumber, tomatoes, pickles, eggs, and ground meat in sections. Drizzle generously with the Lemon Tahini Sauce. Sprinkle with toasted nuts, mint, and sumac if desired. Serve with lemon wedges (if using) and enjoy!

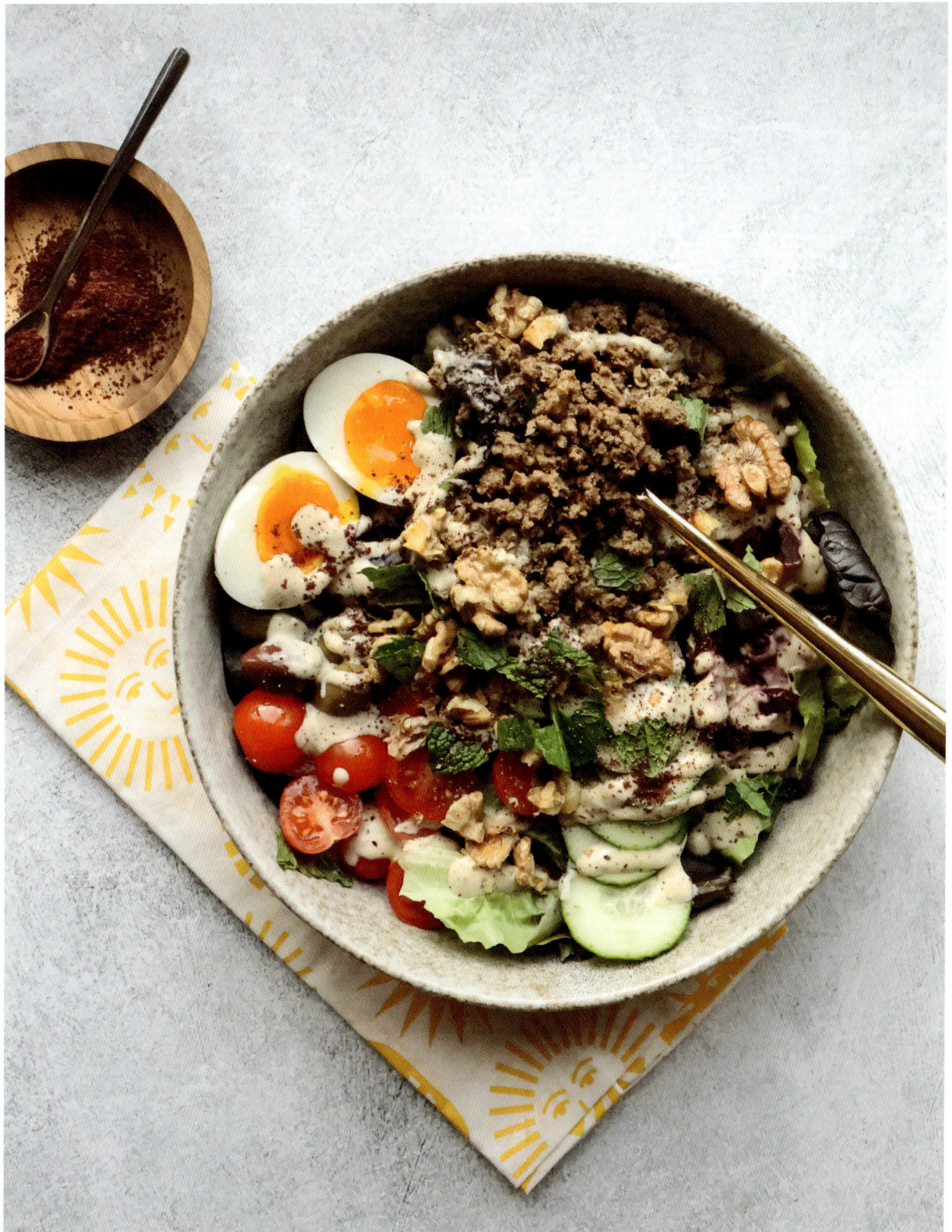

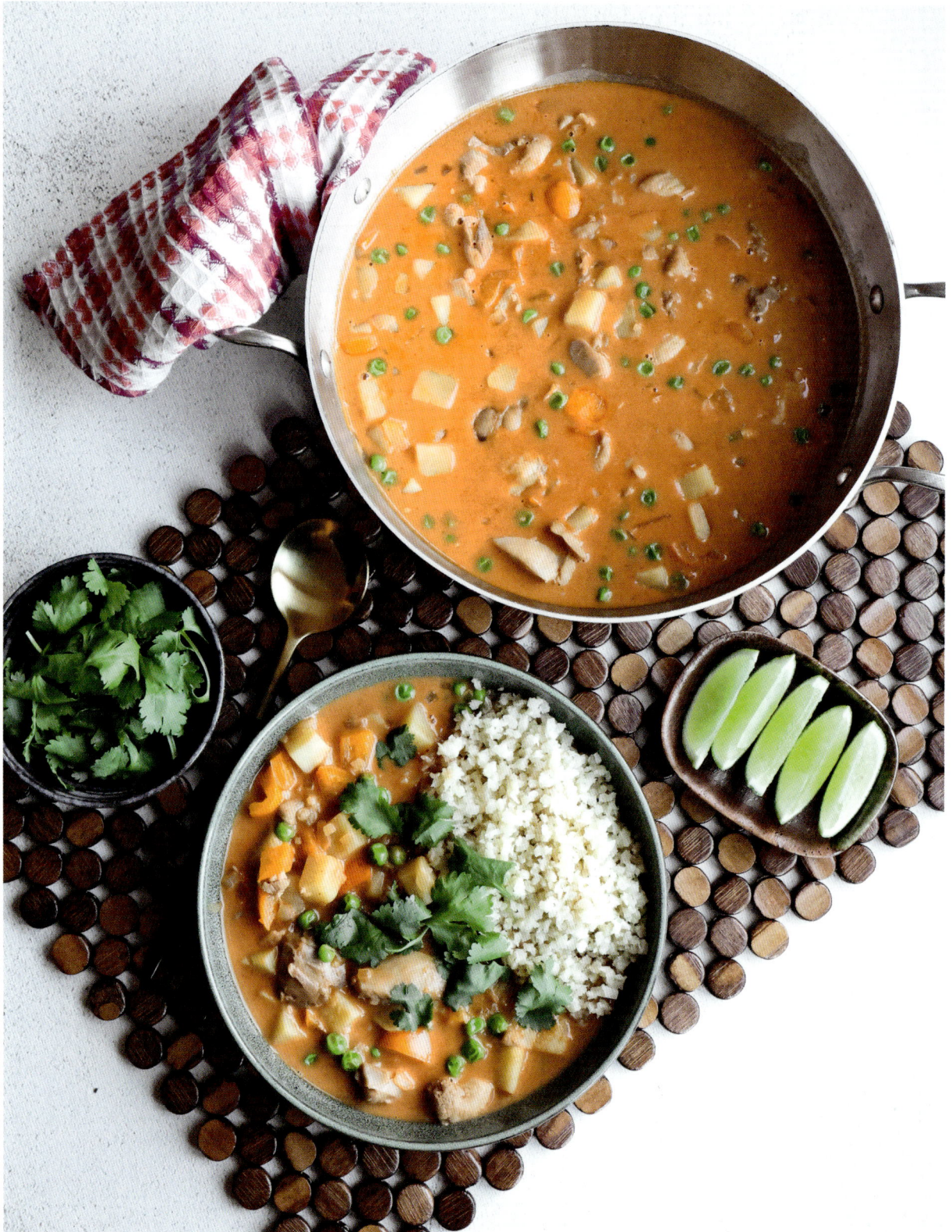

THAI-STYLE CHICKEN (OR SHRIMP) RED CURRY

Thai-style curries are quick and satisfying staple meals, ideal for both weeknight dinners and weekend feasts. You can make your own curry paste if you like, but store-bought options are decent, time-saving, and usually made from whole food ingredients. The spice level seems to vary drastically between brands of red curry paste, though, so I recommend starting with a small amount: With one brand, you might be able to add more than half the jar, while doing that with another could really send spice levels soaring! For a shrimp variation, see the substitution instructions below.

● **GLUTEN-FREE**   ◐ **DAIRY-FREE**   ● **PALEO**

DIETARY LEVELS 1, 2

SERVINGS 4
PREP TIME 20 minutes
COOK TIME 20 minutes
TOTAL TIME 40 minutes

1 tablespoon (14 g) organic, unrefined coconut oil

⅓ cup (53 g) (about 1 large) minced shallot

2 tablespoons (12 g) minced or grated ginger

1 tablespoon (10 g) minced garlic

2 cups (220 g) diced orange or white sweet potatoes

Fine sea salt, to taste

1 red, orange, or yellow bell pepper, diced

1 (14-ounce [392 g]) can full-fat coconut milk

1 cup (237 ml) Easy Homemade Chicken Bone Broth (page 218) or store-bought

1–2 tablespoons (15–30 g) red curry paste

2 makrut lime leaves or 1 teaspoon lime zest

1 tablespoon (9 g) coconut sugar

2 tablespoons (30 ml) paleo-compliant fish sauce, plus more as needed

Pinch white pepper

1 pound (454 g) boneless, skinless chicken thighs, cut into bite-size pieces, or shrimp

⅔ cup (87 g) frozen peas (sub 2 cups [60 g] freshly chopped baby spinach for paleo)

1 tablespoon (15 ml) fresh lime juice, plus more as needed

Cooked rice (sub cauliflower rice for paleo)

OPTIONAL GARNISHES

Chopped fresh cilantro

Green onion

Lime wedges

1. Melt the coconut oil in a large (5-quart [4.7 L]) soup pot or Dutch oven over medium heat. Add the shallot, ginger, and garlic and sauté until fragrant, about 1 minute. Add the sweet potato and season lightly with salt. Cook, stirring occasionally, for about 5 minutes. Add the bell pepper and cook for 3 minutes more or until just beginning to soften.

2. Pour in the coconut milk and chicken broth. Add the curry paste (start with 1 tablespoon [15 g] as some brands are very spicy), lime leaves or zest, coconut sugar, fish sauce, and white pepper. Bring to a simmer and cook for 3 minutes, stirring to fully dissolve the curry paste. Taste and add more curry paste for additional heat, if desired.

3. Add the chicken (or see shrimp instructions below), bring to a boil, reduce heat, cover, and simmer for 10 to 15 minutes or until the chicken is cooked through and the sweet potatoes are tender and can easily be pierced with a fork but aren't falling apart.

   To substitute shrimp, use 1 pound (454 g) of raw shrimp, peeled and deveined. Add it during the last 2 minutes of cooking, once the sweet potatoes are tender. Simmer just until pink and opaque to avoid overcooking.

4. Stir in the frozen peas or spinach during the last minute of cooking. Remove from the heat and stir in 1 tablespoon (15 ml) fresh lime juice. Taste and adjust seasonings by adding extra fish sauce, sea salt, or lime juice for balance. Aim for a harmony of spicy, salty, sour, and sweet flavors.

5. Serve over rice or cauliflower rice, garnished with cilantro, green onion, and lime wedges, if desired.

SERVING SUGGESTIONS
GF/DF (Level 1) Option: Serve atop steamed white rice.
Paleo (Level 2) Option: Serve atop cauliflower rice.

SAUSAGE, BEANS, AND GREENS PASTA

This nutrient-dense comfort-food dish requires minimal prep and comes together quickly. The crispy garlic chips are always the first thing to disappear at our table, and they serve a double purpose, adding extra flavor by creating a garlic-infused oil. Adding gluten-free or grain-free pasta is a great way to bulk up this dish to feed a family or ensure leftovers, but you can also omit it for a lower-carb version. Just be sure to adjust the seasoning accordingly if you do.

● **GLUTEN-FREE**   ● **DAIRY-FREE**

DIETARY LEVELS 1

SERVINGS: 4
PREP TIME 20 minutes
COOK TIME 20 minutes
TOTAL TIME 40 minutes

1 pound (454 g) sweet Italian sausage, loose or casings removed

3 tablespoons (45 ml) extra-virgin olive oil, plus more as needed

4 large garlic cloves, sliced thinly into coins

¼ teaspoon chile flakes, or more to taste

1½ cups (273 g) cooked cannellini or great northern beans, rinsed and drained

Fine sea salt, to taste

Freshly ground black pepper, to taste

2 bunches Lacinato kale, stemmed and chopped (about ¾ pound [340 g])

1 cup (237 ml) Easy Homemade Chicken Bone Broth (page 218) or store-bought

12 ounces (340 g) gluten-free or grain-free pasta

Zest and juice of ½ lemon

1. Brown the Italian sausage in a large, heavy-bottomed skillet. Remove from the skillet, drain excess fat if necessary, and set aside.

2. Add 3 tablespoons (45 ml) of olive oil to the skillet over medium heat. Add the garlic to the pan and cook, stirring, until lightly golden brown. Watch carefully to avoid scorching. As soon as the garlic coins are toasted, use a slotted spoon to remove them from the oil and set aside, leaving the garlic-infused oil in the skillet.

3. Add the chile flakes and cook for 1 minute or until fragrant. Add the beans and season liberally with salt and pepper. Remove from the skillet and set aside.

4. Add the kale and chicken broth to the skillet and cook, stirring occasionally, until liquid is reduced and greens are wilted and tender, about 5 to 7 minutes. Meanwhile, cook the pasta according to package instructions until al dente.

5. Return the sausage and beans to the skillet and stir to combine. Taste and adjust the seasoning: It should be fairly salty to balance out the pasta.

6. After the pasta is cooked, drain and add it to the skillet. Add the lemon zest and juice and an extra drizzle of olive oil, and toss to combine. Again, taste and adjust the seasoning as needed before serving. Garnish with the toasted garlic coins, and enjoy!

NOTE
For compliant pasta options, check out these suggestions:
GF/DF: Brown rice pasta or your favorite gluten-free pasta
Paleo/AIP: Spaghetti squash, zoodles, or a cassava pasta.

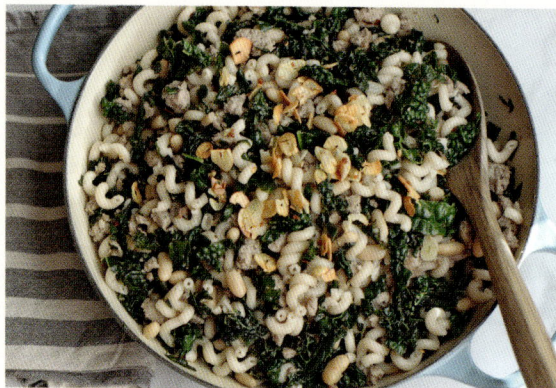

SAVORY KOREAN-STYLE CHUCK ROAST

This is one of the most flavorful yet low-maintenance pot roasts you'll ever make. A few pantry ingredients like coconut aminos, fish sauce, and vinegar, plus staples like garlic and ginger, create a simple "marinade" for the beef that turns into a sumptuous, umami-packed gravy in the oven. The result is a sweet-and-savory triumph. Serve it over fluffy white rice or cauliflower rice (for paleo or AIP) and pair it with the Japanese-Style Cucumber Salad on page 144 for a perfectly balanced meal.

● GLUTEN-FREE　　● DAIRY-FREE　　● PALEO　　● AIP-FRIENDLY

DIETARY LEVELS 1, 2, 3

SERVINGS 6
PREP TIME 15 minutes
COOK TIME 3½ hours
TOTAL TIME About 4 hours

1 (3-pound [1.4 kg]) grass-finished beef chuck roast, excess fat trimmed

1 cup (237 ml) beef broth

⅓ cup (79 ml) coconut aminos

1 tablespoon (15 ml) AIP-compliant fish sauce

2 tablespoons (18 g) coconut sugar

½ onion, roughly chopped

3 green onions, roughly chopped

6 cloves garlic, peeled

1-inch (2.5 cm) piece ginger root, peeled and sliced into coins

2 tablespoons (30 ml) cider vinegar

1 ripe Asian or Bosc pear or 1 tart apple, peeled and roughly chopped

OPTIONAL GARNISHES

Sliced green onions

Chopped fresh cilantro

Sesame seeds (omit for AIP)

1. Preheat the oven to 325°F (163°C). Place the chuck roast in a 5-quart (4.7 L) Dutch oven with a tight-fitting lid.

2. Combine the broth, coconut aminos, fish sauce, coconut sugar, onion, green onions, garlic, ginger, vinegar, and pear or apple in a blender and process until smooth. Pour the mixture over the roast.

3. Cover the Dutch oven, place in the center of the oven, and cook for 3 to 3½ hours or until the beef shreds easily with a fork. Note that the meat does not need to be fully submerged in the liquid to cook, but it's a good idea to flip it once or twice to help distribute the flavors and ensure even cooking.

4. Remove the roast from the pot and set it on a plate to cool slightly, leaving the cooking liquid in the pot. Use a spoon, ladle, or gravy separator to skim the excess fat from the top of the cooking liquid and discard.

5. Use 2 forks or a carving fork and knife to pull the beef into bite-size hunks, removing any excess fat or gristle. Return the beef to the pot and toss gently to coat with the remaining cooking liquid. Garnish with sliced green onions, chopped cilantro, or sesame seeds, if desired.

CURRIED LAMB MEATBALLS IN TOMATO SAUCE

This richly spiced twist on meatballs in tomato sauce is easy to love. This is one of those recipes that makes glorious leftovers and tastes even better after a day or two in the fridge thanks to its warming, aromatic spices, so it's perfect for meal prep. For maximum meals with minimal effort, make a double batch and freeze the extras for those "I don't feel like cooking" days. To take the flavors and colors over the top, add a pinch of saffron threads to your side or accompaniment of choice when cooking!

● GLUTEN-FREE ● DAIRY-FREE ● PALEO

DIETARY LEVELS 1, 2

SERVINGS 6
PREP TIME 20 minutes
COOK TIME 40 minutes
TOTAL TIME 1 hour

FOR MEATBALLS

2 pounds (907 g) ground lamb or grass-finished beef

1 teaspoon ground fennel

1 tablespoon (6 g) curry powder

1 medium shallot, minced

2 cloves garlic, minced

1 egg

1 teaspoon fine sea salt

Freshly ground black pepper, to taste

1 tablespoon (14 g) grass-fed ghee or (15 ml) extra-virgin olive oil

FOR SAUCE

½ medium onion, diced

1 teaspoon ground ginger

1 teaspoon ground cumin

1 teaspoon ground cinnamon

1 teaspoon fine sea salt

1 (28-ounce [800 g]) can crushed tomatoes

Cooked rice, cauliflower rice, or quinoa

OPTIONAL GARNISHES

Fresh parsley

Fresh mint leaves

Toasted pine nuts

To Make the Meatballs

1. Combine all the meatball ingredients except the ghee or oil in a large mixing bowl and mix just until blended. Form into 1½-inch (3.8 cm) meatballs.

2. Melt the ghee in or add oil to a large, deep skillet, a pot, or a big Dutch oven over medium-high heat. Add the meatballs and brown, undisturbed, about 5 minutes, working in batches if necessary. Flip and brown the other side for 5 minutes more, then remove meatballs to a plate and set aside.

To Make the Sauce

3. Drain excess fat from the skillet, leaving about 2 tablespoons (30 ml). Add the onion and cook over medium heat until soft and translucent. Add the spices and salt to the onions and cook, stirring, just until fragrant, about 1 minute. Add the crushed tomatoes to the skillet and stir to combine.

4. Return the meatballs to the skillet. Bring to a simmer and reduce the heat. Simmer for 20 to 25 minutes, uncovered, or until the meatballs are cooked through and the sauce has thickened slightly.

5. Serve over rice, cauliflower rice, or quinoa. Garnish with fresh parsley, fresh mint leaves, or toasted pine nuts, if desired, and enjoy!

CLASSIC SHEPHERD'S PIE

This family-friendly comfort food delivers savory meat in rich gravy, built-in veggies, and a crispy mashed potato topping. Fresh rosemary, thyme, tomato paste, and our Homemade Worcestershire (page 222) add deep flavor. For a subtle twist, swap 1 pound (0.5 kg) of potato for celery root, or stick with the classic.

🟤 **GLUTEN-FREE**   🟡 **DAIRY-FREE**

DIETARY LEVELS 1

SERVINGS 6–8
PREP TIME 30 minutes
COOK TIME 30 minutes
TOTAL TIME 1 hour

Ghee or olive oil for greasing

FOR MASHED POTATO TOPPING

3½ pounds (1.6 kg) (about 4 large) russet potatoes, peeled and cut into 1-inch (2.5 cm) chunks (or replace 1 pound [0.5 kg] with celery root, optional)

½ cup (118 ml) Easy Homemade Chicken Bone Broth (page 218) or store-bought

3 tablespoons (42 g) ghee or (44 ml) extra-virgin olive oil

1 teaspoon fine sea salt

Pinch white pepper, or more to taste

1 raw egg yolk

FOR FILLING

1 tablespoon (15 ml) extra-virgin olive oil

1 large onion, finely diced

4 large carrots, finely diced

4 cloves garlic, minced

2 pounds (907 g) ground lamb or grass-finished beef or bison

1 teaspoon fine sea salt, or more to taste

Freshly ground black pepper, to taste

2 tablespoons (14 g) cassava flour

2 tablespoons (32 g) tomato paste

1½ cups (355 ml) Easy Homemade Chicken Bone Broth (page 218) or store-bought

2 tablespoons (30 ml) Homemade Worcestershire Sauce (page 222)

2 teaspoons finely chopped fresh rosemary

2 teaspoons finely chopped fresh thyme

1 cup (130 g) frozen peas

1. Preheat the oven to 400°F (200°C). Grease a deep 9 x 13-inch (22.9 x 33 cm) baking dish with ghee or olive oil.

To Make the Mashed Potato Topping

2. Place the potatoes in a large saucepan and cover with water by 1–2 inches (2.5–5.1 cm). Place over high heat, bring to a boil, reduce the heat, and continue boiling for 8 to 10 minutes or until fork-tender. (Note: If using celery root, follow the same cooking method as the potatoes, but boil in a separate pot, as celery root takes slightly longer to cook.)

3. Drain potatoes (and celery root, if using) and return to the pot. Add the chicken broth, ghee or olive oil, sea salt, and white pepper. Mash with a potato masher until blended; to avoid gluey potatoes, do not overmash. Taste and adjust seasoning as needed. Stir in the egg yolk and set aside.

To Make the Filling

4. Heat the olive oil in a large, deep skillet over medium-high heat. Add the onion and carrot and sauté until tender, about 5 to 7 minutes. Stir in the garlic and cook 2 minutes more. Add the meat to the skillet and cook until no longer pink, breaking it up with a spatula, about 5 to 7 minutes. If there is a lot of rendered fat in the pan, tilt the pan and spoon off excess grease.

5. Add the salt, pepper, and cassava flour, and stir to coat the meat. Add the tomato paste, chicken broth, Worcestershire sauce, and fresh herbs. Cook, stirring, until the mixture starts to bubble and thicken to a gravylike consistency, about 2 to 3 minutes. Stir in the peas and remove from the heat. Taste and adjust seasoning as needed.

6. Transfer the filling to the prepared dish and smooth the top. Place dollops of mashed potatoes across the top of the filling and spread into an even layer. Leave a little space at the edges to allow steam to escape. Use a fork to create a textured pattern on top for extra crispness.

7. Bake for 30 minutes or until the top is just beginning to brown. Serve with a simple green salad, and enjoy!

BALSAMIC-MARINATED CHICKEN BREASTS

This is one of those delicious, versatile staple recipes you'll come back to again and again. After marinating the chicken, you can bake, grill, or pan-sear it. For an easy high-protein meal prep staple, bake it in the oven, then slice it or shred it with two forks along with the collected pan juices. It's especially good with sides like Rainbow Roasted Root Vegetables (page 204) or Roasted Brussels Sprouts with Bacon (page 195), and it also plays a starring role in the Beet Salad with Chicken and Maple Mustard Vinaigrette on page 131.

● **GLUTEN-FREE**　● **DAIRY-FREE**　● **PALEO**　● **AIP-FRIENDLY**

DIETARY LEVELS 1, 2, 3

SERVINGS 6

PREP TIME 15 minutes

COOK TIME 25 minutes

TOTAL TIME 40 minutes, plus 1–2 hours optional marinating time

¼ cup (59 ml) extra-virgin olive oil

2 teaspoons honey or pure maple syrup (optional)

1 teaspoon herbes de Provence or Italian herb blend

2 cloves garlic, minced

2 tablespoons (30 ml) balsamic vinegar (additive-free for AIP: see note)

2 teaspoons Homemade Worcestershire Sauce (page 222) (optional)

1 teaspoon fine sea salt, or more to taste

¼ teaspoon freshly ground black pepper (omit for AIP)

2 pounds (907 g) (about 4 medium) pasture-raised boneless, skinless chicken breasts

OPTIONAL GARNISHES

Chopped fresh parsley

Chopped fresh rosemary

Chopped fresh thyme

1. Combine the olive oil, honey or maple syrup (if using), dried herbs, garlic, balsamic vinegar, Worcestershire sauce (if using), sea salt, and freshly ground pepper. Whisk until well blended.

2. Rinse and pat dry the chicken breasts with paper towels. Add the chicken to the marinade, flipping to coat evenly. Cover and refrigerate for up to 2 hours. Marinating is optional, but will enhance flavor and tenderness.

3. Remove the chicken from the fridge while you preheat the oven to 400°F (200°C).

4. Transfer the chicken and marinade to a 9 x 13-inch (22.9 x 33 cm) baking dish. Arrange the breasts so they are not touching, allowing heat to circulate for even cooking. Transfer to the center of the oven and bake for 25 minutes or until the thickest part of the largest breast reaches 165°F (74°C) with an instant-read thermometer.

5. Remove from the oven and let rest for 5 minutes. Sprinkle with fresh parsley, rosemary, or thyme, if desired, and serve drizzled with the pan juices.

NOTE

Not all balsamic vinegars are created equal. Some producers use additives like caramel color, molasses, corn syrup, guar gum, or artificial flavoring to color, thicken, and sweeten their imitation balsamic vinegars. Ideally, the ingredient list should only say grape must, cooked grape must, or wine vinegar. Sulfites are also a common ingredient, even in true balsamic, but they are not considered paleo or AIP-compliant, so careful label reading is important. Look for the Whole30-Approved or Certified Paleo stamp on the label to ensure you're getting a product that fits your dietary requirements.

SPICE-RUBBED SLAMMIN' SALMON

I had help from my bold and zesty hubby on this one! In fact, Noah is all over this book: He and I cook side by side most evenings. While I specialize in sneaking in extra vegetables and making healthy meals delicious, he's the one adding bacon to everything, embarking on multiday "meat projects," and spicing things up with his bold flavors. He created this "Slammin' Salmon Rub" during our years in Alaska, and it has been our go-to ever since. It pairs perfectly with fatty, anti-inflammatory wild salmon. Best of all, though, this whole recipe can be whipped up in just 20 minutes from start to finish.

● **GLUTEN-FREE**　　● **DAIRY-FREE**　　● **PALEO**

DIETARY LEVELS 1, 2

SERVINGS 4
PREP TIME 10 minutes
COOK TIME 10 minutes
TOTAL TIME 20 minutes

FOR SPICE RUB

1 teaspoon ground fennel

½ teaspoon ground coriander

½ teaspoon garlic powder

½ teaspoon freshly ground black pepper

¾ teaspoon fine sea salt

FOR SALMON

1½ pounds (680 g) wild salmon fillet, cut into 4 equal pieces

1 tablespoon (15 ml) avocado oil

1. Adjust the oven rack to the middle position and preheat the broiler.

To Make the Spice Rub

2. Combine the spice rub ingredients in a small dish and stir to combine. Note that the rub recipe makes enough for about 2 pounds (907 g) of salmon fillets.

To Make the Salmon

3. Brush the salmon lightly on both sides with avocado oil and place skin-side down on a rimmed baking sheet. Sprinkle the top of the salmon fillets liberally with the spice mixture (for 1½ pounds [680 g], you'll use about three-quarters of the rub). Transfer to the middle rack of the oven and broil for 8 to 12 minutes or until the seasonings have formed a light crust and the fish has browned on top and can be flaked easily with a fork.

4. Remove from the oven and let rest for 3 to 5 minutes before serving. Use a spatula to separate the salmon from the skin before plating. Serve warm with your favorite sides!

NOTE
Pair with the Eat the Rainbow Chopped Salad (page 130), Cowboy Caviar Quinoa Salad (page 139), Lemony Cauliflower Pasta (page 196), or Roasted Brussels Sprouts with Bacon (page 195).

VEGGIE-PACKED MEATLOAF MUFFINS

These moist and savory meatloaf muffins are family-friendly, snackable, and loaded with hidden veggies. Homemade Worcestershire Sauce (page 222) gives them oomph, while fresh herbs add aromatic flair. Cassava flour makes a great egg-free and grain-free binder for this recipe. This starchy root vegetable is on the long list of goitrogenic foods, but can be enjoyed in moderation as part of a thyroid-friendly diet, especially when properly cooked and prepared. Serve them alongside the Velvety Truffle Mashed Cauliflower and Sweet Potatoes (page 202) plus a simple green salad for a fun, satisfying, well-balanced meal.

GLUTEN-FREE   DAIRY-FREE   PALEO   AIP-FRIENDLY

DIETARY LEVELS 1, 2, 3

SERVINGS 6
PREP TIME 25 minutes
COOK TIME 25 minutes
TOTAL TIME 50 minutes

Unrefined coconut oil, for greasing

1 tablespoon (15 ml) extra-virgin olive oil

10 ounces (264 g) frozen cauliflower rice (about 2 cups), thawed

1 cup (110 g) grated carrot or zucchini

½ cup (80 g) minced shallot or onion

2 large cloves garlic, minced

2 pounds (907 g) grass-finished ground beef

1 tablespoon (2 g) minced fresh thyme

1 tablespoon (2 g) minced fresh rosemary

1½ teaspoons fine sea salt

½ teaspoon freshly ground black pepper (omit for AIP)

¼ cup (59 ml) Homemade Worcestershire Sauce (page 222)

¼ cup (29 g) cassava flour

1 tablespoon (15 ml) coconut aminos

1 tablespoon (15 ml) balsamic vinegar (additive-free for AIP)

1. Preheat the oven to 375°F (190°C). Lightly grease a 12-cup muffin tin with coconut oil or line with parchment liners. Place on a rimmed baking sheet to catch any drips.

2. Heat the olive oil in a large skillet over medium heat. Add the cauliflower rice, grated carrot or zucchini, minced shallot or onion, and garlic. Cook, stirring occasionally, until the veggies are tender and moisture has evaporated. Remove from the heat and let cool slightly.

3. Add the veggies to a large mixing bowl along with the ground beef, fresh herbs, sea salt, pepper, Worcestershire sauce, and cassava flour. Mix just until combined. Divide the mixture evenly among the muffin cups, pressing gently to smooth the tops.

4. Combine the coconut aminos and balsamic vinegar in a small dish. Brush the muffin tops lightly with this mixture.

5. Bake for 20 to 25 minutes or until muffins are browned on top and cooked through to an internal temperature of 160°F (71°C). Let the muffins rest for about 5 minutes before serving. Leftovers can be stored in an airtight container in the fridge for up to 4 days or frozen for up to 3 months.

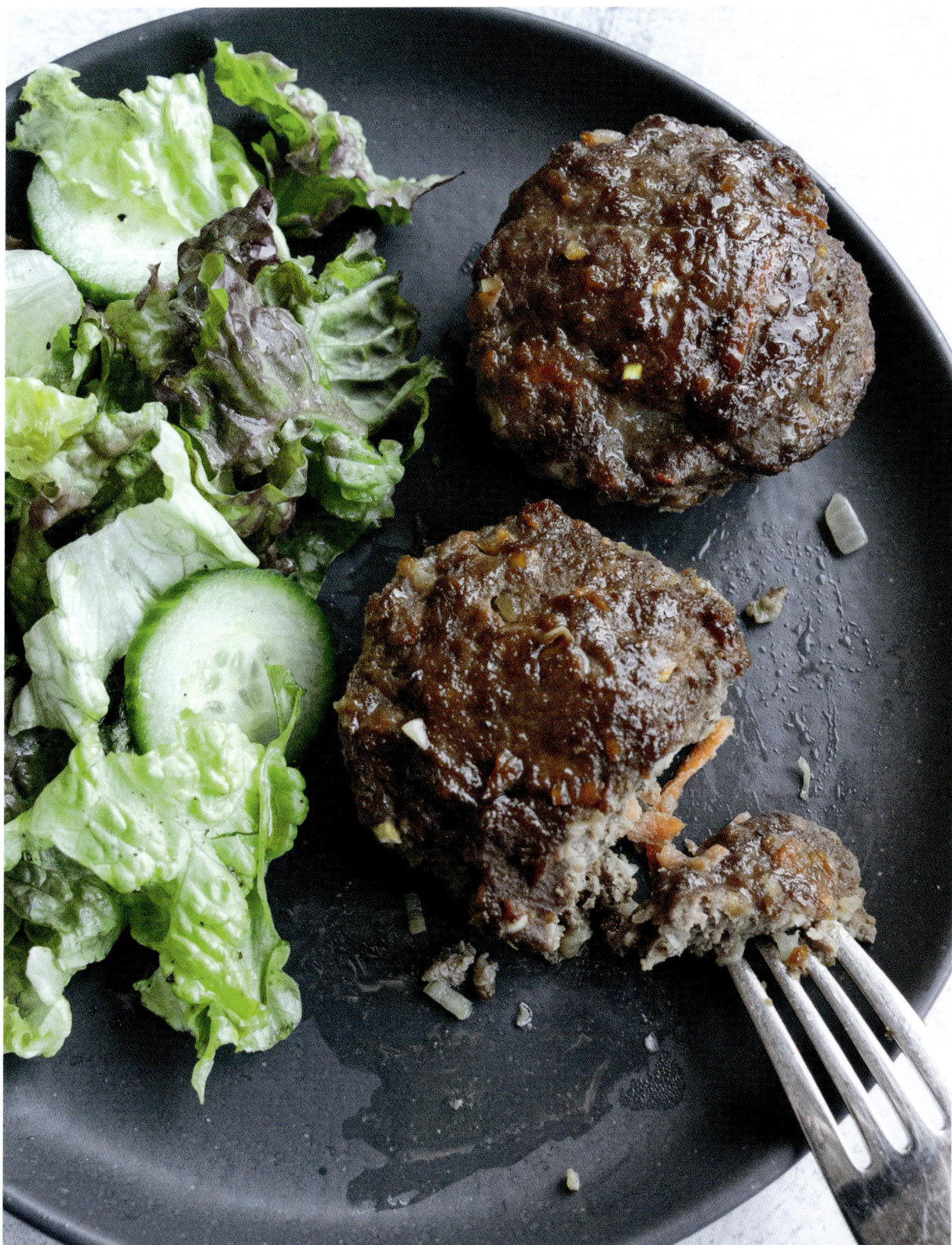

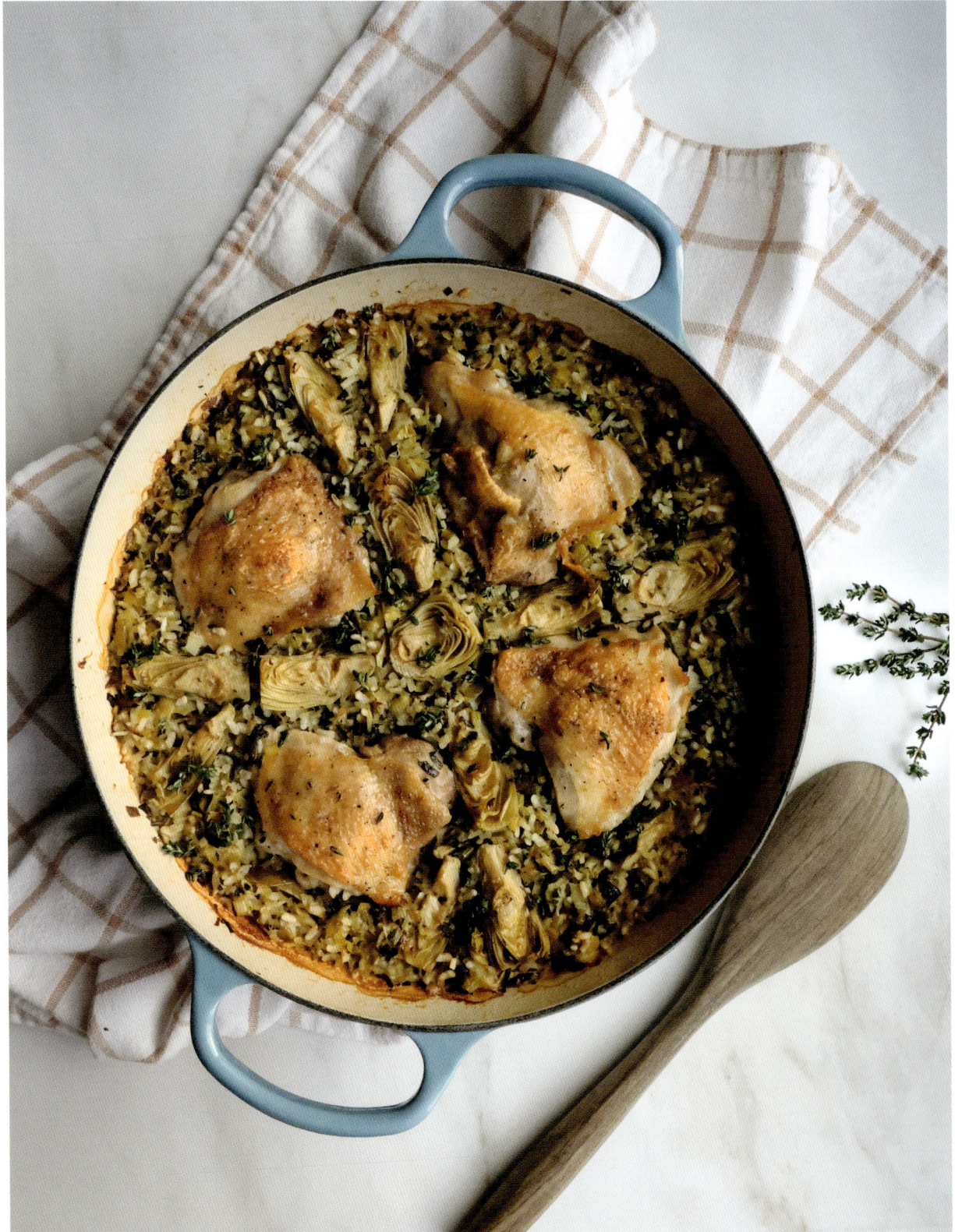

ARTICHOKE CHICKEN AND RICE BAKE

This one-pot meal delivers crispy-skinned chicken thighs nestled into creamy, lemony arborio rice laced with artichokes, leeks, lemon, and greens. I'd like to give a nod to fellow chef and Thyroid Thriver Phoebe Lapine, who has perfected the chicken and rice casserole formula. This is my own riff, inspired by her method and the irresistible flavors of artichoke dip. During testing, it took a more Provençal turn with the addition of white wine and herbes de Provence. If you love artichokes like I do, I think you'll enjoy the results!

● **GLUTEN-FREE**　　◐ **DAIRY-FREE**

DIETARY LEVELS 1

SERVINGS 4
PREP TIME 15 minutes
COOK TIME 45 minutes
TOTAL TIME 1 hour

4 bone-in, skin-on chicken thighs

1½ teaspoons fine sea salt, plus more to taste, divided

Freshly ground black pepper, to taste

2 tablespoons (30 ml) extra-virgin olive oil

1 large leek, white and light green parts only, finely chopped

2 stalks celery, finely chopped

4 cloves garlic, minced

1 cup (185 g) arborio rice

⅓ cup (79 ml) dry white wine

2½ cups (591 ml) Easy Homemade Chicken Bone Broth (page 218) or store-bought

1½ cups (450 g) artichoke hearts, frozen and defrosted, or canned or jarred in water and drained, roughly chopped, divided

3 cups (90 g) roughly chopped spinach or chard

1 teaspoon herbes de Provence

1 teaspoon lemon zest

1 bay leaf

1 tablespoon (9 g) nutritional yeast

2 teaspoons fresh thyme leaves, divided

1 tablespoon (15 ml) fresh lemon juice, plus more for spritzing

OPTIONAL GARNISHES
Brazil Nut "Parmesan" (page 225)
Lemon wedges

1. Preheat the oven to 375°F (190°C). Rinse and pat the chicken thighs dry with paper towels and season on both sides with ½ teaspoon of the salt and the freshly ground pepper to taste.

2. Heat the olive oil in a large oven-safe skillet or Dutch oven over medium-high heat. Sear the chicken, skin-side down, until lightly golden brown, about 5 minutes. Flip and cook for 2 minutes more, then transfer to a plate; the chicken will finish cooking in the oven.

3. Lower the heat to medium and add the leeks and celery, sautéing for 3 to 4 minutes until softened. Stir in the garlic and cook for 30 seconds more, until fragrant. Stir in the arborio rice and cook for 1 minute to lightly toast the grains. Pour in the white wine, scraping up any browned bits from the bottom of the pan. Add the chicken broth and stir to combine. Add half of the artichokes to the pan (reserving the rest for topping).

4. Stir in the greens, herbes de Provence, lemon zest, bay leaf, nutritional yeast, 1 teaspoon of fresh thyme, lemon juice, and the remaining 1 teaspoon of sea salt. Nestle the seared chicken thighs (skin-side up) into the rice mixture, then nestle the remaining artichokes around them.

5. Cover with a lid (or foil) and bake for 25 minutes. Uncover and bake for 10 to 15 minutes more, or until the chicken reaches at least 175°F (80°C) and the rice is tender. For extra crispness and color on the chicken thighs, briefly broil the top.

6. Remove from the oven and let rest for 5 minutes. Discard the bay leaf, spritz generously with lemon juice, and sprinkle with the remaining 1 teaspoon of fresh thyme leaves. Serve with Brazil Nut "Parmesan" (page 225) and extra lemon wedges if desired, and enjoy!

KHAO MAN GAI–INSPIRED CHICKEN AND RICE

This dish is inspired by the comforting flavors of Thai *khao man gai* and Chinese Hainanese chicken, two similar dishes with shared origins. Both feature tender poached chicken, fragrant rice, and nourishing broth. To simplify what can be a long cooking process, this version braises the chicken for deep, rich flavor and fork-tender meat while the rice is toasted pilaf-style in rendered chicken fat, making it incredibly aromatic and flavorful. This meal is nutrient-packed as well as delicious, loaded with collagen, anti-inflammatory aromatics, and thyroid-supportive nutrients like selenium and tyrosine. Serve it alongside my Japanese-Style Cucumber Salad (page 144).

● **GLUTEN-FREE**   ● **DAIRY-FREE**

DIETARY LEVELS 1

SERVINGS 6
PREP TIME 20 minutes
COOK TIME 45 minutes
TOTAL TIME 1 hour, 5 minutes

FOR CHICKEN

1 pound (454 g) bone-in, skin-on chicken thighs

1 pound (454 g) chicken drumsticks

Fine sea salt, to taste

Freshly ground pepper, to taste

1 tablespoon (15 ml) avocado oil

½ cup (80 g) minced shallot

4 cloves garlic

2 tablespoons (12 g) finely minced fresh ginger

4 green onions, white bottoms, finely chopped; green tops, finely chopped, reserved

¼ cup (59 ml) mirin (Japanese sweet rice wine)

1 stalk lemongrass, trimmed, cut into two 6-inch (15.2 cm) pieces and tied together with kitchen twine (optional)

1 small dried Thai chile (optional)

1 tablespoon (15 ml) coconut aminos

2 cups (473 ml) Easy Homemade Chicken Bone Broth (page 218) or store-bought

FOR RICE

2–3 tablespoons (30–44 ml) rendered chicken fat from reserved skin, or avocado oil

1 garlic clove, minced

1 tablespoon (6 g) freshly minced ginger

1½ cups (293 g) jasmine or basmati rice, rinsed

2 cups (473 ml) chicken broth or bone broth

2 tablespoons (30 ml) water

1 tablespoon (15 ml) mirin (Japanese sweet rice wine)

1 tablespoon (15 ml) rice vinegar

½ teaspoon fine sea salt

To Make the Chicken

1. Trim the skin from the chicken thighs and set aside (do not discard). Sprinkle the thighs and drumsticks with sea salt and pepper.

2. Heat the avocado oil in a large, deep skillet or Dutch oven with a tight-fitting lid over medium-high heat. Add the chicken pieces and sear until golden brown on both sides, turning as needed, about 5 minutes per side. Transfer to a plate and set aside.

3. Add the shallot, garlic, ginger, and green onion bottoms to the pan, stirring until fragrant, about 1 minute. Add the mirin and bring to a simmer, scraping up any browned bits from the bottom of the pan.

4. Return the chicken to the pan along with the lemongrass (if using), Thai chile (if using), coconut aminos, and chicken broth. Bring to a simmer, cover, and let the chicken pieces braise for about 45 minutes, flipping halfway through. The chicken is done when it's tender and can easily be pulled away from the bone with a fork. Taste and adjust the broth for seasoning, as desired.

To Make the Rice

5. Heat the reserved chicken skin in a medium saucepan over medium heat, stirring occasionally, until you've got 2–3 tablespoons (30–44 ml) of rendered chicken fat. (To save time, you can substitute avocado oil, but the flavor is best with the chicken fat.) Add the garlic and ginger and cook, stirring, until fragrant, about 1 minute. Add the rice and toast for 1 to 2 minutes, stirring to coat the grains evenly.

6. Add the chicken broth, water, mirin, rice vinegar, and salt. Bring to a boil, reduce the heat to low, cover, and simmer for 20 minutes. Remove from the heat, let rest for 10 minutes, and then fluff with a fork. Keep covered until ready to eat.

7. Scoop the rice into bowls, top with chicken pieces, and ladle the broth over top. Garnish with the reserved green onion tops and serve.

SHEET PAN HARISSA CHICKEN WITH CARROTS AND OLIVES

The North African flavors of this one-dish dinner will fill your kitchen with the most irresistible aromas. This recipe makes good use of our Quick and Easy Harissa (page 220), but a mild store-bought harissa works well too. Just check the ingredients to make sure it meets your dietary requirements. This meal makes four tidy servings with one chicken thigh each, plus ample roasted veggies. To bulk it up and soak up some of those sumptuous pan juices, serve over quinoa (GF/DF/Level 1) or cauliflower rice (Paleo/Level 2).

● **GLUTEN-FREE**   ● **DAIRY-FREE**   ● **PALEO**

DIETARY LEVELS 1, 2

SERVINGS 4
PREP TIME 20 minutes
COOK TIME 40 minutes
TOTAL TIME 1 hour, plus optional marinating time (up to 4 hours)

FOR MARINADE

¼ cup Quick and Easy Harissa (page 220) or store-bought mild harissa

Juice and zest of ½ orange

2 teaspoons fresh lemon juice

1 tablespoon (6 g) minced fresh ginger

2 cloves garlic

½ teaspoon ground cumin

½ teaspoon ground coriander

1½ teaspoons sea salt

½ teaspoon freshly ground black pepper

2 tablespoons (30 ml) extra-virgin olive oil

FOR CHICKEN AND VEGETABLES

4 bone-in, skin-on chicken thighs (about 1½ pounds [680 g])

1 pound (454 g) (about 5 medium) carrots, peeled, halved lengthwise, and cut into 3-inch (7.6 cm) chunks

1 small red onion, cut into ¼-inch (6 mm) wedges

1 small fennel bulb, cut into ¼-inch (6 mm) wedges

½ cup (50 g) pitted green olives (such as Picholine or Castelvetrano), chopped or torn

Chopped fresh parsley or cilantro (optional)

To Make the Marinade

1. Combine all the marinade ingredients in a small bowl and whisk well.

To Make the Chicken and Vegetables

2. Rinse the chicken thighs and pat dry with paper towels. Toss with half of the marinade mixture (about ⅓ cup) in a large bowl. Let the chicken marinate while you prep the remaining ingredients, or refrigerate for up to 4 hours for deeper flavor.

3. Preheat the oven to 425°F (220°C).

4. Combine the carrots, red onion, and fennel with the remaining marinade in a large mixing bowl and toss to combine. Arrange the vegetables on a sheet pan in a single layer. Nestle the marinated chicken thighs between the vegetables, skin-side up.

5. Transfer the pan to the center rack of the oven and roast for 30 minutes. Remove from the oven, sprinkle with olives, and return to the oven for 10 minutes more, or until vegetables are tender and browned in spots, the chicken skin is crisp and golden, and the chicken thighs are cooked through, registering 175°F (80°C) in the thickest part of the chicken. Garnish with fresh parsley or cilantro (if using) and serve immediately, drizzled with the flavorful pan juices.

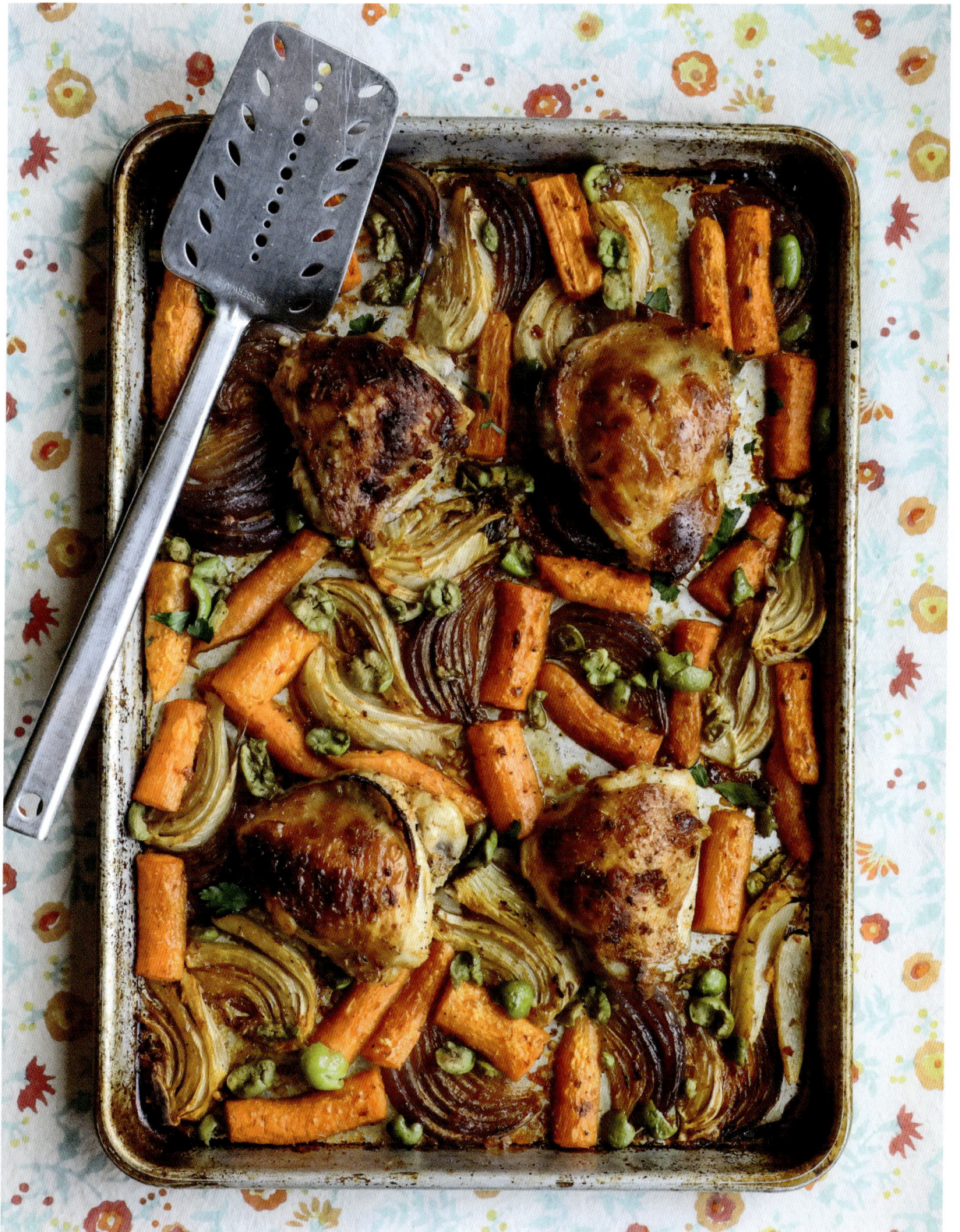

SEARED CHICKEN BREASTS WITH MUSHROOM CAPER PAN SAUCE

This dish highlights one of the simplest chef techniques for showstopping meals: pan sauces. Lightly dust chicken breasts in cassava flour, sear them to golden perfection, then use the flavorful brown bits left in the pan to build a deeply savory mushroom caper sauce—all in the same skillet! (See the note on the opposite page for an AIP-friendly version.) As a bonus, this dish is rich in selenium, a key nutrient for thyroid health that supports hormone conversion and helps protect against inflammation.

Cassava flour is a popular staple in gluten-free and grain-free cooking, and for good reason. Its fine texture and starchy qualities make it behave much like wheat flour in terms of thickening and browning. In this recipe, it creates a lovely crust on the chicken and helps thicken our velvety pan sauce, without any gritty texture or off-putting flavors like some other gluten-free alternatives.

● **GLUTEN-FREE** ● **DAIRY-FREE** ● **PALEO** ● **AIP-FRIENDLY**

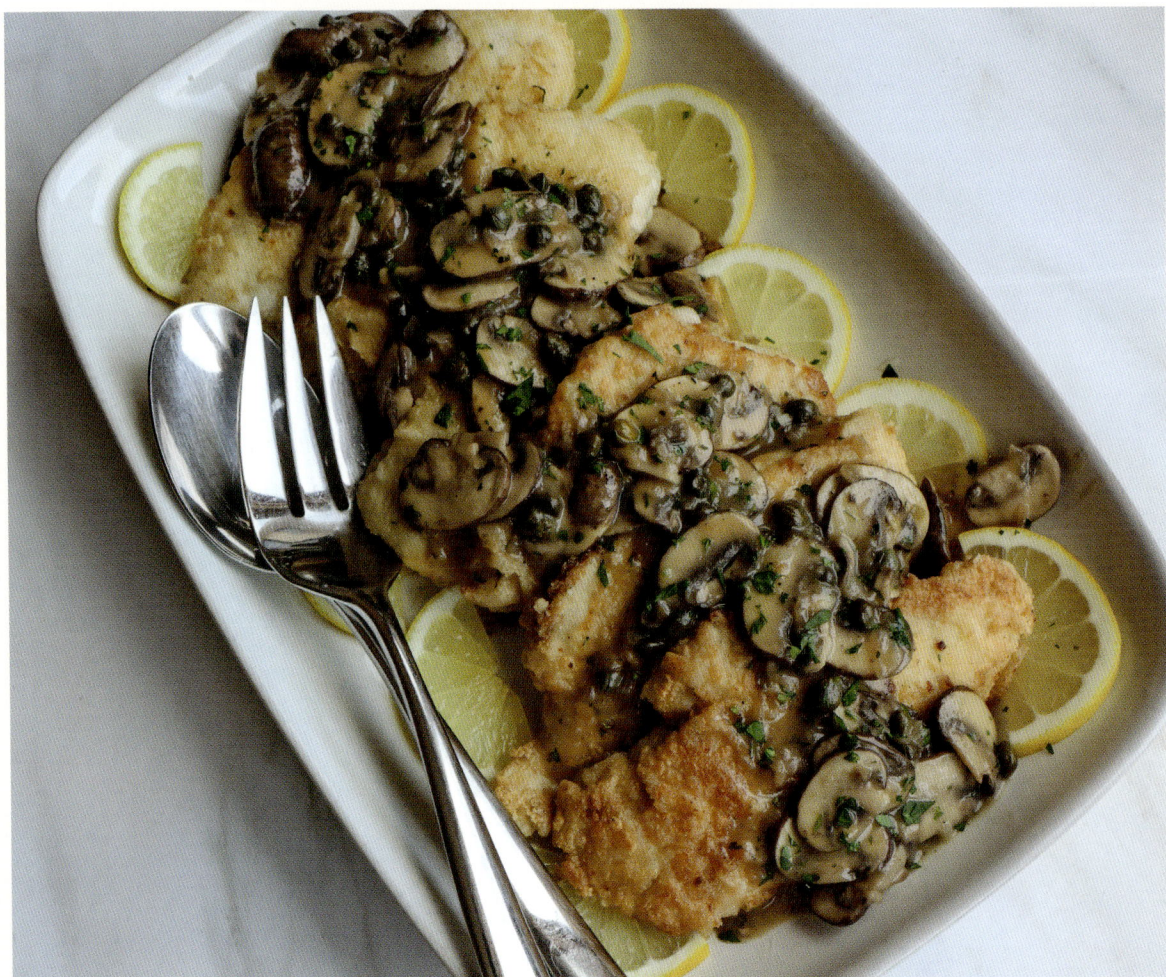

DIETARY LEVELS 1, 2, 3

SERVINGS 4
PREP TIME 20 minutes
COOK TIME 20 minutes
TOTAL TIME 40 minutes

FOR CHICKEN

1½ pounds (680 g) boneless, skinless chicken breasts

¼ cup (60 ml) extra-virgin olive oil, divided

1 tablespoon (15 ml) fresh lemon juice

1 large clove garlic, minced

½ teaspoon fine sea salt

Freshly ground black pepper (omit for AIP)

⅓ cup (38 g) cassava flour

2 tablespoons (28 g) ghee (sub extra-virgin olive oil for AIP)

FOR PAN SAUCE

¼ cup (40 g) minced shallot (about 1 medium)

½ cup (118 ml) dry white wine (sub Easy Homemade Chicken Bone Broth [page 218] or store-bought for AIP)

6 ounces (about 2 cups [140 g]) sliced button or cremini mushrooms

¼ teaspoon fine sea salt

Freshly ground black pepper (omit for AIP)

1 teaspoon cassava flour

2 tablespoons (18 g) drained capers

½ cup (118 ml) Easy Homemade Chicken Bone Broth (page 218) or store-bought

1½ teaspoons finely chopped fresh parsley

1 teaspoon lemon juice (optional)

Lemon slices, for garnish (optional)

To Make the Chicken

1. Preheat the oven to 200°F (93°C). Rinse the chicken breasts and pat dry with paper towels. Combine 2 tablespoons (30 ml) of the olive oil, lemon juice, garlic, salt, and pepper in a medium bowl. Toss the chicken to coat and set aside.

2. Place cassava flour in a shallow dish and dredge the chicken in it, coating all sides. Shake off excess and set aside.

3. Heat the remaining 2 tablespoons (30 ml) of olive oil and the ghee (or more olive oil) in a large stainless steel or enameled cast-iron skillet over medium-high heat. When the oil is shimmering, add the chicken (working in batches if needed to avoid crowding). Sear for 4 to 5 minutes per side or until golden brown and cooked through. Lower the heat if needed to prevent scorching. Transfer the chicken to a baking dish and keep warm in the oven.

To Make the Pan Sauce

4. Return the skillet to medium heat and add the shallots. Cook, stirring, for 2 to 3 minutes until soft and translucent. Pour in the white wine or chicken broth and scrape up the browned bits from the bottom of the pan. Let simmer until reduced by half.

5. Add the mushrooms, salt, and pepper. Cook for 5 to 7 minutes, stirring occasionally, until mushrooms have released their liquid and the pan is nearly dry. Add 1 teaspoon cassava flour and stir to coat. Add the capers and chicken broth and bring to a gentle simmer. Cook for 1 to 2 minutes or until the sauce has thickened slightly. Remove from the heat.

6. Stir in the parsley, then taste and adjust seasonings as needed. (If using chicken broth instead of wine, add a squeeze of fresh lemon juice for acidity.) Spoon the sauce over the chicken, garnish with lemon slices, if desired, and serve.

NOTE

For an AIP-friendly version, omit the black pepper throughout, use olive oil in place of the ghee, and replace the white wine with an equal amount of chicken broth.

A NOTE ON PAN CHOICE

For the best pan sauce, use a stainless steel or enameled cast-iron skillet. These create a beautiful golden crust (known as *fond*) that builds flavor in the sauce. Avoid cast-iron or aluminum, as they can react with acidic ingredients like lemon juice and wine, resulting in a metallic taste.

CRISPY "PARMESAN" CABBAGE AND BRATWURST SHEET PAN MEAL

This unique sheet pan meal draws on the classic pairing of bratwurst and cabbage, but adds a delicious twist: a crispy, savory Brazil Nut "Parmesan" (page 225) topping. By tucking the bratwurst mixture between the cabbage leaves, the flavors meld beautifully as they roast, creating a dish that's deeply savory, caramelized, and packed with texture. For a complete meal, serve it alongside Truffle Mashed Cauliflower and Sweet Potatoes (page 202) and French Carrot Salad with Mint (page 145).

● GLUTEN-FREE   ● DAIRY-FREE   ● PALEO

DIETARY LEVELS 1, 2

SERVINGS 4
PREP TIME 25 minutes
COOK TIME 25 minutes
TOTAL TIME 50 minutes

FOR BRATWURST MIXTURE

1 pound (454 g) ground pork

¾ teaspoon fine sea salt

¼ teaspoon white pepper

¼ teaspoon ground nutmeg

⅛ teaspoon ground ginger

⅛ teaspoon ground mace (or extra nutmeg)

¼ teaspoon dried marjoram

½ teaspoon dried rubbed sage

¼ teaspoon onion powder

¼ teaspoon garlic powder

1 tablespoon (15 ml) sparkling or filtered water

FOR CABBAGE

½ small- to medium-sized cabbage

⅓ cup Brazil Nut "Parmesan" (page 225)

2 cloves garlic, finely minced

1 teaspoon anchovy fillets, finely chopped

3 tablespoons (45 ml) extra-virgin olive oil

Chopped fresh parsley

1. Preheat the oven to 450°F (232°C). Line a rimmed sheet pan with parchment paper.

To Make the Bratwurst Mixture
2. Combine all the sausage ingredients in a medium mixing bowl and mix just until combined.

To Make the Cabbage
3. Cut the cabbage half into 8 equal wedges, leaving the stem/core intact on each wedge to hold it together. Arrange the wedges on the sheet pan, spreading the leaves to open up space between them.

4. Combine the Brazil Nut "Parmesan," garlic, anchovy, and olive oil in a small bowl. Mix to form a paste and set aside.

5. Gently loosen and create space between some of the leaves of each cabbage wedge so you have a few spaces to stuff the bratwurst mixture. Divide the sausage mixture into 8 equal portions, then press 1 portion into each of the 8 cabbage wedges, working the mixture between the leaves. Spread the "Parmesan" paste on top of the sausage-stuffed cabbage wedges. (For a time-saving option, instead of stuffing the cabbage, roll the sausage into 8 equal-sized meatballs and nestle them between the cabbage wedges.)

6. Transfer the pan to the center of oven and roast for about 25 minutes or until the cabbage is tender and browned on the edges and the sausage is cooked through. Garnish with fresh parsley, if desired, and serve!

NOTE

For even cooking, proper caramelization, and juicy sausage, it's important that you use a cabbage that's on the small to medium side. If only large heads are available, peel away some of the outer leaves of each wedge to keep them at a manageable size.

MOLE-INSPIRED PALEO ENCHILADAS

This recipe takes a little time, but the result is a bubbling pan of irresistible chicken enchiladas. Mole-inspired flavors like cacao and cinnamon bring warmth to the chicken, green chile, and sweet potato filling. The sauce is the boss, but you can save time with a paleo-friendly store-bought option. If tolerated, sprinkle with cheese or dairy-free shreds. Otherwise, generous, flavorful garnishes do the trick.

● **GLUTEN-FREE**   ◐ **DAIRY-FREE**   ● **PALEO**

DIETARY LEVELS 1, 2

SERVINGS 6
PREP TIME 1 hour, 10 minutes
COOK TIME 20 minutes
TOTAL TIME 1 hour, 30 minutes

FOR SAUCE

2 tablespoons (30 ml) avocado oil

½ white or yellow onion, diced

4 cloves garlic, minced

1 (14-ounce [400 g]) can crushed tomatoes, blended until smooth

1½ cups (355 ml) Easy Homemade Chicken Bone Broth (page 218) or store-bought

1 tablespoon (5 g) cacao powder

2 tablespoons (32 g) tomato paste

1 teaspoon tahini or almond butter

1 tablespoon (8 g) + 1 teaspoon chile powder

½ teaspoon cumin

½ teaspoon Mexican oregano

¼ teaspoon cinnamon

¾ teaspoon fine sea salt

FOR FILLING

2 tablespoons (30 ml) avocado oil

½ white or yellow onion, finely diced

1 cup (130 g) finely diced sweet potato

1 (4-ounce [113 g]) can diced green chiles, mild

1 tablespoon (8 g) chile powder

⅛ teaspoon chipotle powder (or cayenne pepper), or more to taste

½ teaspoon garlic powder

¾ teaspoon fine sea salt

1 pound (454 g) shredded cooked chicken

Zest and juice of ½ lime

FOR ASSEMBLY

Avocado oil, for pan-frying

10 gluten-free tortillas (see note on page 113)

1 ripe avocado, diced

½ cup (8 g) chopped fresh cilantro

½ cup (50 g) sliced olives

2 green onions, thinly sliced

To Make the Sauce

1. Combine the avocado oil and onion in a large saucepan. Place over medium heat and sauté until the onion is translucent. Add the garlic and cook for 1 to 2 minutes more. Add the crushed tomatoes, chicken broth, cacao, tomato paste, tahini or almond butter, dry spices, and salt. Bring to a gentle boil, then reduce the heat, cover, and simmer for 10 to 15 minutes or until the flavors meld and the sauce thickens. Remove from the heat and let cool slightly.

To Make the Filling

2. Combine the avocado oil and onion in a large skillet over medium-high heat. Cook, stirring occasionally, until the onion is lightly browned. Add the sweet potatoes and cook, stirring until soft and browned in spots, about 5 to 7 minutes. Add the green chiles, chile powder, chipotle powder or cayenne, garlic powder, and salt. Cook, stirring, for 2 to 3 minutes. Add the chicken and lime zest and juice and stir to combine. Taste and adjust seasoning as needed.

To Assemble

3. Preheat the oven to 350°F (177°C). Heat a skillet over medium heat with a small amount of avocado oil. Fry tortillas for about 15 to 20 seconds per side, just until pliable. Set aside on a paper towel–lined plate. Repeat with the remaining tortillas.

4. Spread a thin layer of enchilada sauce in a 9 × 13-inch (22.9 × 33 cm) baking dish. Dunk a tortilla in the sauce, add approximately ⅓ cup (45 g) of filling, roll up, and place seam-side down in the dish. Repeat with the remaining tortillas and filling. Top with the remaining sauce.

5. Bake uncovered for 20 minutes until heated through. Garnish with diced avocado, cilantro, olives, and green onions, and enjoy!

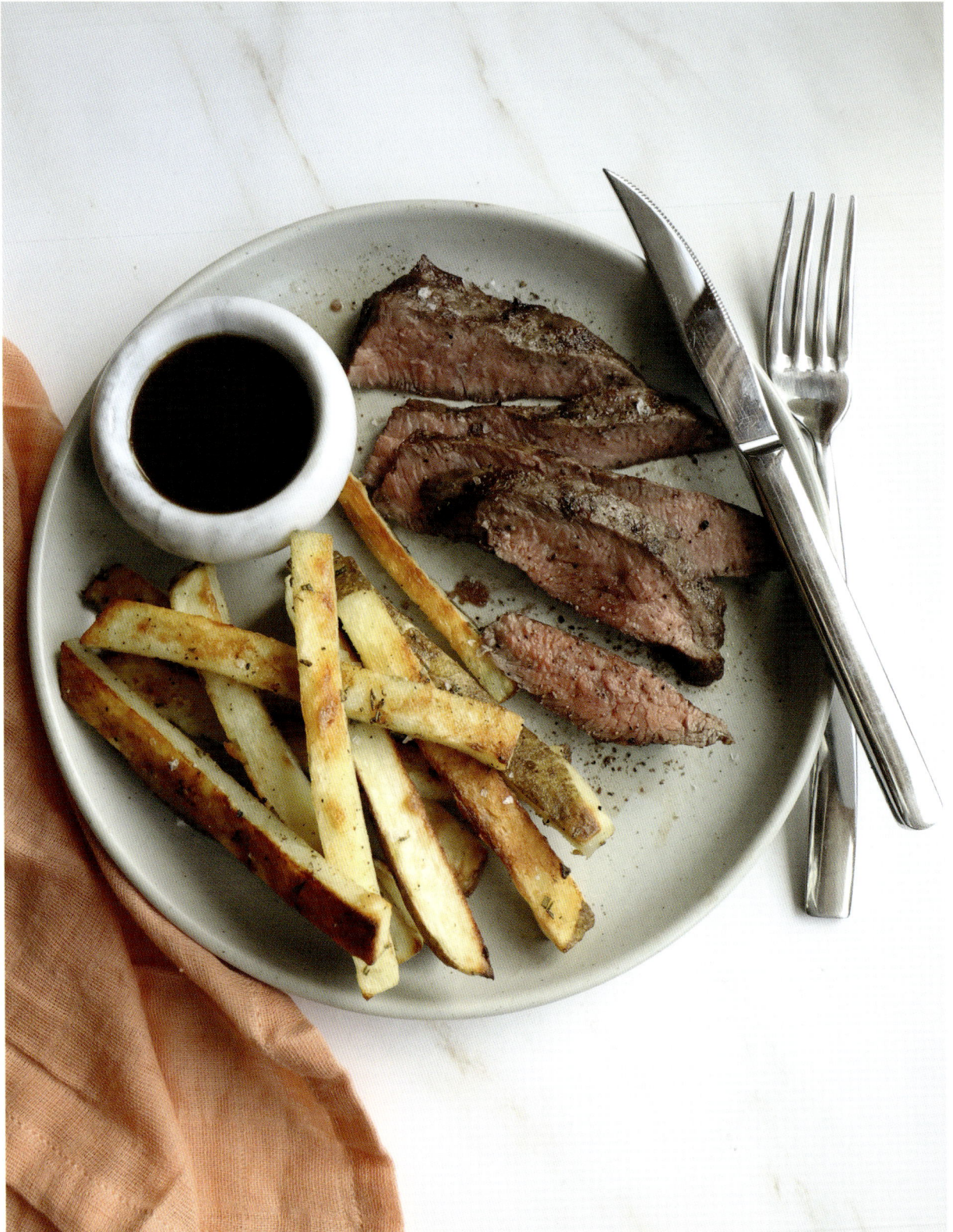

STEAK FRITES WITH HOMEMADE WORCESTERSHIRE SAUCE

The beauty of steak frites lies in its meat-and-potatoes simplicity: Seared steak, crispy fries, and a simple sauce make for a satisfying yet elegant meal. What kind of steak, you ask? Any kind! Flat iron is our family favorite, but hanger, New York, ribeye, or your favorite cut would work just fine.

The Oven-Roasted Garlic Fries (page 194) and Homemade Worcestershire Sauce (page 222) recommended here are suitable for all three dietary levels (GF/DF, Paleo, and AIP), but for an alternative you could also substitute Sweet Potato Fries (page 200, GF/DF, Paleo). The Worcestershire sauce is a lovely, simple dip or drizzle with lots of flavor, but if you're in the mood for something different, try the Parsley Garlic Sauce (page 221).

⬤ **GLUTEN-FREE**　⬤ **DAIRY-FREE**　⬤ **PALEO**　⬤ **AIP-FRIENDLY**

DIETARY LEVELS 1, 2, 3

SERVINGS 4
PREP TIME 5 minutes
COOK TIME 15 minutes
TOTAL TIME 20 minutes

2 pounds (907 g) grass-finished steak

1 tablespoon (15 ml) melted ghee (sub extra-virgin olive oil for AIP)

Fine sea salt, to taste

Freshly ground pepper, to taste (omit for AIP)

1 batch Oven-Roasted Garlic Fries (page 194)

1 batch Homemade Worcestershire Sauce (page 222)

1. Pat the steak dry on both sides and brush with ghee or olive oil. Season with sea salt and freshly ground black pepper.

2. If you haven't done so already, prepare the Oven-Roasted Garlic Fries and Homemade Worcestershire Sauce.

3. Heat a grill to medium-high or heat a cast-iron skillet over medium-high heat. Sear the steak for 5 to 7 minutes per side, depending on thickness, until well-browned and cooked to your desired doneness. For medium-rare (recommended), cook until the steak feels medium-firm to the touch or registers 130°F (54°C) on an instant-read thermometer. Let rest for 5 minutes before slicing across the grain. Serve immediately with the fries and the Worcestershire sauce for dipping or drizzling.

PINEAPPLE TERIYAKI CHICKEN KEBABS

These vibrant, fun-to-eat skewers bring a taste of the tropics to your table. Pineapple not only adds natural sweetness but also contains bromelain, an enzyme that supports digestion—a boon for Thyroid Thrivers, who are often prone to sluggish digestion. Safety tip: If you're using wooden skewers, be sure to soak them in water for at least 30 minutes before roasting to prevent burning.

● **GLUTEN-FREE** ● **DAIRY-FREE** ● **PALEO**

DIETARY LEVELS 1, 2

SERVINGS 4
PREP TIME 30 minutes
COOK TIME 20 minutes
TOTAL TIME 50 minutes

FOR KEBABS

1½ pounds (680 g) boneless, skinless chicken breast cut into 1-inch (2.5 cm) pieces

1 medium pineapple, peeled, cored, and cut into 1-inch (2.5 cm) pieces (about 4 cups [660 g])

1 medium red onion, cut into 1-inch (2.5 cm) pieces

1 medium red bell pepper, cut into 1-inch (2.5 cm) pieces

FOR TERIYAKI SAUCE

1 teaspoon avocado oil

1 tablespoon (6 g) grated fresh ginger

2 cloves garlic, minced

⅓ cup (79 ml) coconut aminos, plus more as needed

2 tablespoons (40 g) honey

¼ teaspoon Chinese five-spice powder (optional, but recommended)

1½ teaspoons arrowroot starch

1 tablespoon (15 ml) water, plus more as needed

To Make the Kebabs

1. Place a rack in the upper third of the oven and preheat to 425°F (220°C). Line a sheet pan with parchment paper.

2. Thread the chicken, pineapple, red onion, and red bell pepper onto skewers, alternating ingredients until all ingredients are used up. Place skewers on the prepared sheet pan.

To Make the Teriyaki Sauce

3. Heat the avocado oil in a small saucepan over medium-high heat. Add the ginger and garlic and cook, stirring, about 1 minute or until fragrant. Stir in the coconut aminos, honey, and five-spice powder. Bring to a simmer and let bubble for 1 to 2 minutes.

4. Combine the arrowroot starch with the water in a small dish and mix with a fork until smooth. Whisking the sauce constantly to prevent lumps, drizzle in the arrowroot slurry. Bring to a low boil, stirring constantly, just until the sauce thickens to a brushable glaze. Immediately remove from the heat. If the sauce becomes too thick, you can thin it with an extra tablespoon (15 ml) of water or coconut aminos.

5. Using a silicone brush, generously coat both sides of the kebabs with the teriyaki glaze. Transfer to the oven and roast for 15 minutes, flipping the kebabs halfway through and brushing with any glaze that has pooled on the sheet pan. Remove from oven when the chicken is fully cooked and the largest cubes have reached an internal temperature of 165°F (74°C).

NOTE

For a complete meal, serve the kebabs with cauliflower rice or zucchini noodles for a paleo-compliant (Level 2) option, or quinoa or white basmati rice for a GF/DF (Level 1) option.

BUTTERNUT, CHARD, AND CHICKEN CURRY

This AIP-approved curry creates sultry, aromatic flavors, without the use of nightshades or seed spices. If you're not on strict AIP, you can substitute 2 to 3 teaspoons of regular curry powder for the dry spices listed below. Serve this on its own as a hearty stew or use it to top rice (GF/DF) or cauliflower rice (Paleo/AIP).

⬤ **GLUTEN-FREE**   ⬤ **DAIRY-FREE**   ⬤ **PALEO**   ⬤ **AIP-FRIENDLY**

DIETARY LEVELS 1, 2, 3

SERVINGS 4
PREP TIME 20 minutes
COOK TIME 30 minutes
TOTAL TIME 50 minutes

1 tablespoon (15 ml) avocado oil or (14 g) unrefined coconut oil

1 small onion, diced

1 stalk lemongrass

2 cloves garlic, minced

1 tablespoon (6 g) minced fresh ginger

1 teaspoon turmeric powder

½ teaspoon cinnamon

¼ teaspoon ground clove

¼ teaspoon ground mace

1 heaping teaspoon fine sea salt

1 (14-ounce [392 g]) can full-fat coconut milk

1 pound (454 g) boneless, skinless chicken thighs, cut into 1-inch (2.5 cm) pieces

3 cups (390 g) peeled, cubed butternut squash or sweet potato

1 tablespoon (15 ml) AIP-compliant fish sauce

3 makrut lime leaves or 1 teaspoon finely grated lime zest

1 bunch Swiss chard, stems removed, roughly chopped

1 tablespoon (15 ml) fresh lime juice (about ½ lime), plus more as needed

½ lime, cut into wedges

1. Heat the avocado or unrefined coconut oil in a large soup pot over medium-high heat. Add the onion and cook, stirring, until golden brown, about 5 to 7 minutes.

2. Meanwhile, place the lemongrass on a cutting board and use a meat mallet or rolling pin to pound and bruise the lemongrass to release its oils. Trim off the dry top section and cut the remaining stalk into 2 pieces approximately 6 inches long. Tie together with kitchen twine and set aside.

3. After the onion is caramelized, add the garlic, ginger, dry spices, and salt. Cook, stirring until fragrant, about 2 minutes. Pour in the coconut milk and stir, scraping up any browned bits from the bottom of the pot. Add the chicken, butternut squash, fish sauce, lime leaves or lime zest, and lemongrass. Bring to a boil, then reduce the heat to a gentle simmer. Cover and simmer for about 15 minutes.

4. Stir in the Swiss chard and simmer for 5 minutes more or until the greens are wilted, the chicken is fully cooked, and the squash is tender when pierced with a fork.

5. Remove the pot from the heat and stir in the lime juice. Taste and adjust seasoning, adding more lime juice or salt if needed. Discard the lime leaves and lemongrass pieces. Serve as desired (see note) with lime wedges and enjoy!

NOTE
If you're following dietary plan Levels 1 (GF/DF) or 2 (Paleo), feel free to serve this with paleo or Whole30-compliant sambal oelek.

CRISPY CHICKEN AND VEGGIE NUGGETS

Loved by kids (and grown-ups) of all ages, these nuggets also happen to be AIP! The sweet potato and broccoli not only add a hidden serving of vegetables but also contribute color, flavor, and a wonderfully tender texture. Crushed plantain chips make the perfect stand-in for panko crumbs, and to get them brown and crisp without overcooking the poultry, we'll pretoast them to a golden brown. The Dairy-Free Ranch Dip (page 213) is a perfect match for these, but I've also included a Zesty Avocado Dip (below) for an AIP option.

● **GLUTEN-FREE**   ● **DAIRY-FREE**   ● **PALEO**   ● **AIP-FRIENDLY**

DIETARY LEVELS 1, 2, 3

SERVINGS 4 (makes about 20 nuggets)
PREP TIME 30 minutes
COOK TIME 15 minutes
TOTAL TIME 45 minutes

FOR NUGGET MIXTURE

1 tablespoon (15 ml) extra-virgin olive oil, plus more for brushing

1 cup (130 g) diced white or orange sweet potato

1 cup (71 g) finely chopped broccoli florets

½ teaspoon onion powder

½ teaspoon garlic powder

½ teaspoon fine sea salt

Freshly ground black pepper, to taste (omit for AIP)

1 pound (454 g) ground chicken or turkey

FOR CRUMB COATING

2 cups (300 g) AIP-compliant plantain chips

1 teaspoon sea salt

1 teaspoon garlic powder

1½ teaspoons extra-virgin olive oil

FOR ZESTY AVOCADO DIP

1 medium avocado

2–3 tablespoons (30–44 ml) fresh lemon juice

½ teaspoon garlic powder

½ teaspoon onion powder

¾ teaspoon fine sea salt

1 tablespoon (15 ml) extra-virgin olive oil

2 tablespoons (30 ml) water

Pinch white pepper (omit for AIP)

To Make the Nugget Mixture

1. Preheat the oven to 375°F (190°C). Place a baking rack on a rimmed baking sheet lined with parchment paper. Brush the baking rack with olive oil to prevent sticking.

2. Fit a small saucepan with a steamer basket and add about 1 inch (2.5 cm) of water to the pan. Bring to a boil over high heat. Add the sweet potatoes, cover, reduce the heat to medium, and steam for 10 minutes. Add the chopped broccoli on top of the sweet potatoes and steam for 5 minutes more. Remove from the heat and let cool slightly.

3. Place the veggies in a medium mixing bowl with the onion powder, garlic powder, salt, pepper, and olive oil. Use a potato masher to mash and mix thoroughly. Add the ground chicken or turkey and stir to combine.

To Make the Crumb Coating

4. Combine the plantain chips, sea salt, garlic powder, and olive oil in a small food processor and grind to a fine crumb.

5. To prebrown the crumb coating, transfer the crumbs to a dry skillet and cook, stirring constantly, over medium heat until golden brown, about 3 to 5 minutes. Immediately transfer to a wide, shallow dish such as a pie dish to avoid scorching and to cool. A less hands-on alternative is to toast the crumbs on a rimmed baking sheet in a 300°F (149°C) oven for 5 to 10 minutes, watching closely to avoid scorching.

6. Form the nugget mixture into balls, about 1 tablespoon each. Roll the balls in the crumb mixture, then press gently into nugget shapes. Arrange nuggets on the prepared baking rack so they're not touching. Carefully transfer to the center of the oven and bake for 15 minutes or until firm to the touch and the filling is cooked through.

To Make the Zesty Avocado Dip

7. Combine all the dip ingredients in a small food processor and blend into a smooth paste. Taste and adjust seasonings. Serve the nuggets fresh from the oven with the Zesty Avocado Dip or your favorite dipping sauce.

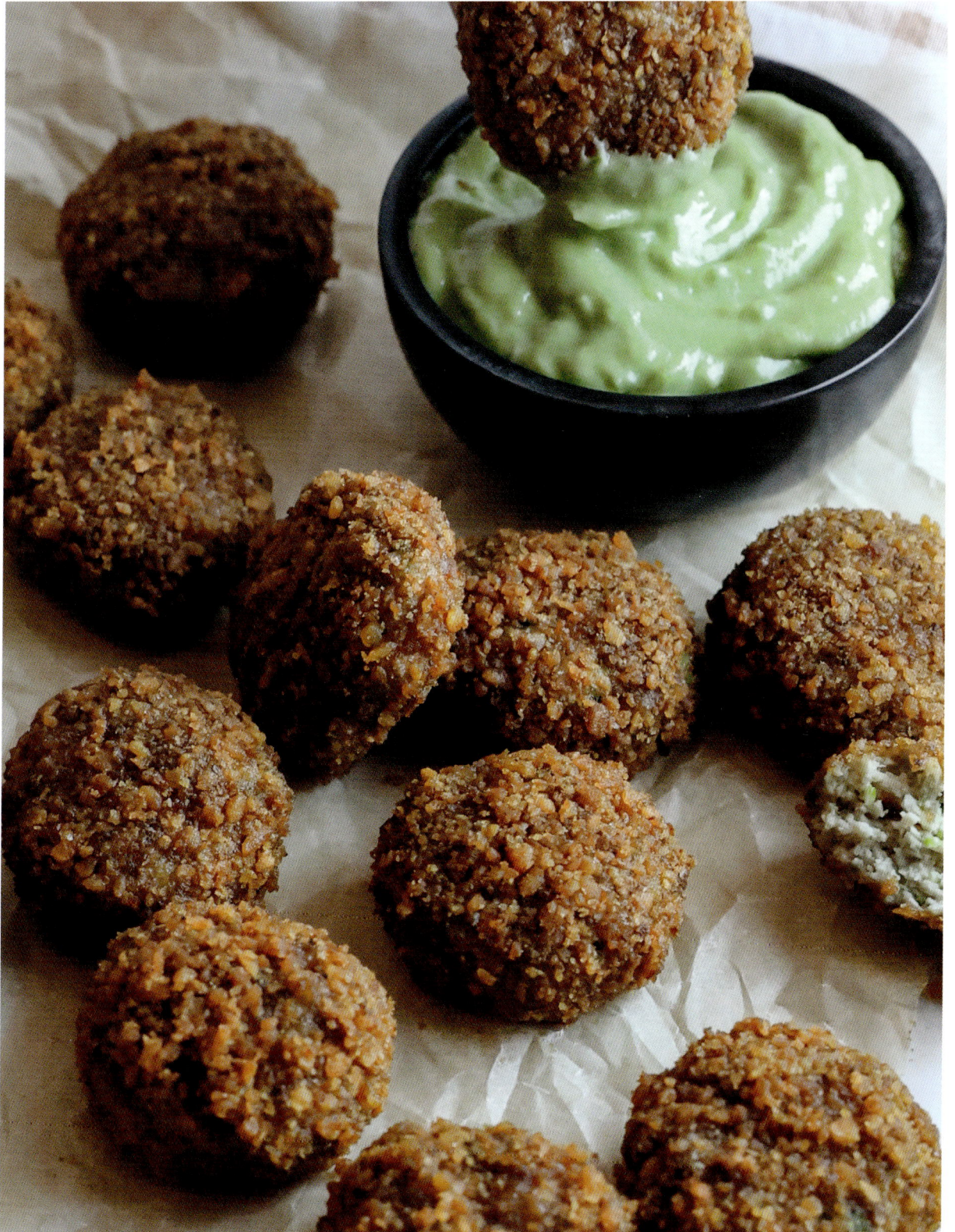

PASTA WITH WHITE BOLOGNESE SAUCE

This is a savory, nightshade-free twist on the classic tomato-based pasta sauce. A rich blend of pancetta, beef, pork (or veal), and mushrooms creates a deep, umami-packed base, while nutritional yeast adds a subtle cheesy flavor—minus the dairy, of course. The result? A comforting, velvety sauce that's both flavorful and AIP-friendly.

● GLUTEN-FREE   ● DAIRY-FREE   ● PALEO   ● AIP-FRIENDLY

DIETARY LEVELS 1, 2, 3

SERVINGS 6
PREP TIME 20 minutes
COOK TIME 40 minutes
TOTAL TIME 1 hour

2 ounces (57 g) compliant pancetta or bacon, finely chopped

2 tablespoons (30 ml) extra-virgin olive oil

1 medium onion, finely chopped

1 large carrot, finely chopped

2 stalks celery, finely chopped

4 ounces (113 g) button mushrooms, finely chopped

3 cloves garlic, minced

1 pound (454 g) ground grass-finished beef (sub veal if desired)

1 pound (454 g) pasture-raised ground pork (sub veal if desired)

3 tablespoons (22 g) cassava flour

1 cup (237 ml) dry white wine (sub additional chicken bone broth for AIP)

2 cups (473 ml) Easy Homemade Chicken Bone Broth (page 218) or store-bought

¼ cup (36 g) nutritional yeast

2 bay leaves

2 teaspoons chopped fresh rosemary

2 teaspoons chopped fresh thyme

1 teaspoon dried rubbed sage

¼ teaspoon garlic powder

⅛ teaspoon ground cloves

1½–2 teaspoons fine sea salt, to taste

Freshly ground black pepper, to taste (omit for AIP)

Fresh lemon juice, to taste (optional)

16 ounces (454 g) GF, paleo, or AIP pasta (see note on page 156)

OPTIONAL TOPPINGS

Brazil Nut "Parmesan" (page 225; omit for AIP)

Chopped fresh parsley

1. Cook the pancetta or bacon in a large Dutch oven over medium heat until its fat is rendered and it is beginning to crisp. Add the olive oil, onion, carrot, celery, mushrooms, and garlic. Cook, stirring occasionally, until tender, about 5 to 7 minutes.

2. Add the ground beef and pork or veal to the pan and cook, breaking up the meat with a spatula, until it is browned and the liquid has reduced, about 5 to 7 minutes. If the meat renders excess fat, tilt the pot and skim some off with a spoon.

3. Sprinkle the cassava flour onto the meat mixture and stir to coat evenly. Cook, stirring, for about 2 minutes. Add the white wine or additional chicken broth, and cook, stirring, until the liquid has thickened. Add the 2 cups (473 ml) chicken broth, nutritional yeast, bay leaves, rosemary, thyme, sage, garlic powder, cloves, sea salt, and pepper. Bring to a simmer, reduce the heat to low, cover, and cook for 20 to 30 minutes.

4. Meanwhile, prepare your pasta of choice (see note).

5. Taste the sauce and adjust the seasoning as desired. If you're omitting the white wine, finish the sauce with a spritz of fresh lemon juice to brighten the flavors.

6. Top the pasta with the sauce and sprinkle with Brazil Nut "Parmesan" (if using) or parsley, if desired.

CLASSIC CLEAN FAJITAS (BEEF OR CHICKEN)

This vibrant and flavorful crowd-pleaser is easy to adapt to your needs and preferences. It's one of those back-pocket meals I make on repeat and is perfect for gatherings where dietary needs vary. Gluten-free? Dairy-free? Paleo? No problem. Just set out an array of toppings and let everyone build their own. Both steak and chicken work well here, but remember to slice the meat across the grain for maximum tenderness.

● **GLUTEN-FREE**   ● **DAIRY-FREE**   ● **PALEO**

DIETARY LEVELS 1, 2

SERVINGS 4–6

PREP TIME 20 minutes (plus 30 minutes to 4 hours for marinating)

COOK TIME 20

TOTAL TIME 40 minutes + marinating time

4 cloves garlic, minced

2 teaspoons chile powder

½ teaspoon ground cumin

½ teaspoon smoked paprika

⅛ teaspoon cinnamon

⅛ teaspoon chipotle or cayenne pepper powder

Freshly ground black pepper, to taste

1½ teaspoons fine sea salt, divided

Zest of 1 medium lime

2 tablespoons (30 ml) avocado oil

1½ pounds (680 g) steak (flank, flat iron, or skirt) or boneless, skinless chicken breasts, sliced into thin strips across the grain

1 red bell pepper, sliced into thin strips

1 yellow bell pepper, sliced into thin strips

1 medium red onion, julienned

2 ripe avocados, mashed

Juice of ½–1 medium lime

10–12 medium gluten-free or grain-free tortillas (see note on page 113)

1 small lime, cut into wedges

Paleo-compliant hot sauce (optional)

1. Combine the garlic, dry spices, 1 teaspoon of the fine sea salt, lime zest, and avocado oil in a medium mixing bowl and whisk well. Add the steak or chicken strips and toss until well-coated. Cover, refrigerate, and marinate for at least 30 minutes or up to 4 hours for maximum flavor.

2. Heat a 12-inch (30 cm) heavy-bottomed skillet over medium-high heat and add the meat. Cook, stirring occasionally, until the meat is cooked through. For steak, cook to your desired degree of doneness. For chicken, cook thoroughly until no longer pink inside. Remove the meat and pan juices, leaving about 2 tablespoons (30 ml) of the juices in the skillet.

3. Add the sliced peppers and onion to the skillet and cook over medium-high heat, stirring frequently, for about 5 to 7 minutes or until the veggies are well-browned in spots but still crisp-tender. If the skillet starts to dry out or darken, lower heat slightly and deglaze by adding about 2 tablespoons (30 ml) of the reserved juices at a time, scraping up any browned bits from the bottom.

4. Add the cooked meat and remaining juices back to the skillet with the veggies over medium heat. Stir to combine and cook until everything is heated through, about 2 minutes. Taste and adjust the seasoning as desired with additional salt, pepper, lime juice, or hot sauce. Reduce the heat to the lowest setting to keep warm.

5. Mash the avocados with a fork in a small bowl. Stir in the juice of half the lime and the remaining ½ teaspoon of sea salt. Taste and adjust seasoning as desired with additional lime juice or salt.

6. Heat the tortillas according to package instructions. Spoon the fajita mixture into tortillas and top each with a dollop of guacamole. Serve with lime wedges and your favorite compliant hot sauce, if desired.

CHILE LIME SHRIMP (OR FISH) TACOS

Shrimp and fish tacos are all over restaurant menus these days, but they're so easy to make at home. This version calls for a super simple, homemade pico de gallo salsa; for a sweet, tropical flair, swap the tomatoes for fresh pineapple. If you're not a fan of shrimp, no worries: These are just as delicious with salmon, cod, or halibut.

● GLUTEN-FREE ● DAIRY-FREE ● PALEO

DIETARY LEVELS 1, 2

SERVINGS 4
PREP TIME 30 minutes
COOK TIME 10 minutes
TOTAL TIME 40 minutes

FOR SHRIMP

1 large clove garlic, finely minced

Zest and juice of ½ lime

1 teaspoon chile powder

½ teaspoon ground cumin

½ teaspoon fine sea salt

Pinch cayenne pepper, or to taste

1½ teaspoons avocado oil or extra-virgin olive oil

1 pound (454 g) shrimp, peeled, deveined, and cut into 1-inch (2.5 cm) pieces

FOR SALSA

1 pint (284 g) cherry tomatoes, diced small (or 2 cups [310 g] diced pineapple)

½ cup diced white onion (about ½ small onion)

¼ cup (8 g) chopped fresh cilantro

Juice of ½–1 lime

1 jalapeño, seeded and finely chopped

Pinch cayenne pepper

1 teaspoon extra-virgin olive oil

¾ teaspoon fine sea salt

Freshly ground black pepper, to taste

FOR CREMA

½ cup (115 g) paleo or Whole30-compliant mayonnaise

Zest and juice of ½ lime

½ teaspoon ground cumin

½ teaspoon garlic powder

Up to 1 tablespoon (15 ml) of paleo-compliant hot sauce

½ teaspoon fine sea salt

FOR BLACK BEANS

1 (14-ounce [400 g]) can black beans, undrained (omit for strict paleo)

Pinch fine sea salt

1 tablespoon (15 ml) olive oil

Sprig cilantro

FOR ASSEMBLY

8 small tortillas (see note on page 113)

1 small lime, cut into wedges

OPTIONAL GARNISHES

Shredded cabbage

Shredded lettuce

Fresh cilantro

Sliced avocado

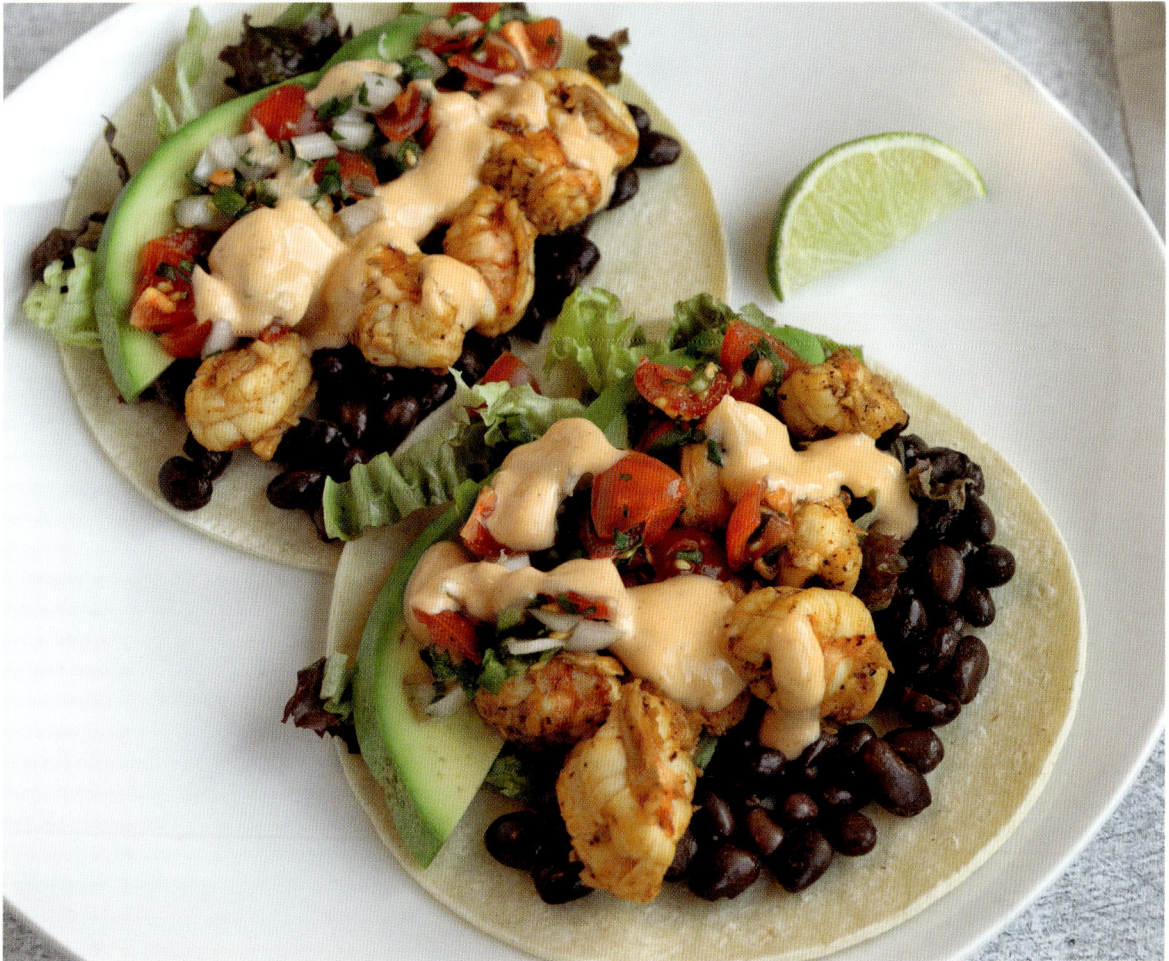

To Make the Shrimp

1. Combine the garlic, lime zest and juice, chile powder, cumin, salt, cayenne, and oil in a medium mixing bowl and stir well. Add the shrimp and toss to coat. Marinate for up to 30 minutes; marinating for any longer may toughen the shrimp.

To Make the Salsa

2. Combine the salsa ingredients in a separate medium mixing bowl and stir to combine. Start with the juice of ½ lime and adjust with additional lime juice and seasonings to taste. Set aside.

To Make the Crema

3. Combine the crema ingredients in a small mixing bowl. Taste and adjust seasonings as desired and set aside.

To Make the Black Beans

4. Reheat the black beans and their juices in a small saucepan over medium heat with a pinch of salt, olive oil, and a sprig or 2 of cilantro.

To Assemble

5. Heat the tortillas according to package directions.

6. Heat a medium skillet over medium-high heat and add the shrimp along with the marinade, stirring constantly until pink and just cooked through, about 3 minutes.

7. Serve the tacos buffet-style with the salsa, crema, black beans, lime wedges, and garnishes.

SPICED RED LENTIL STEW

This cozy, spiced red lentil stew is one of my favorite bang-for-your-buck meals. Inspired by traditional Indian dal, it's not an authentic preparation, but it delivers the same comfort, warmth, and gently spiced flavor in a porridge-like texture that's especially soothing and satisfying. Packed with flavor, fiber, and plant-based protein, it's made from simple, affordable ingredients and involves minimal effort. Enjoy it by the bowlful, spooned over mashed sweet potatoes or rice, or topped with a fried egg for breakfast.

● GLUTEN-FREE   ● DAIRY-FREE   ● VEGAN

DIETARY LEVELS 1

SERVINGS 6

PREP TIME 20 minutes,
plus 2 to 4 hours soaking time

COOK TIME 20 minutes

TOTAL TIME 40 minutes,
plus 2 to 4 hours soaking time

1 cup (192 g) red lentils

1 tablespoon (15 ml) apple cider vinegar or lemon juice

2 tablespoons (28 g) unrefined coconut oil

1 medium onion, finely diced

1 tablespoon (10 g) minced garlic

1 tablespoon (6 g) minced fresh ginger

2 teaspoons ground cumin

2 teaspoons ground coriander

2 teaspoons curry powder

2 cups (473 ml) water or vegetable broth

1 (14-ounce [400 g]) can diced tomatoes with green chiles

¾ cup (168 g) full-fat coconut milk (about ½ of a 13.5-ounce [383 g] can)

1 teaspoon fine sea salt, or to taste

Up to 1 tablespoon (15 ml) fresh lemon juice, for brightness

Fresh cilantro leaves, for garnish

1. Presoak the lentils (optional, but recommended: see note). Place the lentils in a fine-mesh strainer and rinse thoroughly to remove any dust or debris. Transfer to a medium mixing bowl and cover with filtered water by 2 or 3 inches (5.1–7.6 cm). Add apple cider vinegar or lemon juice and soak at room temperature for 2 to 4 hours (red lentils don't require as much soaking time as some other varieties). Drain and rinse the soaked lentils in a fine-mesh strainer and set aside.

2. Melt the coconut oil over medium-high heat in a 3-quart (2.8 L) lidded pot or Dutch oven. Add the onion and cook, stirring occasionally, until golden brown in spots, about 10 minutes.

3. Add the garlic, ginger, cumin, coriander, and curry powder. Stir constantly for 1 to 2 minutes, just until the spices are lightly toasted and fragrant (but not burned).

4. Add the lentils, water or vegetable broth, and diced tomatoes with chiles. Bring to a boil, then reduce the heat, cover, and simmer for 20 minutes or until the lentils are soft and beginning to break down. Stir occasionally, lowering the heat as needed as the mixture thickens.

5. Stir in the coconut milk, sea salt, and up to 1 tablespoon (15 ml) lemon juice for added brightness. Taste and adjust seasoning as needed. Serve warm, topped with fresh cilantro.

NOTE

Presoaking the lentils is an easy, effective way to improve their digestibility. This can be especially helpful for Thyroid Thrivers with sensitive digestion or for those who are healing gut issues. Adding a touch of acidity, like apple cider vinegar or lemon juice, to the soaking water supports the breakdown of phytic acid (a naturally occurring antinutrient), making the beneficial minerals in lentils more absorbable. Note that if you decide to skip this step, the lentils will take 30 to 40 percent longer to cook, and the recipe will require up to twice the amount of water or broth. For red and yellow lentils, 2 hours of soaking time is sufficient. For green, black, and brown lentils, soak for 6 to 8 hours.

PESTO CHICKEN SALAD WRAPS

This simple, high-protein meal-prep staple gets plenty of flavor from a zingy, dairy-free pesto that uses nutritional yeast in place of Parmesan for plenty of cheesy umami flavor. Serve it on romaine leaves, gluten-free or grain-free tortillas, or your favorite gluten-free or grain-free crackers. Garnish with halved grapes, ground black pepper, and freshly torn basil leaves for extra flair.

●GLUTEN-FREE   ●DAIRY-FREE   ●PALEO

DIETARY LEVELS 1, 2

SERVINGS 4
PREP TIME 10 minutes
COOK TIME 20 minutes
TOTAL TIME 30 minutes

FOR DAIRY-FREE LEMON PESTO

1 cup (40 g) basil leaves, loosely packed, large stems removed, and roughly chopped

2 tablespoons (18 g) pine nuts, lightly toasted

1 teaspoon nutritional yeast

1–2 tablespoons (15–30 ml) extra-virgin olive oil

¼ teaspoon fine sea salt

1 teaspoon lemon zest

2 teaspoons fresh lemon juice

1 large clove garlic, peeled and roughly chopped

FOR CHICKEN SALAD

Aromatic herbs, like bay leaves, peppercorns, and salt (optional)

1 pound (454 g) boneless, skinless chicken breasts or 2½–3 cups [350–420 g] cooked, shredded chicken

¼ cup (65 g) Dairy-Free Lemon Pesto

¼ cup (60 g) paleo or Whole30-compliant mayonnaise

1 teaspoon fresh lemon juice

¼ cup (30 g) chopped walnuts (optional)

Sea salt, to taste

Freshly ground black pepper, to taste

FOR ASSEMBLY

8 whole Romaine leaves or small grain-free tortillas (see note on page 113)

2 cups (110 g) fresh arugula or other baby greens (if using tortillas)

OPTIONAL GARNISHES

Halved grapes

Fresh basil leaves

To Make the Dairy-Free Lemon Pesto

1. Combine all the pesto ingredients in a small food processor and blend to a fine paste. Set aside.

To Make the Chicken Salad

2. If cooking your own chicken, fill a medium saucepan halfway with water and bring it to a boil. If desired, add aromatics like bay leaves, peppercorns, and salt to the water. Add the chicken breasts, reduce the heat, and cook at a low simmer for 15 to 20 minutes or until the chicken is cooked through and reaches an internal temperature of 165°F (74°C). To avoid dryness, do not overcook. Transfer the chicken to a plate and set aside to cool slightly.

3. When the chicken has cooled, use 2 forks to shred it. Add to a medium mixing bowl along with ¼ cup (65 g) of the Dairy-Free Lemon Pesto, mayo, lemon juice, walnuts (if using), and seasoning to taste. Stir well, taste, and adjust seasoning as desired.

To Assemble

4. Divide the chicken salad evenly among lettuce leaves or tortillas. If using tortillas, add a small handful of greens. Top with halved grapes and freshly torn basil leaves, if desired, and enjoy! Store leftover chicken salad in an airtight container in the refrigerator for up to 5 days.

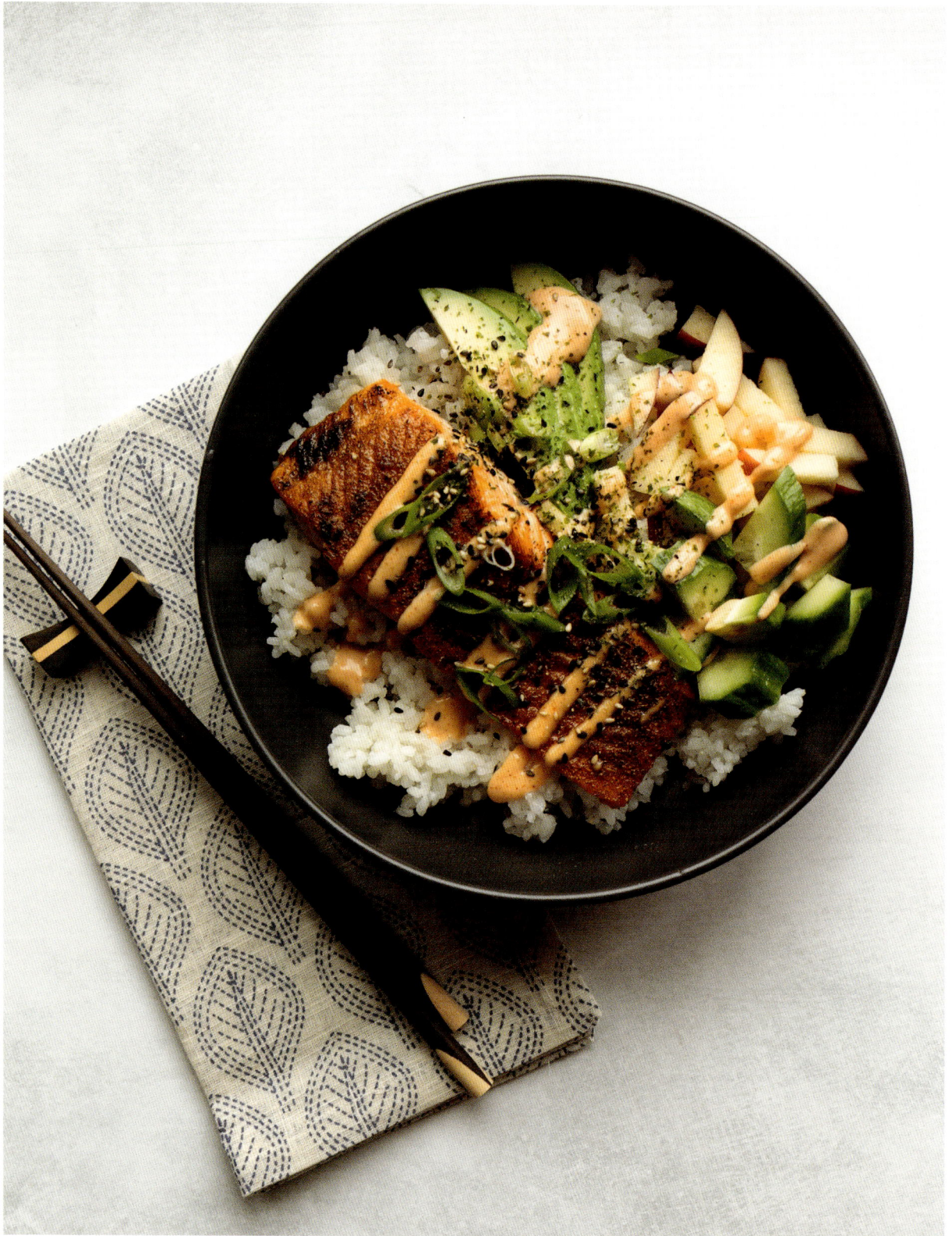

SUSHI-STYLE BUDDHA BOWL

If you have leftover fish or rice to use up, this is the recipe you're looking for. (We're using cooked fish here for ease of sourcing, but if you prefer to use raw fish for a more authentic sushi-style bowl, be sure to use high-quality, sushi-grade fish from a trusted source.) These Buddha Bowls call for just a handful of simple ingredients. Yes, I know the apple might sound out of place, but trust me on this one: It adds just the right sweet, juicy twist and brings all the other flavors together beautifully. Serve as is or mix everything together and wrap in sheets of nori seaweed for a fun, sushi-style wrap!

● **GLUTEN-FREE**   ● **DAIRY-FREE**

DIETARY LEVELS 1

SERVINGS 4
PREP TIME 15 minutes
TOTAL TIME 15 minutes

FOR SRIRACHA MAYO

½ cup (115 g) paleo or Whole30-compliant mayonnaise

¼ teaspoon garlic powder

1–3 teaspoons sriracha or sambal oelek, according to spice preference

1 teaspoon toasted sesame oil

¼ teaspoon fine sea salt

1 teaspoon fresh lemon juice

FOR ASSEMBLY

4 cups (660 g) cooked white rice, ideally sushi rice

1–1½ pounds (454–680 g) cooked or canned wild salmon, low-mercury tuna, or yellowtail

1 avocado, sliced

1 cup (135 g) diced cucumber

1 cup (152 g) diced apple

¼ cup (59 ml) coconut aminos, or to taste

2 green onions, thinly sliced

2 teaspoons (16 g) furikake, dulse, kelp flakes, or sesame seeds

To Make the Sriracha Mayo
1. Whisk together the ingredients for the sriracha mayo in a small bowl. Taste and adjust flavor as desired, and set aside.

To Assemble
2. Divide the rice evenly among 4 bowls. Top each with 4–6 ounces of fish, ¼ avocado, ¼ cup (34 g) diced cucumber, and ¼ cup (38 g) diced apple. Drizzle with coconut aminos and Sriracha Mayo to taste. Garnish with sliced green onions and sprinkle with furikake, kelp flakes, dulse, or sesame seeds for extra umami and enjoy!

THAI BEEF LETTUCE WRAPS

Inspired by Thai beef salad and the bold flavors of *larb gai*, a Thai ground chicken salad, these Thai Beef Lettuce Wraps are bursting with fresh herbs, salty fish sauce, and citrusy brightness. They're quick, flexible, and ideal for a weeknight dinner or light meal prep. Add white rice, cauliflower rice, or sliced cucumbers to bulk up your meal.

● **GLUTEN-FREE**   ● **DAIRY-FREE**   ● **PALEO**

DIETARY LEVELS 1, 2

SERVINGS 6
PREP TIME 20 minutes
COOK TIME 10 minutes
TOTAL TIME 30 minutes

1 tablespoon (15 ml) avocado oil

2 pounds (907 g) grass-fed ground beef

½ teaspoon fine sea salt

Freshly ground black pepper, to taste

¾ cup (120 g) thinly sliced shallots, divided

3 tablespoons (45 ml) paleo-compliant fish sauce

1 cup (150 g) finely diced red bell pepper

1 cup (110 g) coarsely grated carrot

1 tablespoon (15 g) sambal oelek or ½ teaspoon chile flakes

3 tablespoons (45 ml) fresh lime juice

1 tablespoon (9 g) coconut sugar or maple syrup

4 green onions, thinly sliced

½ cup (8 g) chopped fresh cilantro

¼ cup (24 g) chopped fresh mint, plus extra for garnish

½ cup (75 g) chopped dry-roasted roasted peanuts (sub macadamia nuts for paleo)

1 large head butter, romaine, or leaf lettuce, separated into leaves

1. Heat the avocado oil in a large skillet over medium-high heat. Add the ground beef, seasoning, and half the sliced shallots. Cook, breaking up the meat with a spatula, until browned and cooked through, about 7 to 8 minutes. If needed, tilt the skillet, spoon off excess fat, and discard.

2. Add the fish sauce, stir to combine, and cook for 2 to 3 minutes or until liquid is reduced. Add the bell pepper, carrot, and sambal oelek or chile flakes. Cook for 1 to 2 minutes more or until the veggies are slightly softened.

3. Remove the skillet from the heat. Stir in the lime juice, coconut sugar or maple syrup, remaining shallots, green onions, cilantro, and mint. Stir to combine. Taste and adjust the seasoning, adding more lime juice, fish sauce, or sambal oelek, as desired.

4. Sprinkle the chopped nuts on top of the warm beef mixture. To serve, spoon into lettuce cups, fold like a taco, and enjoy!

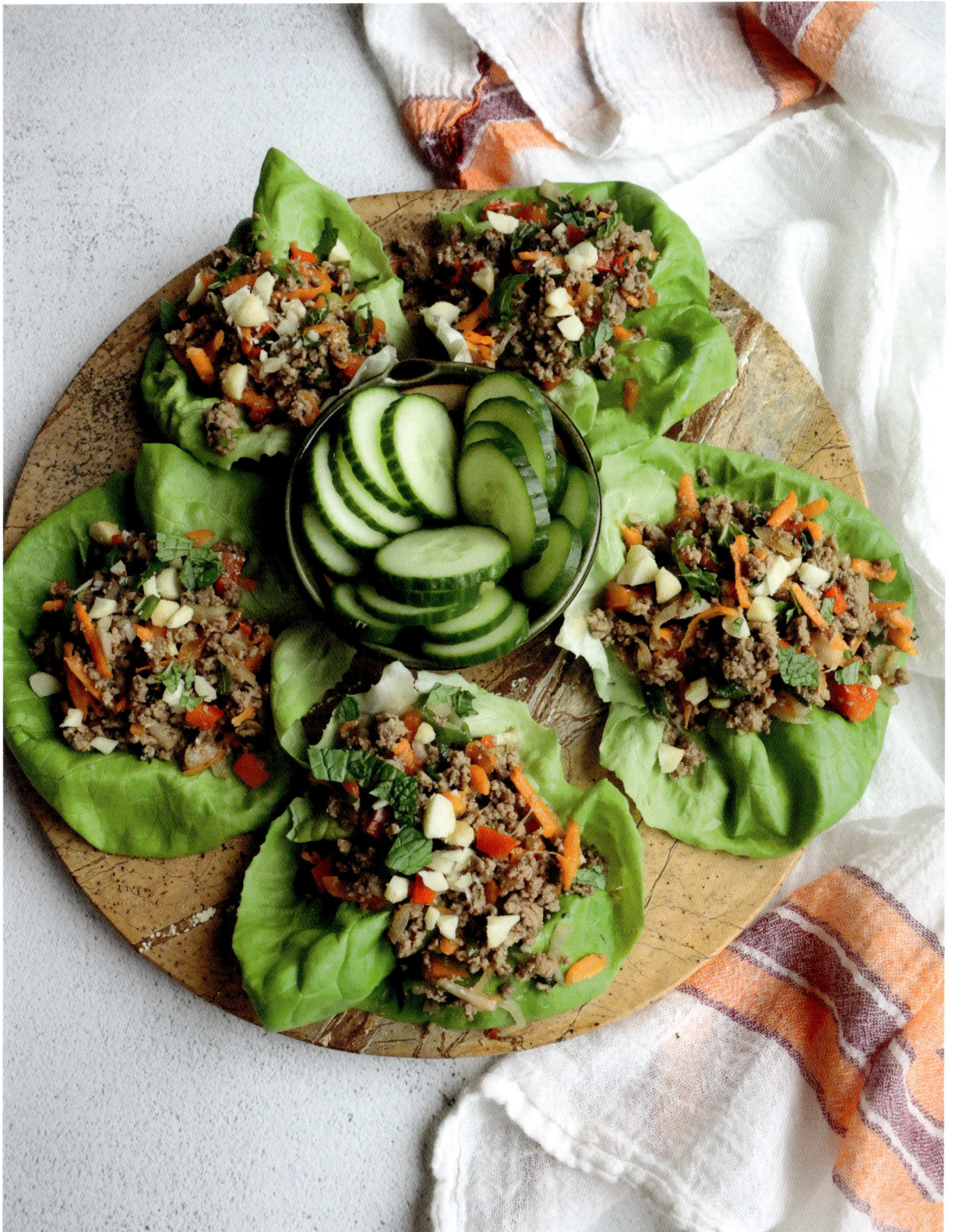

BLAT WRAPS

This riff on the classic BLT (plus avocado) makes for a quick, fresh, and mouthwatering lunch. For a GF/DF (Level 1) version, you can use your favorite gluten-free bread instead of lettuce for a more traditional sandwich experience. But I have to say that this combo takes particularly well to a lettuce wrap, concentrating the flavors and doubling the crunchy/juicy factor. While these are best when the bacon is fresh and crisp, they're also meal prep–friendly. Cook all the bacon at once, wash and dry your lettuce leaves, and slice your tomato ahead of time—just wait to cut the avocado until serving to avoid browning.

● **GLUTEN-FREE**   ● **DAIRY-FREE**   ● **PALEO**

DIETARY LEVELS 1, 2

SERVINGS 4
PREP TIME 10 minutes
COOK TIME 20 minutes
TOTAL TIME 30 minutes

1 pound (454 g) compliant bacon

8 large leaves romaine lettuce (from about 1 romaine heart)

½ cup (115 g) paleo or Whole30-compliant mayonnaise

2 medium beefsteak tomatoes, sliced

2 medium ripe avocados, sliced

Flaky sea salt, to taste

Freshly ground pepper, to taste

1. First, cook the bacon using 1 of these 2 methods:

   Stovetop method: Cook the bacon in batches in a large skillet over medium heat, flipping as needed, until crisp. Transfer to a paper towel–lined plate.

   Oven method: Preheat the oven to 375°F (191°C). Line a rimmed baking sheet with parchment paper and set a baking rack on top. Lay the bacon strips side by side on the rack. Transfer to the oven and bake for 15 to 20 minutes, rotating the pan halfway through for even crisping. Remove from oven when bacon is brown and crisp to your liking, and transfer to a paper towel–lined plate. (Note: You may need to cook the bacon in 2 batches if preparing the entire pound at once.)

2. Wash and pat the romaine leaves dry, keeping them whole. Smear each romaine leaf with mayo, then lay 2 to 3 strips of bacon on each leaf. Top with tomato and avocado slices and season to taste with flaky sea salt and freshly ground pepper, if desired. Fold like a taco and enjoy!

NOTE
For meal prep and leftovers: Store lettuce, bacon, and sliced tomato in separate airtight containers in the fridge. Slice the avocado just before serving. Assemble wraps when ready to eat.

HERB-MARINATED PORK TENDERLOIN WITH FENNEL-OLIVE SAUCE

This elegant yet approachable pork tenderloin is bursting with Mediterranean flavor: A simple garlic and herb marinade adds depth, while the warm fennel-olive sauce brings briny brightness, aromatic sweetness, and savory richness. Finally, just a touch of our AIP-friendly Homemade Worcestershire Sauce (page 222) gives it that crave-worthy umami. For an AIP recipe, this one's a stunner! Serve it with Roasted Brussels Sprouts with Bacon (page 195), or Velvety Truffle Mashed Cauliflower and Sweet Potato (page 202) for a complete AIP-compliant meal.

● GLUTEN-FREE   ● DAIRY-FREE   ● PALEO   ● AIP-FRIENDLY

DIETARY LEVELS 1, 2, 3

SERVINGS 4

PREP TIME 15 minutes, plus 1–4 hours optional marinating time

COOK TIME 25 minutes

TOTAL TIME 40 minutes, plus optional marinating time

FOR PORK

1 tablespoon (15 ml) extra-virgin olive oil, plus more as needed

1 tablespoon (15 ml) Homemade Worcestershire Sauce (page 222)

2 cloves garlic, minced

1 tablespoon (2 g) finely chopped fresh rosemary, or 1 teaspoon dried rosemary

1 tablespoon (3 g) fresh thyme leaves, or 1 teaspoon dried thyme

1 teaspoon lemon zest

1 teaspoon fine sea salt

2-pound (907 g) pasture-raised pork tenderloin, trimmed

FOR FENNEL-OLIVE SAUCE

2 tablespoons (30 ml) extra-virgin olive oil

1 small fennel bulb, finely diced (about 1½ cups [240 g])

2 cloves garlic, minced

½ cup (50 g) pitted green olives, such as Picholine or Castelvetrano, chopped

¼ cup (25 g) pitted Kalamata olives, chopped

2 tablespoons (18 g) capers, rinsed and chopped

1 teaspoon Homemade Worcestershire Sauce (page 222)

¼ teaspoon fine sea salt, or to taste

1 tablespoon (15 ml) fresh lemon juice, plus more as needed

Chopped fresh parsley or fennel fronds (optional)

To Make the Pork

1. Whisk together the olive oil, Worcestershire sauce, garlic, rosemary, thyme, lemon zest, and sea salt in a medium mixing bowl. Add the pork loin and toss to coat. Marinating is optional, but if you'd like to do so, cover and refrigerate for 1 to 4 hours.

2. Preheat the oven to 400°F (200°C). Heat a large oven-safe skillet over medium-high heat. Add a drizzle of olive oil and sear the pork on all sides until golden, about 2 to 3 minutes per side. Transfer the skillet to the oven and roast for 15 to 20 minutes, or until the internal temperature reaches 145°F (°63 C). Remove from the oven and let rest 5 to 10 minutes before slicing.

To Make the Fennel-Olive Sauce

3. While the pork roasts, heat the olive oil in a medium skillet over medium heat. Add the fennel and sauté for 6 to 8 minutes until softened and lightly golden. Add the garlic and cook for 30 seconds more, until fragrant.

4. Stir in the olives, capers, Worcestershire sauce, and salt. Cook for 1 to 2 minutes to warm through. Remove from the heat and add fresh lemon juice. Taste and adjust the seasoning with more lemon juice or salt, if needed. Cover to keep warm until ready to serve.

5. To serve, slice the pork tenderloin into medallions and spoon the warm sauce over the top. Garnish with fresh parsley or fennel fronds if desired. Serve immediately.

Sweet Potato Fries
with Fry Sauce,
page 200

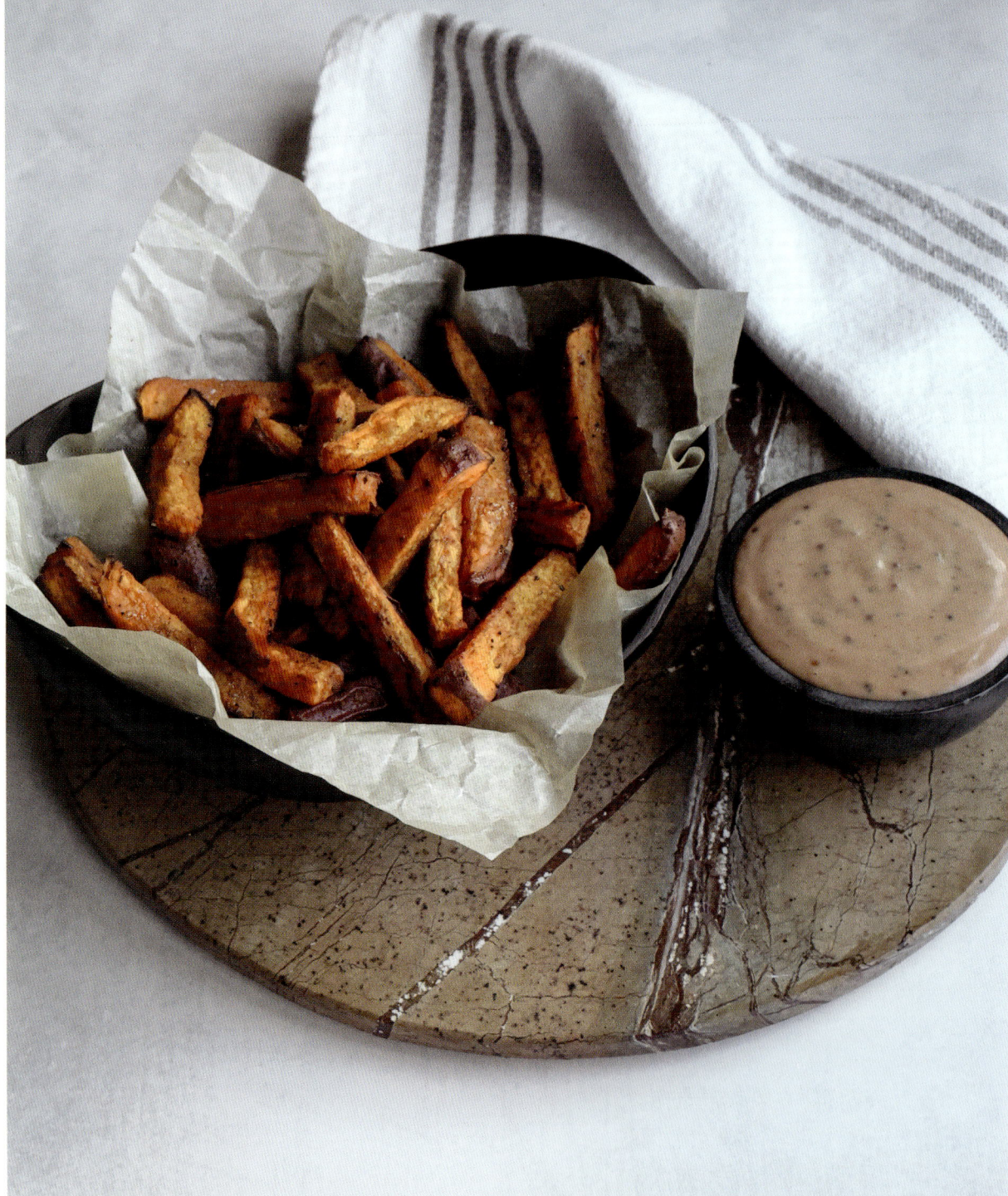

13

Sides

Some people think of sides as an afterthought—a way to get those obligatory veggies dutifully down. I like to flip the script and let veggies play a starring role, bringing you back bite after bite to those mineral-rich greens, detoxifying beets, warming winter squashes, and boldly flavored crucifers. The sides in this chapter pull double duty, adding flavor, color, and variety to your plate while also delivering essential nutrients like fiber, antioxidants, and complex carbohydrates. Whether roasted, sautéed, or sheet-pan simple, we'll use flavor-boosting cooking techniques to make them as easy to prepare as they are to love. Whether you're craving something savory, zesty, or just a little crispy on the edges, this chapter has you covered.

OVEN-ROASTED GARLIC FRIES

These easy oven fries (pictured with the Steak Frites on page 175) are a surefire crowd-pleaser. Truffle salt is optional here but highly recommended, especially if you're using rutabaga or parsnips: It's a great way to enhance flavor while keeping the recipe nightshade-free. Rutabaga has a tough and bitter outer skin that needs to be peeled and the same goes for larger parsnips, but if you're using smaller, younger parsnips or russet potatoes, try leaving the skin on for added flavor, fiber, and nutrients.

● **GLUTEN-FREE**　　● **DAIRY-FREE**　　● **PALEO**　　● **AIP-FRIENDLY**　　● **VEGAN**

DIETARY LEVELS 1, 2, 3

SERVINGS 4
PREP TIME 15 minutes
COOK TIME 25–30 minutes
TOTAL TIME 40–45 minutes

1½ pounds (1.4 kg) russet potatoes (sub rutabaga or parsnips for paleo and AIP)

3 tablespoons (45 ml) avocado oil

1 teaspoon garlic powder

½ teaspoon fine sea salt

Freshly ground black pepper, to taste (omit for AIP)

1 teaspoon minced fresh rosemary

¼ teaspoon truffle salt or fine sea salt

Truffle salt for garnish (optional)

1. Preheat the oven to 450°F (230°C). Line a rimmed sheet pan with parchment paper.

2. If using russet potatoes or smaller parsnips, you can peel them or not, as desired. If using rutabaga or larger parsnips, peel them now. Slice the potatoes, rutabaga, or parsnips into ¼-inch (6 mm) batons (french fry shapes).

3. Combine the batons with oil, garlic powder, fine sea salt, and pepper in a large mixing bowl. Toss until evenly coated.

4. Spread the fries evenly across the sheet pan to ensure even crisping. Transfer to the oven and roast for 25 to 30 minutes, stirring halfway through, until golden brown and crispy on the edges. Remove from the oven and sprinkle immediately with the rosemary and truffle salt or additional sea salt. Toss again and serve immediately for the best taste and texture.

SERVING SUGGESTION
A quick garlic aioli makes a delicious GF/DF/paleo-compliant dipping sauce for these fries. Finely mince a clove of garlic with a hefty pinch of salt to mellow the garlic's bite. Add this to about ½ cup (115 g) of your favorite paleo or Whole30-compliant mayo, plus freshly ground black pepper, a few shakes of garlic powder, about 1 teaspoon of extra-virgin olive oil, a pinch of lemon zest, and a spritz of fresh lemon juice. Taste and adjust seasoning as desired, and for best results, let sit for 15 to 30 minutes before serving. Chef's kiss!

ROASTED BRUSSELS SPROUTS WITH BACON

With Brussels sprouts, the right preparation makes all the difference. Here, we're roasting them until crispy and caramelized, creating a delicious contrast between the tender sprouts and chewy-crisp bacon bits. And nestled inside all that texture and flavor is one of the most detox-supporting veggies you can eat: The sulfur-containing compounds (glucosinolates) in Brussels sprouts support liver detoxification and the production of glutathione, one of the body's master antioxidants. This is one of those sides that's as much at home in a weeknight dinner as it is on a holiday buffet. When choosing bacon, make sure it's compliant with your dietary level: See the note on page 115 for tips.

● GLUTEN-FREE　　● DAIRY-FREE　　● PALEO　　● AIP-FRIENDLY

DIETARY LEVELS 1, 2, 3

SERVINGS 6
PREP TIME 20 minutes
COOK TIME 30 minutes
TOTAL TIME 50 minutes

2 pounds (907 g) Brussels sprouts

6 ounces (170 g) raw compliant bacon, diced

3 tablespoons (45 ml) extra-virgin olive oil

Fine sea salt, to taste

Freshly ground pepper, to taste (omit for AIP)

1. Preheat the oven to 400°F (200°C).

2. Wash and trim the Brussels sprouts, removing any brown or bruised outer leaves, and cut them in half through the stem end. Place in a large mixing bowl along with the bacon, olive oil, a generous pinch of sea salt, and freshly ground pepper to taste.

3. Spread evenly across a rimmed baking sheet. Transfer to the oven and roast for 15 minutes. Remove from the oven, toss with a spatula, and spread out the mixture evenly again. Return to the oven for 10 to 15 minutes or until the sprouts are brown and blistered in spots and the bacon is chewy-crisp. Serve.

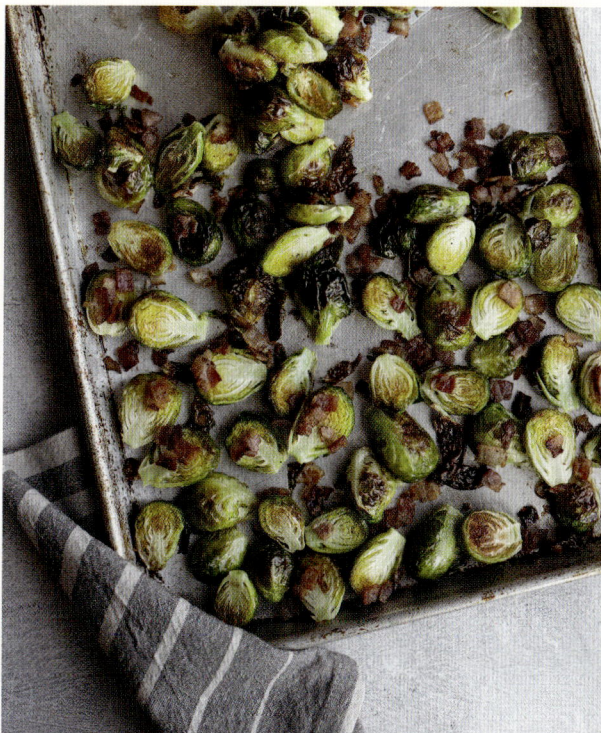

LEMONY CAULIFLOWER PASTA

I love how these zippy, briny flavors come together for a fresh take on cauliflower. You're going to want to dig right in, but before serving, take an extra moment to taste and adjust the seasonings—whether it's a spritz of lemon juice, a drizzle of olive oil, or a pinch of sea salt—to bring those flavors and textures into perfect balance. Plus, this pasta goes with almost everything: Try it with Spice-Rubbed Slammin' Salmon (page 161), Balsamic-Marinated Chicken Breasts (page 160), or Veggie-Packed Meatloaf Muffins (page 162).

● **GLUTEN-FREE**   ● **DAIRY-FREE**   ● **PALEO**   ● **AIP-FRIENDLY**

DIETARY LEVELS 1, 2, 3

SERVINGS 4
(as a side dish)

PREP TIME 15 minutes

COOK TIME 15 minutes

TOTAL TIME 30 minutes

4 ounces (113 g) gluten-free or grain-free pasta (see note on page 156)

1½ teaspoons sea salt, divided, plus more to taste

3 tablespoons (45 ml) olive oil, divided, plus more for drizzling

½ large head cauliflower, cut into bite-size florets

2 tablespoons (30 ml) water

Freshly ground black pepper, to taste (omit for AIP)

3 garlic cloves, minced

2 tablespoons (18 g) capers, drained

Pinch crushed red pepper flakes (omit for AIP)

Zest and juice of ½ lemon, plus more to taste

2 tablespoons (8 g) chopped fresh parsley

1. Bring a large pot of water to a boil, then add 1 teaspoon of the salt. Cook the pasta according to package instructions until al dente. Set aside ½ cup (118 ml) of the cooking water before draining. Drain the pasta, toss with 1 tablespoon (15 ml) of the olive oil to prevent sticking, and set aside.

2. Heat 1 tablespoon (15 ml) of the olive oil in a large skillet over medium heat. Add the cauliflower florets and water and season with the remaining ½ teaspoon of salt and black pepper. Cover and steam for 2 minutes, then uncover and cook, stirring occasionally, for 5 to 7 minutes or until the cauliflower is tender and golden brown in spots. Transfer to a plate and set aside.

3. Heat the remaining 1 tablespoon (15 ml) of olive oil in the same skillet over medium heat. Add the garlic, capers, and chile flakes and cook, stirring, for about 1 minute or until the garlic is just starting to turn golden. Add the lemon zest and juice and parsley, and if needed, a splash of the reserved pasta water, to moisten. Add the cooked cauliflower and pasta to the skillet and toss to combine. If needed, add more pasta water to moisten. Taste and adjust the seasoning with additional lemon juice and seasoning.

4. Plate the pasta, top with desired garnishes (see note), and enjoy!

OPTIONAL GARNISHES:
For GF/DF/Paleo (Level 1 or 2 only) options: toasted pine nuts or a sprinkling of Brazil Nut "Parmesan" (page 225)

For GF/DF/Paleo/AIP (Levels 1, 2, or 3) options: fresh parsley, extra capers, a drizzle of olive oil, and lemon wedges

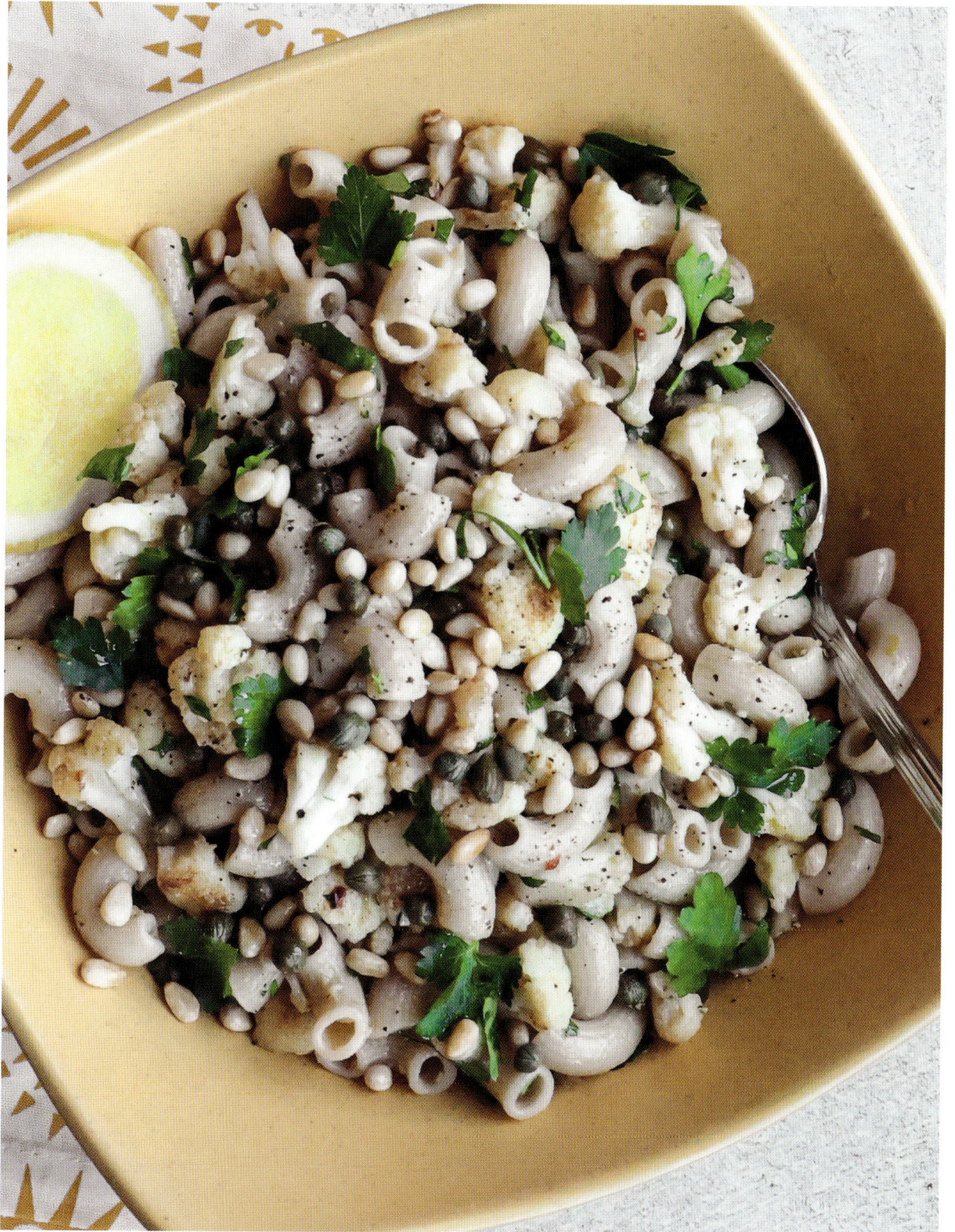

SLOW-ROASTED MISO-BUTTER SWEET POTATOES

This recipe uses just a few simple toppings—buttery, grass-fed ghee, chickpea miso paste, and a touch of tahini—to transform roasted sweet potatoes into an umami-packed delight. The combination is also powerfully gut-supportive, because it pairs prebiotic-rich sweet potatoes with a probiotic topping. The other magic trick here is slow-roasting the sweet potatoes at a lower temperature. This hands-off approach concentrates their natural sweetness while locking in moisture for the silkiest, most sumptuous sweet potatoes you've ever tasted. Pair them with your favorite protein and a simple green salad for an easy, satisfying meal.

● GLUTEN-FREE   ● DAIRY-FREE

DIETARY LEVELS 1

SERVINGS 4
PREP TIME 5 minutes
COOK TIME 2 hours
TOTAL TIME 2 hours, 5 minutes

2 medium orange-fleshed sweet potatoes, such as garnet or jewel yams, unpeeled

¼ cup (54 g) grass-fed ghee

¼ cup (64 g) chickpea miso (see note)

2 teaspoons tahini

Fine sea salt, to taste

Freshly ground black pepper, to taste

1. Preheat the oven to 300°F (150°C).

2. Arrange the sweet potatoes directly on the center rack of the oven, placing a rimmed, parchment paper–lined baking sheet on the rack directly below to catch any drips. Do not pierce the skin: Keeping them intact locks in moisture and prevents drying out. Roast for 1¾ to 2 hours, depending on size. They're done when a paring knife slides in with little to no resistance.

   Optional Step for Extra Moisture: Remove the sweet potatoes from oven and wrap loosely in a clean kitchen towel, letting them rest for about 10 minutes to trap the steam and make the flesh even silkier.

3. Combine the ghee, chickpea miso, and tahini in a small bowl and use a fork to mash everything together, creating a soft and spreadable mix.

4. Cut each sweet potato in half lengthwise and score the soft flesh with a fork to maximize flavor absorption. Smear each half generously with the miso mixture. Taste and adjust the seasoning, if needed. (Keep in mind that miso is naturally salty, so you may not need extra salt!) Serve immediately.

ABOUT MISO

Miso is a delicious, salty-umami seasoning paste made from beans or grains fermented with "koji," a starter culture that imbues it with probiotic bacteria. There are many types and flavors of miso out there, most of them made with soy. Chickpea miso is the ideal choice here, not only because it has a light and mild flavor that doesn't overpower the sweet potato the way a darker miso paste might, but also because it's soy-free and gluten-free, making it one of the most thyroid-friendly choices.

Can't find chickpea miso? A mellow white miso will also work. Be sure to check labels carefully, as many miso pastes contain soy or gluten-containing grains such as barley, which some thyroid patients may need to avoid due to sensitivities or allergies.

CITRUS-GLAZED BEETS

These slow-roasted, honey-glazed beets get a few strategic touches from fresh herbs, orange juice, and a bright splash of vinegar, and the result is a side dish that will brighten up any meal. Yes, the roasting time is long, but it's worth it: It's what makes them so incredibly yum.

● GLUTEN-FREE   ● DAIRY-FREE   ● PALEO   ● AIP-FRIENDLY

DIETARY LEVELS 1, 2, 3

SERVINGS 6
PREP TIME 20 minutes
COOK TIME 1½ hours
TOTAL TIME 1 hour,
50 minutes

4 large (about 2 pounds)
(907 g) red or golden beets

2 tablespoons (30 ml)
extra-virgin olive oil

¾ teaspoon fine sea salt

Freshly ground black
pepper, to taste (omit
for AIP)

2 teaspoons honey

Juice of 1 medium orange

1 teaspoon chopped
fresh rosemary, plus
more as needed

1 teaspoon chopped
fresh thyme, plus more
as needed

1½ teaspoons champagne
vinegar or apple cider
vinegar

1. Preheat the oven to 350°F (177°C).

2. Peel the beets and cut them into bite-size wedges. Add to a 9 x 13-inch (22.9 x 33 cm) baking dish and toss with the remaining ingredients. Bake for 1¼ to 1½ hours, stirring halfway through. Beets are done when fork-tender and caramelized, and when the liquid is almost completely evaporated. Note that honey burns easily, so watch closely during the last 15 minutes of roasting to avoid scorching.

3. Garnish with fresh thyme and rosemary, if desired, and enjoy!

SWEET POTATO FRIES WITH FRY SAUCE

Level up your burger night with these addictive sweet potato fries. No deep fryer required: Just a sheet pan and a hot oven will do the trick! Dunk them in a sweet and tangy homemade sauce and serve them with the Lamb Burger Salad (page 140), the Crispy Chicken and Veggie Nuggets (page 178), or as a stand-in for the frites in Steak Frites (page 175).

● **GLUTEN-FREE**　● **DAIRY-FREE**　● **PALEO**

DIETARY LEVELS 1, 2

SERVINGS 4
PREP TIME 20 minutes
COOK TIME 35 minutes
TOTAL TIME 55 minutes

FOR FRIES

2 tablespoons (30 ml) avocado oil or melted, unrefined coconut oil

½ teaspoon smoked paprika

¼ teaspoon garlic powder

½ teaspoon fine sea salt

Freshly ground black pepper, to taste

2 teaspoons maple syrup

1½ pounds (1.4 kg) sweet potatoes, peeled or unpeeled

FOR FRY SAUCE

½ cup (115 g) paleo or Whole30-compliant mayonnaise

3 tablespoons (33 g) stone-ground mustard

1 tablespoon (20 g) honey

1 tablespoon (16 g) tomato paste

2 teaspoons white wine vinegar

¼ teaspoon kosher salt, plus more to taste

Freshly ground black pepper, to taste

A few shakes of paleo-compliant Louisiana-style hot sauce

To Make the Fries

1. Preheat the oven to 450°F (230°C). Line a rimmed baking sheet with parchment paper.

2. Combine the oil, smoked paprika, garlic powder, sea salt, pepper, and maple syrup in a large mixing bowl. Whisk to combine.

3. Slice the sweet potatoes into ¼-inch (6 mm) batons (french fry shapes), add to the bowl, and toss until evenly coated.

4. Spread the fries in a single layer on the prepared baking sheet, leaving space between them for better crisping. Transfer to the oven and roast for 30 to 35 minutes, stirring halfway through. The fries are done when they are golden brown and crispy on the edges.

To Make the Fry Sauce

5. Combine all the ingredients for the sauce in a small mixing bowl. Stir well and adjust seasoning to taste.

6. Serve the fries alongside the Fry Sauce while hot and crisp.

GARLICKY SHEET PAN BROCCOLI

If you're looking for creative ways to jazz up veggie sides, this crispy, garlicky roasted broccoli is just the ticket. It makes excellent use of the Brazil Nut "Parmesan" (page 225), which gets tucked into all of the broccoli's nooks and crannies, creating pockets of flavor between those irresistible caramelized branches.

● GLUTEN-FREE   ● DAIRY-FREE   ● PALEO   ● VEGAN

DIETARY LEVELS 1, 2

SERVINGS 4
PREP TIME 10 minutes
COOK TIME 20 minutes
TOTAL TIME 30 minutes

1½ pounds (680 g) (about 2 medium heads) broccoli, cut into bite-size florets

3 tablespoons (45 ml) extra-virgin olive oil

3 cloves garlic, minced

¼ teaspoon fine sea salt, or to taste

Freshly ground black pepper, to taste

¼ teaspoon crushed red pepper flakes (optional)

½ teaspoon lemon zest

¼ cup Brazil Nut "Parmesan" (page 225)

Juice of ½ lemon

1. Preheat the oven to 425°F (218°C). Line a sheet pan with parchment paper for easy cleanup.

2. Combine the broccoli florets with the oil, garlic, salt, pepper, red pepper flakes, lemon zest, and Brazil Nut "Parmesan" in a large mixing bowl. Toss to coat. Spread the broccoli on the prepared sheet pan in an even layer to ensure even crisping.

3. Transfer to the oven and roast for 15 to 20 minutes or until the broccoli is browned and crispy on the edges. Remove from the oven and immediately spritz with fresh lemon juice. Serve warm and enjoy!

VELVETY TRUFFLE MASHED CAULIFLOWER AND SWEET POTATOES

This sumptuous mash combines the mild sweetness of white-fleshed sweet potatoes with the light, creamy texture of cauliflower. Infused with rosemary, garlic, and a luxurious hint of truffle, this side dish feels restaurant-worthy yet simple enough for a weeknight meal. Not a truffle fan? Simply omit it for a classic version of this dish.

● **GLUTEN-FREE**   ● **DAIRY-FREE**   ● **PALEO**   ● **AIP-FRIENDLY**   ● **VEGAN**

DIETARY LEVELS 1, 2, 3

SERVINGS 6
PREP TIME 20 minutes
COOK TIME 20 minutes
TOTAL TIME 40 minutes

2 pounds (907 g) (about 3 medium) white-fleshed sweet potatoes, peeled and cut into 1-inch (2.5 cm) cubes

6 cloves garlic, smashed and peeled

2½ teaspoons fine sea salt, divided

½ head (about 1 pound [454 g]) cauliflower, cut into florets

¼ cup (59 ml) extra-virgin olive oil

1 teaspoon chopped fresh rosemary

½ teaspoon truffle salt or fine sea salt

1 teaspoon fresh lemon juice, plus more as needed

Pinch white pepper (omit for AIP)

1 teaspoon truffle oil or extra-virgin olive oil for drizzling

1. Combine the cubed sweet potato, garlic cloves, and 2 teaspoons of the sea salt in a medium pot. Cover with cool water by 2 inches (5.1 cm). Bring to a boil, reduce the heat, and simmer, covered, for 8 minutes.

2. Add the cauliflower to the pot and return to a boil. Cook for 8 minutes more or until the cauliflower and sweet potatoes are both very tender. Reserve 1 cup (237 ml) of cooking liquid. Drain the vegetables and garlic in a colander.

3. Add the vegetables and garlic to a food processor (or return to the pot and use an immersion blender) along with the oil, rosemary, the remaining ½ teaspoon of sea salt, truffle salt or additional sea salt, lemon juice, and white pepper. Puree until smooth, adding the reserved cooking liquid as needed to reach your desired consistency.

4. Taste and adjust the seasoning, adding more salt, truffle salt, lemon juice, or white pepper, if needed. Drizzle lightly with truffle oil or olive oil to serve, and enjoy!

SERVING SUGGESTION
Pair this mash with grilled steak, roasted chicken, or pan-seared fish. For an extra special accompaniment, serve alongside sautéed mushrooms with garlic and herbs.

WILTED GREENS WITH TOASTED GARLIC CHIPS

This simple side dish pairs tender wilted greens with garlic-infused oil, crispy garlic chips, and a lemony finish. One pound (454 g) of greens may seem like a lot, but they cook down significantly, so this is a quick and easy way to get your daily greens in with plenty of flavor and no fuss. Serve alongside just about any protein, top with an egg (non-AIP), or toss into Samurai Breakfast Bowls with Steel-Cut Oats (page 115) for a boost of color and nutrients. Or partner it with Herb-Marinated Pork Tenderloin with Fennel-Olive Sauce (page 191), Spice-Rubbed Slammin' Salmon (page 161), or Balsamic-Marinated Chicken Breasts (page 160) for a complete meal.

● GLUTEN-FREE   ● DAIRY-FREE   ● PALEO   ● AIP-FRIENDLY   ● VEGAN

DIETARY LEVELS 1, 2, 3

SERVINGS 4–6
PREP TIME 10 minutes
COOK TIME 5–10 minutes
TOTAL TIME 15–20 minutes

3 tablespoons (45 ml) extra-virgin olive oil

3 cloves garlic, thinly sliced into coins

⅛–¼ teaspoon dried chile flakes (optional, omit for AIP)

16 ounces (454 g) roughly chopped spinach, chard, or kale, stems removed

Fine sea salt, to taste

Freshly ground black pepper, to taste (omit for AIP)

1–2 teaspoons fresh lemon juice, to taste

1. Warm the olive oil in a large skillet over medium-high heat. Add the sliced garlic and cook, stirring frequently, until lightly golden, about 2 to 3 minutes. Watch closely to avoid overbrowning, which can make the garlic bitter. Use a slotted spoon to transfer the garlic chips to a paper towel–lined plate. Set aside.

2. If using chile flakes, stir them into the hot oil and cook for about 1 minute to infuse the oil with flavor.

3. Working in batches, add the greens to the skillet, stirring as they wilt and cook down. Cook until the greens are just tender and vibrant in color, about 5 to 10 minutes depending on the variety (spinach cooks quickly; kale takes longer). Season to taste with sea salt and pepper.

4. Remove the skillet from the heat. Lightly spritz the greens with lemon juice and toss to combine. Taste and adjust the salt and acidity as needed. Transfer to a serving dish and sprinkle with the reserved crispy garlic chips. Serve warm.

RAINBOW ROASTED ROOT VEGGIES

This staple side dish highlights the natural flavors of these energy-boosting root vegetables through the simple magic of caramelization in a hot oven. A touch of apple cider vinegar brightens them up, making it a versatile and colorful accompaniment to your favorite protein, salads, or bowls. You can easily shift the flavor profile with your choice of oil too: Coconut oil enhances the veggies' natural sweetness, while extra-virgin olive oil adds a more savory touch. Finally, don't worry about separating the beets (if using): They'll tint the other veggies slightly pink, but the result is a beautiful, sunset-hued color palette.

● GLUTEN-FREE   ● DAIRY-FREE   ● PALEO   ● AIP-FRIENDLY   ● VEGAN

DIETARY LEVELS 1, 2, 3

SERVINGS 4–6

PREP TIME 15 minutes

COOK TIME 40–45 minutes

TOTAL TIME 55–60 minutes

2 pounds (907 g) assorted root vegetables, such as carrots, parsnips, beets, golden beets, turnips, or celery root

3 tablespoons (45 ml) melted unrefined coconut oil or extra-virgin olive oil

2 teaspoons apple cider vinegar

1 teaspoon fine sea salt

Freshly cracked pepper, to taste (omit for AIP)

1 teaspoon fresh thyme leaves (optional)

1. Preheat the oven to 400°F (200°C). Prepare a large, rimmed baking sheet with parchment paper. Peel the root veggies and cut them into ½-inch (1.3 cm) cubes. Place in a medium mixing bowl and add the oil, vinegar, salt, and pepper and toss well to coat.

2. Spread the vegetables out in a single layer on the baking sheet. Roast for 35 to 40 minutes, flipping halfway through, until tender and golden brown in spots. Taste and adjust the seasoning as needed. Sprinkle with fresh thyme, if using, and serve warm.

CARAMELIZED CAULIFLOWER WITH PARSLEY GARLIC SAUCE

Deeply roasted, nutty cauliflower is pretty irresistible on its own—almost like veggie popcorn. This recipe takes it to the next level with a punchy Parsley Garlic Sauce (page 221) that brings fresh herbs, garlic, and lemon to the party. It's the perfect contrast to all that caramelized richness. For extra texture and a little crunch, feel free to top it off with toasted pine nuts or walnuts (just remember to skip those if you're on AIP/Level 3).

● GLUTEN-FREE ● DAIRY-FREE ● PALEO ● AIP-FRIENDLY ● VEGAN

DIETARY LEVELS 1, 2, 3

SERVINGS 4
PREP TIME 20 minutes
COOK TIME 30 minutes
TOTAL TIME 50 minutes

1 medium head cauliflower, cut into florets

2–3 tablespoons (30–45 ml) avocado oil

½ teaspoon fine sea salt

Freshly ground black pepper, to taste (omit for AIP)

About ½ batch Parsley Garlic Sauce (page 221)

¼ cup (30 g) lightly toasted pine nuts or chopped walnuts (optional, omit for AIP)

1. Roast the cauliflower. Preheat the oven to 425°F (220°C). Line a rimmed baking sheet with parchment paper for easy cleanup.

2. Toss the cauliflower florets with the oil, salt, and pepper in a large mixing bowl. Spread in a single layer on the prepared baking sheet. Transfer to the center rack of the oven and roast for 25 to 30 minutes, flipping halfway through. The cauliflower is done when it's deep golden brown and caramelized on the edges.

3. While the cauliflower is roasting, prepare the Parsley Garlic Sauce.

4. Transfer the roasted cauliflower to a serving dish. Drizzle generously with the Parsley Garlic Sauce or serve it on the side. Garnish with toasted nuts, if using.

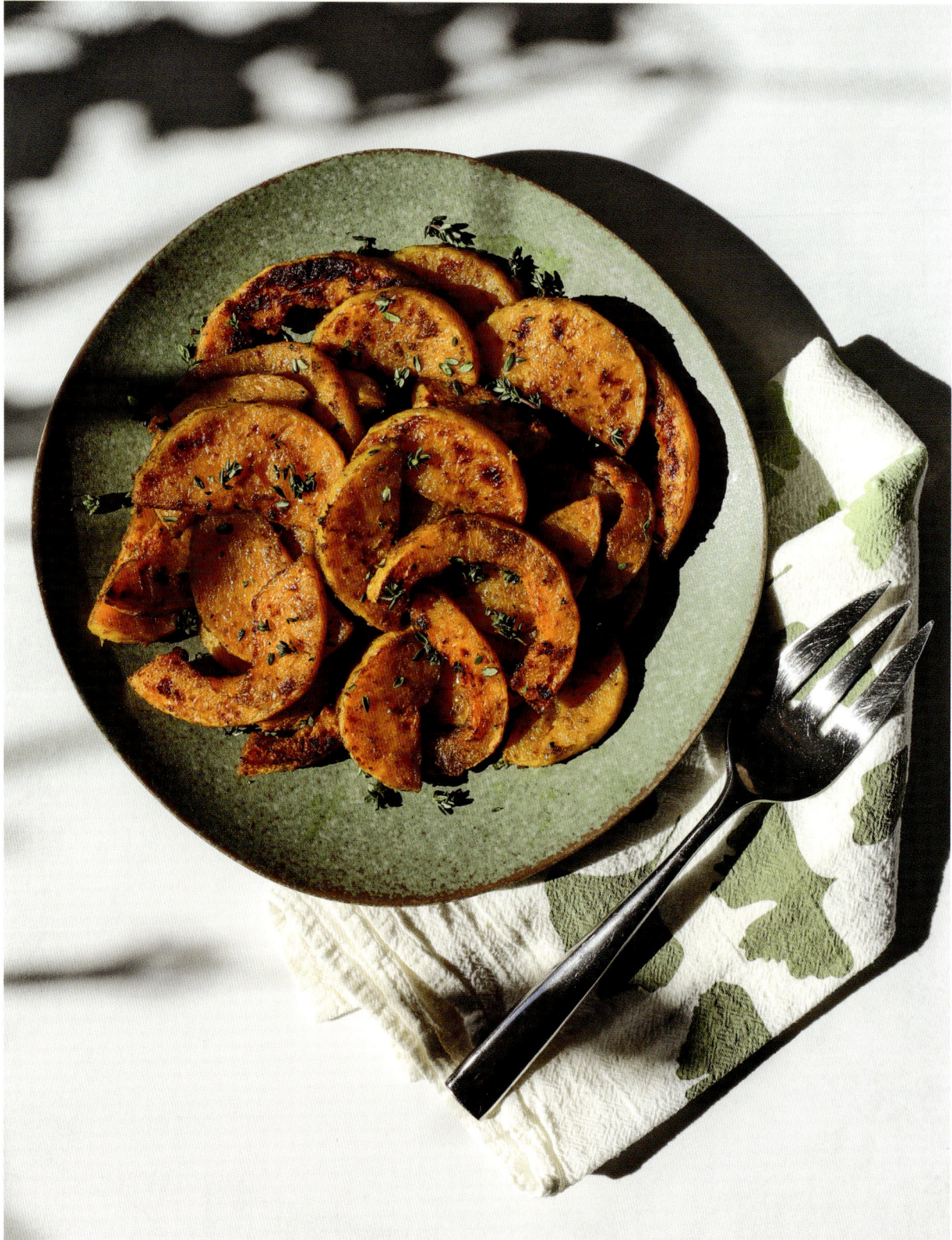

SAVORY BUTTERNUT SLICES

A blend of seasonings lights up this sheet pan winter squash with savory, sweet, and aromatic elements, while oven roasting gives the squash those deliciously blistered brown spots that nobody can resist. Serve this alongside Spice-Rubbed Slammin' Salmon (page 161), Sausage, Beans and Greens Pasta (page 156), or Balsamic-Marinated Chicken Breasts (page 160).

● GLUTEN-FREE   ● DAIRY-FREE   ● PALEO   ● AIP-FRIENDLY   ● VEGAN

DIETARY LEVELS 1, 2, 3

SERVINGS 4–6
PREP TIME 15 minutes
COOK TIME 25–30 minutes
TOTAL TIME 45 minutes

¾ teaspoon garlic powder

¾ teaspoon onion powder

¼ teaspoon ground ginger

¼ teaspoon ground turmeric

¼ teaspoon ground allspice (sub cinnamon for AIP)

¾ teaspoon fine sea salt

Freshly ground black pepper, to taste (omit for AIP)

1 small (about 2 pounds) (907 g) butternut squash, peeled, seeded, and cut into ¼-inch (6 mm) half-moons

1 tablespoon (15 ml) melted unrefined coconut oil

Fresh thyme, rosemary, or parsley (optional)

1. Preheat the oven to 450°F (230°C) and line a large, rimmed sheet pan with parchment paper.

2. Combine the garlic powder, onion powder, ground ginger, turmeric, allspice or cinnamon, sea salt, and pepper in a small bowl. Set aside.

3. Toss the squash with the melted coconut oil in a large bowl. Sprinkle with the seasoning mix and toss to coat evenly.

4. Arrange the squash slices in a single layer on the prepared sheet pan. Transfer the pan to the middle rack of the oven and roast for 15 minutes, then remove from the oven and carefully flip each slice using tongs or a small spatula to ensure even browning. Return to the oven and roast for 10 to 15 minutes more or until the squash is tender and browned in spots. Check the underside of the slices to avoid scorching. Remove from the oven, garnish with fresh thyme or parsley, if desired, and enjoy!

Roasted
Garlic and
White Bean
Dip, page 214

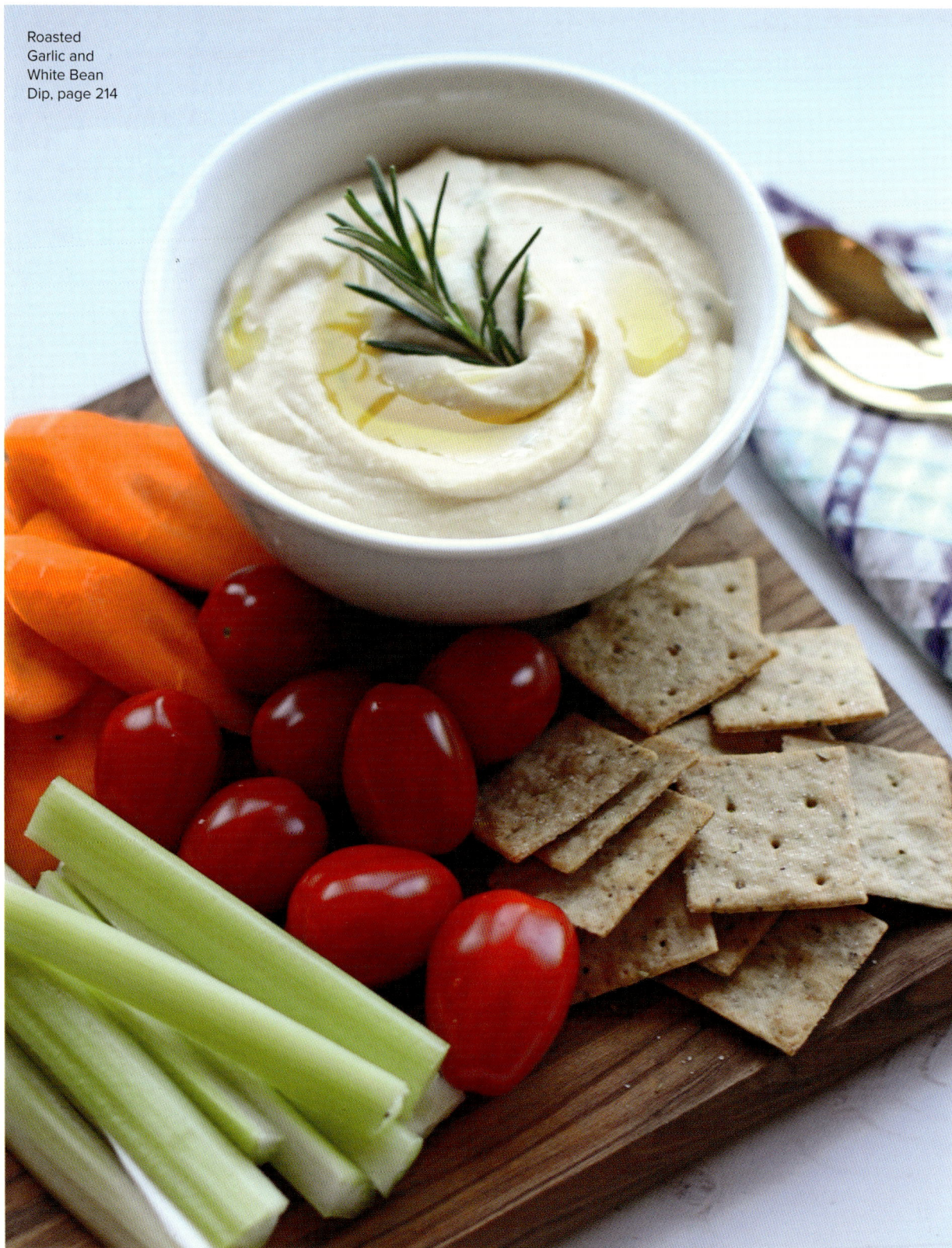

14

Snacks and Staples

Elevating thyroid-friendly cooking from good to great is all about the details—those finishing touches, flavor-boosting condiments, and nourishing snacks that keep you going between meals—and that's what this chapter is all about. Whether you need a quick bite to curb your hunger, a vibrant dip or sauce to liven up a meal, or a simple vinaigrette for dressing your leafy greens, I've got you covered.

From crispy kale chips even picky eaters will devour to probiotic-packed carrot hummus, soothing bone broth, and my always-on-hand staples like easy Homemade Worcestershire Sauce and Brazil Nut "Parmesan," these recipes are crafted with thyroid-friendly ingredients that support your wellness goals. They're quick to prepare, easy to keep on hand, and perfect for pulling together a meal or tiding you over until the next one.

These finishes, flourishes, and snacks are more than just extras; they're a key strategy for making thyroid-friendly eating doable, delicious, and successful throughout your THYROID30 wellness adventure and beyond.

BAKED "PARMESAN" ZUCCHINI ROUNDS

This fun, family-friendly way to enjoy zucchini delivers a crispness plus a hit of "cheesy" flavor (minus the dairy) in every bite. Thanks to the Brazil Nut "Parmesan" (page 225), you'll also get a healthy dose of thyroid-supportive selenium. Serve these as a snack, side, or appetizer with marinara sauce or, if you're feeling indulgent, my Dairy-Free Ranch Dip (page 213).

● **GLUTEN-FREE**　● **DAIRY-FREE**　● **PALEO**　● **VEGAN**

DIETARY LEVELS 1, 2

SERVINGS 4
PREP TIME 15 minutes
COOK TIME 30 minutes
TOTAL TIME 45 minutes

2 medium zucchini

1 tablespoon (15 ml) extra-virgin olive oil

¼ teaspoon garlic powder

¼ teaspoon Italian herb blend

Freshly ground black pepper

½ batch Brazil Nut "Parmesan" (page 225)

Marinara sauce or Dairy-Free Ranch Dip (page 213) for dipping (optional)

1. Preheat the oven to 425°F (218°C), using convection mode if available for even crisping. Place a baking rack on a rimmed baking sheet.

2. Slice the zucchinis into ¼-inch (6 mm)-thick rounds. Combine the olive oil, garlic powder, herb blend, and pepper in a medium mixing bowl. Whisk to blend. Add the zucchini and toss to coat.

3. Place the Brazil Nut "Parmesan" in a small shallow bowl and lightly press the zucchini rounds into the mixture to coat. Aim for a thin, even coating (not thick or cakey). Place the rounds on the prepared baking rack, transfer to the oven, and bake for 20 minutes. Rotate the pan, return to the center rack of the oven, and switch the oven to broil mode. Broil for approximately 5 minutes or until the tops are golden brown, watching closely to avoid scorching.

4. Serve, pairing with dips, if desired, and enjoy!

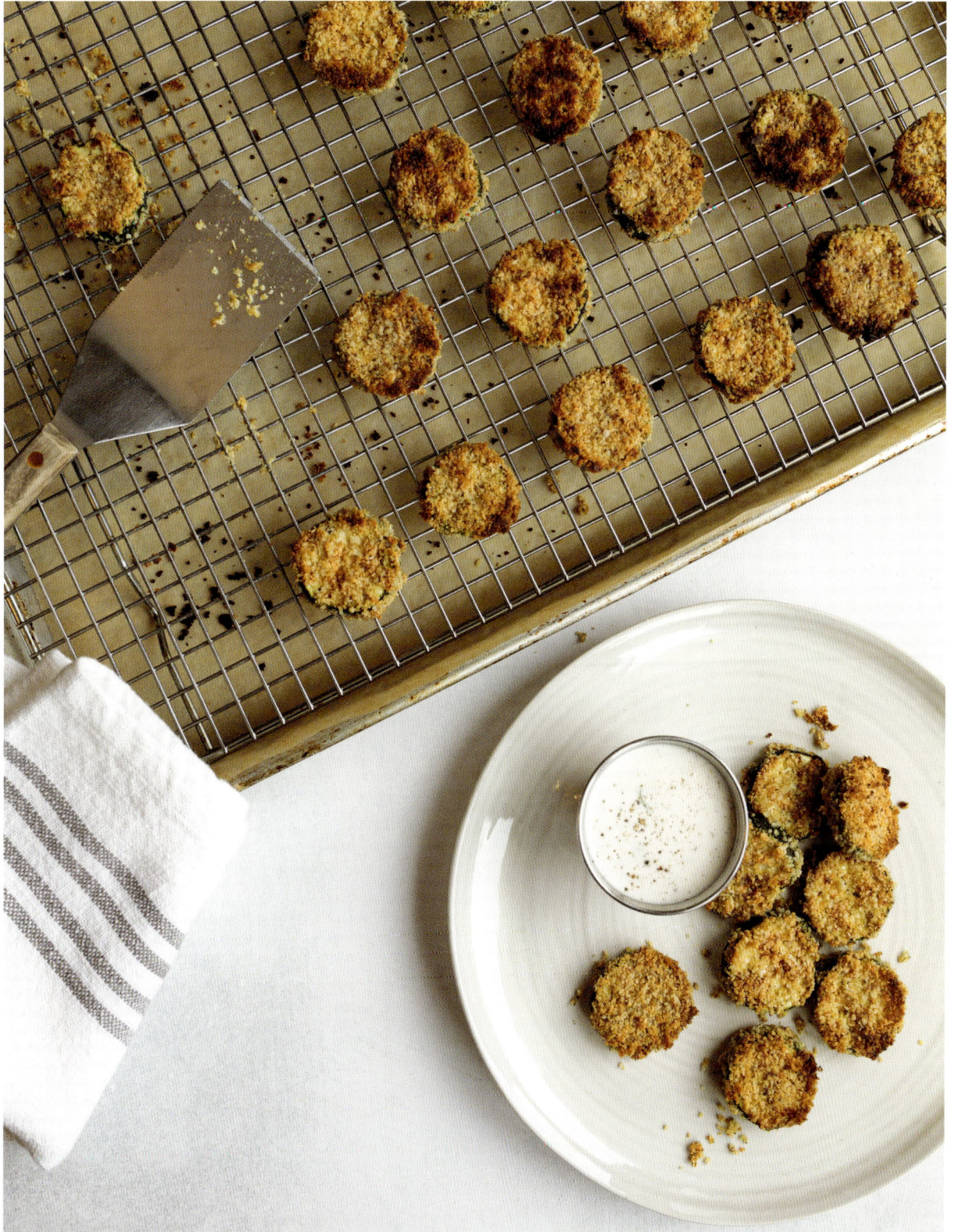

"CHEESY" KALE CHIPS

Ready to watch the kids (and adults) in your life devour kale? I hope so, because these nacho cheese–flavored kale chips will convert even the pickiest eaters. The secret to crispy, light chips is starting with bone-dry kale, so take the extra step to wash, spin, and air-dry the leaves completely before seasoning. The "cheesy" flavor comes from the perfect blend of nutritional yeast (a.k.a. "nooch"), savory seasonings, and creamy tahini. Don't worry if this looks like too much kale: It'll shrink a *lot* during baking, so you'll end up with about 6 cups of cooled, crisped chips.

● **GLUTEN-FREE**   ○ **DAIRY-FREE**   ● **PALEO**   ● **VEGAN**

DIETARY LEVELS 1, 2

SERVINGS 6

PREP TIME 15 minutes
(plus drying time for
the kale)

COOK TIME 30 minutes

TOTAL TIME 45 minutes
(plus drying time for
the kale)

2 bunches curly kale

2 tablespoons (30 ml)
avocado or extra-virgin
olive oil

2 tablespoons (30 g) tahini

1 tablespoon (15 ml) fresh
lemon juice

1 tablespoon (15 ml)
coconut aminos

½ teaspoon garlic powder

½ teaspoon onion powder

¾–1 teaspoon fine sea salt

2 tablespoons (18 g)
nutritional yeast

1 pinch cayenne pepper

1. Remove the kale leaves from the stems and tear into pieces. Thoroughly wash and dry the kale. Preheat the oven to 300°F (150°C). You'll need 2 rimmed baking sheets.

2. Make the "cheese" sauce. Combine the oil, tahini, lemon juice, coconut aminos, garlic powder, onion powder, sea salt, nutritional yeast, and cayenne pepper in a small food processor. Blend to a paste.

3. Place the kale leaves in a large mixing bowl. Add the tahini mixture to the kale and massage the sauce into the leaves with your hands, ensuring every piece is well-coated and no lumps remain.

4. Spread the kale in a single layer on the 2 baking sheets. Place the baking sheets on the upper- and lower-third oven racks. Bake for 20 minutes, rotating the pans halfway through and gently tossing the kale to ensure even drying.

5. After 20 minutes, remove the kale from the oven and toss again. Turn the oven off and return the kale to the oven for 10 minutes more to ensure maximum crispness.

6. Remove the kale chips from the oven and let them cool completely on the baking sheets. They will continue to crisp up as they cool. If they're still chewy, return them to the warm oven for another 5 to 10 minutes or until they're crisp when cool. Cool completely and store in an airtight container at room temperature for up to 3 days.

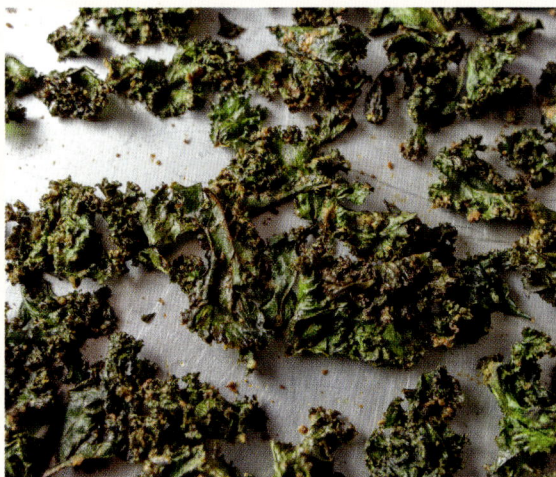

DAIRY-FREE RANCH DIP OR DRESSING

Go ahead and enjoy this dairy-free rendition of a beloved staple condiment as a dip or dressing. Serve with your favorite crudités, drizzled on your dinner salad, or with the "Parmesan" Zucchini Rounds on page 210.

● **GLUTEN-FREE**   ● **DAIRY-FREE**   ● **PALEO**   ● **VEGAN**

DIETARY LEVELS 1, 2

SERVINGS 8
PREP TIME 10 minutes
TOTAL TIME 10 minutes

¼ cup (59 ml) paleo or Whole30-compliant almond milk

¾ cup (175 g) paleo or Whole30-compliant mayo (sub vegenaise for vegan, see note)

1 tablespoon (15 ml) fresh lemon juice

1 teaspoon garlic powder

1 teaspoon onion powder

1 large green onion, finely minced

¼ teaspoon fine sea salt, or more to taste

¼ teaspoon ground black pepper

Combine all the ingredients in a medium mixing bowl and whisk well. For best flavor, make at least 30 minutes in advance. Store in an airtight container in the refrigerator for up to 1 week.

NOTE
To avoid ultra-processed ingredients, look for mayo labeled paleo or Whole30-Approved. See THYROID30 Support and Resources on page 246 for recommended brands.

ROASTED GARLIC AND WHITE BEAN DIP

Sometimes the simplest recipes are the best. Here, we combine just a few basic ingredients to create a mouthwatering snack or party appetizer to serve with your favorite veggie dippers or gluten-free crackers. You can also use it as a flavorful spread for a protein- and veggie-packed lettuce wrap.

● **GLUTEN-FREE**   ● **DAIRY-FREE**   ● **VEGAN**

DIETARY LEVELS 1

SERVINGS 6–8

PREP TIME 15 minutes

COOK TIME Up to 1½ hours

TOTAL TIME Up to 1 hour, 45 minutes

1 bulb garlic

1 tablespoon (15 ml) water

3 tablespoons (45 ml) extra-virgin olive oil, divided

1½ cups (273 g) (or one 14-ounce jar or can) cannellini or great northern beans, cooked, drained, and rinsed

1 teaspoon finely chopped fresh rosemary or sage

1–2 teaspoons fresh lemon juice, to taste

½–¾ teaspoon fine sea salt, or to taste

1. Preheat the oven to 350°F (177°C).

2. Cut the top ¼-inch (6 mm) off the garlic bulb and place in a small baking dish, cut-side up. Add water to the bottom of the dish and drizzle the garlic with 1 tablespoon (15 ml) of the olive oil. Cover or wrap tightly with foil and bake for 1 to 1½ hours or until the garlic is tender and golden brown in spots. Remove from the oven and let sit until cool enough to handle.

3. Combine the beans, rosemary or sage, lemon juice, sea salt, and the remaining 2 tablespoons (30 ml) of olive oil in a small food processor or blender.

4. Squeeze the roasted garlic cloves from their papery skins and add to the bean mixture. Mix until smooth and well blended. Taste and adjust seasoning as desired. Serve with your favorite veggie dippers—peppers, snap peas, carrots, cucumber, zucchini, cherry tomatoes, celery, and so on—or gluten-free or grain-free crackers of choice.

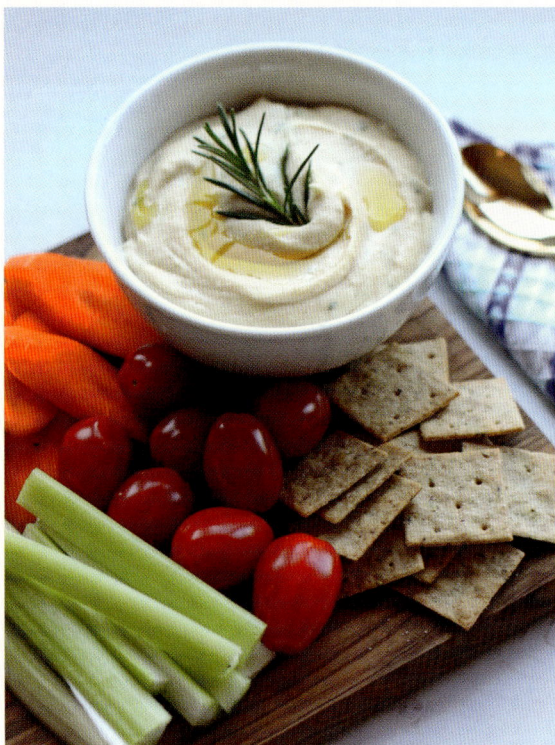

PROBIOTIC CARROT HUMMUS

This bright and zesty carrot hummus is packed with gut-supportive ingredients. A scoop of fermented sauerkraut brings the flavors to life (literally!), adding the benefits of live and active cultures. Along with the natural prebiotic fiber in the carrots, this dip delivers a one-two punch of nourishment for your microbiome. For a bold (and equally irresistible) variation, try adding a spoonful of Quick and Easy Harissa (page 220) to the mix.

● **GLUTEN-FREE** ● **DAIRY-FREE** ● **VEGAN**

DIETARY LEVELS 1

SERVINGS 6–8 (about 2 cups [480 g])
PREP TIME 10 minutes
COOK TIME 20 minutes
TOTAL TIME 30 minutes

FOR ROASTED CARROTS

5 medium (about 1 pound [454 g]) carrots, peeled and sliced into ¼-inch (6 mm) rounds

1 tablespoon (15 ml) extra-virgin olive oil

½ teaspoon ground cumin

½ teaspoon ground coriander

¼ teaspoon smoked paprika

Pinch cayenne pepper (optional)

½ teaspoon fine sea salt

Freshly ground black pepper, to taste

FOR HUMMUS

1 cup (240 g) cooked chickpeas (drained and rinsed, if using canned)

1 teaspoon lemon zest

3 tablespoons (45 ml) fresh lemon juice, plus more as needed

3 tablespoons (45 g) tahini

3 tablespoons (45 ml) extra-virgin olive oil, plus extra for drizzling

1 garlic clove, minced

1 teaspoon fine sea salt, or to taste

¼ cup (36 g) fermented sauerkraut (optional, but recommended)

Up to 3 tablespoons (45 ml) water

Sesame seeds (optional)

To Make the Roasted Carrots

1. Preheat the oven to 400°F (200°C) and line a sheet pan with parchment paper for easy cleanup.

2. Toss the carrots with the olive oil, spices, salt, and pepper in a medium mixing bowl until evenly coated. Spread in a single layer on the prepared baking sheet and roast for 20 minutes, stirring halfway through, until tender and golden in spots. Remove from the oven and let cool slightly.

To Make the Hummus

3. Combine the chickpeas, lemon zest and juice, tahini, olive oil, garlic, salt, sauerkraut, and roasted carrots in a small food processor. Blend until smooth, scraping down the sides as needed. If the hummus is too thick, you can add up to 3 tablespoons (45 ml) of water to adjust the consistency. Taste and adjust with additional salt or lemon juice, if needed.

4. Transfer the carrot hummus to a serving bowl. Drizzle with olive oil and sprinkle with sesame seeds, if desired. Serve with fresh vegetables, grain-free or gluten-free crackers, or use as a spread in wraps and sandwiches. Store in an airtight container in the refrigerator for up to 5 days.

STICKY THAI-STYLE ZINGY WINGS

If you like flavors that pop, you're going to love these zingy chicken wings. They're incredibly easy to make and feature a three-ingredient glaze that comes together in a flash. Pro tip: A touch of baking soda on the wings ensures crisp and crackling skin.

● GLUTEN-FREE   ● DAIRY-FREE   ● PALEO   ● AIP-FRIENDLY

DIETARY LEVELS 1, 2, 3

SERVINGS 4
PREP TIME 10 minutes
COOK TIME 45 minutes
TOTAL TIME 55 minutes

Coconut or avocado oil

2 pounds (907 g) pasture-raised chicken wings

½ teaspoon baking soda

½ teaspoon fine sea salt

Freshly black cracked pepper, to taste (omit for AIP)

1 tablespoon (15 ml) AIP-compliant fish sauce

1 tablespoon (15 ml) fresh lime juice

1 tablespoon (9 g) coconut sugar

1 lime wedge, for spritzing

Fresh cilantro leaves (optional)

1. Place an oven rack in the upper third of oven and preheat to 425°F (218°C). Line a rimmed baking sheet with parchment paper and place a wire rack on top. Spray or brush the wire rack with coconut or avocado oil to prevent sticking.

2. Pat the wings thoroughly dry with paper towels and place in a large mixing bowl. Toss with baking soda, salt, and pepper. Let sit for 10 to 15 minutes (this is optional, but it improves crispiness).

3. Arrange the wings on the wire rack skin-side down, ensuring they're not touching. Transfer to the oven and bake for 20 minutes. Remove from the oven, flip the wings over, and bake for 20 minutes more or until golden and crisp.

4. During the last 5 minutes of baking, combine the fish sauce, lime juice, and coconut sugar in a small skillet or saucepan and bring to a boil over medium-high heat. Simmer until the sugar is melted and bubbles coat the surface, about 1 to 2 minutes. Remove from the heat and set aside.

5. After the wings are crisp, remove them from the oven and transfer them to a large mixing bowl. Toss with the glaze while they're still hot, using a heat-proof spatula to scrape every bit of glaze from the pan. Transfer to a serving dish, spritz with juice from the lime wedge, garnish with fresh cilantro, if desired, and enjoy!

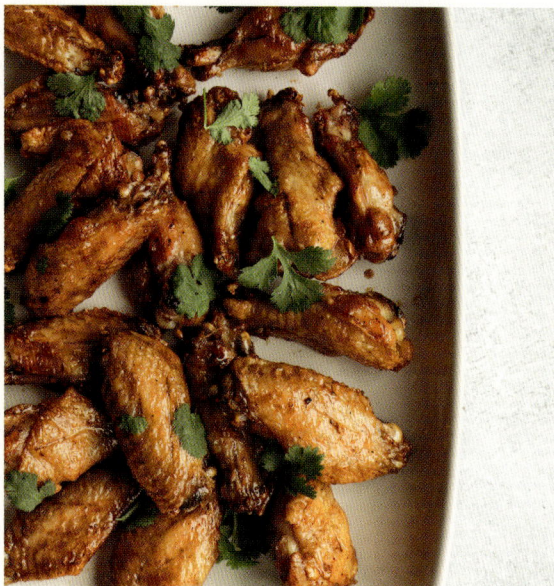

AVOCADO BOATS WITH TAHINI LIME DRESSING

This recipe comes together fast and requires no cooking—perfect for a quick, nutrient-packed meal or snack. Creamy avocado halves are stuffed with shredded carrots, cucumbers, beets, or radishes, then drizzled with a tahini lime dressing that's so good you might want to drink it through a straw. That's partially thanks to sumac, a dried brick-red spice made from ground sumac berries. Its tart, tangy flavor is bright, citrusy, and easy to fall in love with. It's optional for this recipe, but if you can get your hands on some, it's a phenomenal flavor booster that adds a little magic to lots of recipes.

● **GLUTEN-FREE**   ◌ **DAIRY-FREE**   ● **PALEO**   ● **VEGAN**

DIETARY LEVELS 1, 2

SERVINGS 4
PREP TIME 10 minutes
TOTAL TIME 10 minutes

FOR DRESSING

3 tablespoons (45 g) tahini

3 tablespoons (45 ml) fresh lime juice

1 tablespoon (6 g) finely minced
fresh ginger

1 tablespoon (15 ml) coconut aminos

1 tablespoon (15 ml) water

½ teaspoon ground sumac, plus more as
needed (optional, but recommended)

¼ teaspoon fine sea salt, or to taste

Freshly ground black pepper, to taste

¼ cup (59 ml) avocado, walnut, or
macadamia oil

FOR AVOCADO BOATS

2 ripe avocados, halved and pitted

1½ cups (165 g) grated beet, carrot,
cucumber, or radish

2 tablespoons (20 g) raw pumpkin or
sunflower seeds

Sprouts

Hemp hearts (optional)

To Make the Dressing

1. Combine the tahini, lime juice, ginger, coconut aminos, water, and sumac (if using) in a 2-cup (473 ml) glass measuring cup or small mixing bowl. Season with salt and pepper to taste. Whisk with a fork to combine. Drizzle in the oil, whisking continuously to blend. Taste and adjust the seasoning as desired. The recipe makes about ¾ cup (177 ml).

To Make the Avocado Boats

2. Scoop out the avocado halves from their peels using a soup spoon and discard the peels. Stabilize the avocado halves by slicing a thin sliver from the underside of each to create a flat base: This helps prevent them from rolling around on the plate.

3. Stuff each avocado half with the grated vegetables. Drizzle generously with the tahini dressing and top with pumpkin or sunflower seeds and sprouts. Garnish with hemp hearts and sumac (if using). Enjoy as a snack or serve with your favorite protein for a complete meal.

SERVING SUGGESTIONS

Pair this with Zesty Homemade Breakfast Sausage Patties (page 107), Balsamic-Marinated Chicken Breasts (page 160), or Spice-Rubbed Slammin' Salmon (page 161).

EASY HOMEMADE BONE BROTH

Homemade bone broth is a nutrient-packed staple, rich in gut-nourishing collagen, gelatin, and trace minerals. This big-batch recipe creates a deep, flavorful broth that's perfect for sipping or using as a base for soups, stews, and sauces. The long, slow simmer, plus a splash of apple cider vinegar, ensures maximum nutrient extraction from the bones and connective tissue, while aromatic veggies and herbs add layers of flavor. Feel free to mix your bones (poultry, beef, lamb, pork): I find the best-tasting broths use a combination. Find more bone broth tips in the FAQ section on the next page!

● **GLUTEN-FREE**   ● **DAIRY-FREE**   ● **PALEO**   ● **AIP-FRIENDLY**

DIETARY LEVELS 1, 2, 3

SERVINGS 12
(about 3 quarts [2.8 L])

PREP TIME 20 minutes

COOK TIME 24 hours

TOTAL TIME 24 hours
plus 20 minutes

2–3 pounds (0.9–1.4 kg) bones (raw or cooked), such as chicken carcasses, wings, drumsticks, necks, or feet; or beef, lamb, or pork bones like marrow bones, knuckle bones, or meaty rib bones

2–3 ribs celery, chopped

3–4 large carrots, unpeeled and chopped

1 yellow onion, roughly chopped, skin on

2–3 cloves garlic, smashed

½ teaspoon dried turmeric or 2–3 coins fresh turmeric root

1 teaspoon fine sea salt or Himalayan salt

2–3 bay leaves

½ teaspoon whole black peppercorns (omit for AIP)

1–2 tablespoons (15–30 ml) apple cider vinegar

12–14 cups (2.8–3.3 L) filtered water, or enough to cover the ingredients

1. Combine all the ingredients in a large stock pot or slow cooker (see the FAQ on next page). Bring to a simmer, cover, and cook over low heat for approximately 24 hours. To extract maximum nutrients, do not boil. The occasional small bubble rising to the surface indicates a good temperature for bone broth.

2. After 24 hours, strain the broth into another large pot or mixing bowl.

3. To chill the broth, fill a clean sink with ice and a few inches (cm) of water and carefully lower the pot or bowl of broth into the ice bath. Let sit to chill, stirring occasionally, for up to 30 minutes.

4. Cover and store the broth in the refrigerator overnight, allowing the layer of rendered fat on top to harden. Remove and discard this fat (see FAQ on next page). If you don't have time to chill it overnight, you can just skim the fat from the top with a spoon or gravy separator.

5. Set aside any stock you may want for immediate use, and freeze the rest in glass or ceramic containers. Be sure to label and date them (see FAQ on next page).

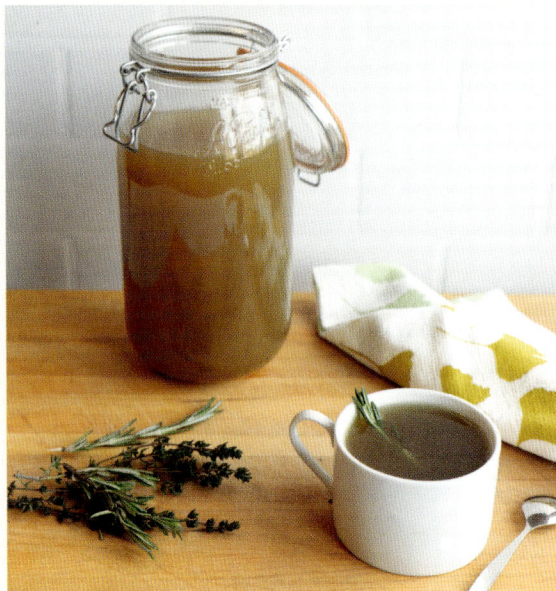

BONE BROTH FAQS

What's the best kind of cooking vessel for bone broth? Since bone broth cooks for so long, it's best to use nontoxic cookware and avoid Teflon or nonstick coatings. A stainless-steel stockpot or ceramic slow cooker works best. An 8-quart (7.6 L) slow cooker is ideal, but a 6-quart (5.7 L) one can work if you don't have extra ingredients. For the stovetop, an 8- to 12-quart (7.6–11.4 L) stockpot should provide plenty of room.

How do you come up with bones for the stockpot? Ask your butcher or check the freezer aisle for soup bones. You can also substitute 2 pounds (907 g) of chicken wings or drumsticks, which are both rich in connective tissue, and the added chicken meat will give your broth amazing flavor. I like to collect scraps in the freezer in a large silicone freezer bag: roast chicken carcasses, necks from the giblet bag (gold!), pot roast bones, and veggie scraps too—onion skins, leek tops, fennel stalks, celery leaves, carrot peels, mushroom stems. Once you've got a good stash, toss them in a pot with water and a splash of vinegar. Simmer and done!

How do you safely cook bone broth for 24 hours? The safest way to do this is in a slow cooker. These are ideal because they maintain a steady, safe temperature overnight. Induction cooktops are also generally safe for overnight use as they don't involve open flame or high external heat. Gas stoves are not recommended for overnight simmering due to open flames and toxic gas emissions. Electric stoves may also pose a risk as the heating element can cause scorching if left unattended.

Can you make bone broth in a pressure cooker? Absolutely, and this can be a great way to shorten cooking time and still get a rich, gelatinous broth. Add ingredients and water (don't exceed the max fill line), then cook on high pressure for 2 to 3 hours. Let the pressure release naturally before straining and storing.

Why do you recommend chilling the broth in an ice bath? Hot broth takes hours to cool in the fridge, sitting in the "danger zone" (40°F to 140°F [4°C to 60°C]). An ice bath brings the temp down faster and eases the workload on your fridge. The broth may not reach fully safe temps in the ice bath alone, but cooling it first will allow it to chill faster and more safely once refrigerated.

My bone broth jiggles now that it's cooled. Is that normal? Yes! That's a great sign. It means you have a wonderfully rich bone broth that's loaded with healing gelatin and collagen. That gelatinous texture is the naturally rendered gelatin at work. Don't worry: It will liquefy as soon as it's heated. Gelling and stickiness signify that you've made a really excellent batch of bone broth—high five!

Should you skim the fat after it's cooled? While rendered fat can be wonderful to cook with, broth fat cooked this long may oxidize, forming inflammatory compounds. I recommend chilling the broth overnight to harden the fat, then remove and discard.

What's the best way to store bone broth? To avoid thyroid and endocrine-disrupting toxins, use glass or ceramic containers with tight-fitting lids. Bone broth can be refrigerated for up to 5 days or frozen for several months. If freezing, be sure to leave headroom in your containers to allow for the liquid to expand. Avoid freezing bone broth in canning jars, as they tend to break as the liquid freezes and expands.

QUICK AND EASY HARISSA

This versatile, beguiling Tunisian condiment traditionally calls for roasting, steaming, and peeling the red peppers. My version cuts corners by sautéing the peppers and onions until richly caramelized to mimic that smoky-sweet flavor. Aleppo pepper adds a mild earthy heat to this spice paste: If you can't find it, you can substitute up to half the amount of chile flakes, adjusting according to your spice tolerance. Enjoy it smeared on the Scrambled Egg Breakfast Tacos (page 111), toss it with roasted veggies, serve it alongside grilled seafood, or stir it into the Probiotic Carrot Hummus (page 215).

● GLUTEN-FREE ● DAIRY-FREE ● PALEO ● VEGAN

DIETARY LEVELS 1, 2

SERVINGS Makes about 1 cup (235 g)

PREP TIME 10 minutes

COOK TIME 20 minutes

TOTAL TIME 30 minutes

2 tablespoons (30 ml) avocado oil

3–4 cloves garlic, minced

2 red bell peppers, diced

1 large shallot or small red onion, diced

1 teaspoon fine sea salt

1 tablespoon (16 g) tomato paste

1–1½ teaspoons Aleppo pepper (or up to ½ teaspoon chile flakes)

1 teaspoon ground coriander

1 teaspoon ground cumin

½ teaspoon caraway seeds

2 tablespoons (30 ml) fresh lemon juice

1 tablespoon (15 ml) extra-virgin olive oil

Cayenne pepper, to taste (optional)

1. Heat the avocado oil in a medium skillet over medium-high heat. Add the garlic and cook, stirring until fragrant, about 1 minute. Add the peppers, shallot or onion, and salt and cook, stirring occasionally, until moisture has evaporated and the vegetables are browned in spots, about 10 to 12 minutes.

2. Add the tomato paste and spices to the pan. Cook, stirring, for another 2 to 3 minutes, allowing the spices to bloom and the tomato paste to cook off its raw flavor.

3. Remove from the heat and let cool. Add the mixture to a small food processor along with the lemon juice and olive oil and process until smooth. Taste and adjust seasoning with more lemon juice, olive oil, salt, or cayenne for desired flavor and consistency. Store in an airtight container in the fridge for up to 2 weeks. Use as a condiment, dip, or flavor booster in your favorite dishes.

PARSLEY GARLIC SAUCE

As a Thyroid Thriver, it's essential to have a good green sauce in your back pocket. This one can jazz up countless meals and is perfect for meal prep. Drizzle it over a quinoa or cauliflower rice bowl with shredded chicken; serve it alongside grilled seafood, fish, or steak; or use it to add brightness to roasted vegetables like cauliflower or root veggies. The possibilities are endless! See it in action in our Caramelized Cauliflower (page 205).

- GLUTEN-FREE
- DAIRY-FREE
- PALEO
- AIP-FRIENDLY
- VEGAN

DIETARY LEVELS 1, 2, 3

SERVINGS 6–8 (makes ¾–1 cup [175–235 ml])

PREP TIME 15 minutes

TOTAL TIME 15 minutes

2 cups (180 g) roughly chopped, loosely packed flat-leaf parsley (1 large or 2 small bunches)

Zest and juice of 1 large lemon, plus more as needed

⅓ cup (79 ml) extra-virgin olive oil

4 cloves garlic, peeled and roughly chopped

2 teaspoons Italian herb blend

½–1 teaspoon fine sea salt, plus more as needed

Freshly ground black pepper, to taste (omit for AIP)

1 tablespoon (15 ml) filtered water

Combine all sauce ingredients in a mini food processor or blender. Pulse to blend and mix until you reach a rustic sauce consistency (not pureed or overly smooth). Taste and adjust with additional salt, pepper, or lemon juice as needed. Store in an airtight container in the refrigerator for up to 5 days or freeze for up to 3 months.

HOMEMADE WORCESTERSHIRE SAUCE

You'll love having this homemade Worcestershire on hand to give your recipes a blast of flavor. It's so easy to make, comes together quickly, and tastes way better than store-bought. Not to mention, it is difficult to find a store-bought version that is additive-free and paleo/AIP-compliant. Add it to marinades, sauces, dressings, and more! Whenever I make a batch, I stash the leftovers in the freezer (for up to 3 months). Time works its magic on these flavors, and they get better and better with age. Pro tip: This is a recipe where measurements matter, so grab those measuring spoons and stick to the exact amounts for best results.

● **GLUTEN-FREE**   ● **DAIRY-FREE**   ● **PALEO**   ● **AIP-FRIENDLY**

DIETARY LEVELS 1, 2, 3

SERVINGS About 8 (approximately ½ cup)

PREP TIME 5 minutes

COOK TIME 7 minutes

TOTAL TIME 12 minutes

½ cup (118 ml) apple cider vinegar

2 tablespoons (30 ml) coconut aminos

2 tablespoons (30 ml) filtered water

2 teaspoons blackstrap molasses

1 heaping teaspoon minced anchovy fillets

¼ teaspoon ground ginger

¼ teaspoon mustard powder (omit for AIP)

¼ teaspoon onion powder

¼ teaspoon garlic powder

⅛ teaspoon cinnamon

⅛ teaspoon ground cloves

¼ teaspoon freshly ground pepper (sub ground mace for AIP)

½ teaspoon fine sea salt

1. Combine all ingredients in a small saucepan and whisk thoroughly to combine. Place over medium heat and bring to a simmer. Cook for 5 to 7 minutes or until the sauce has thickened slightly. Remove from the heat and let cool. Pour through a fine-mesh sieve to strain.

2. Transfer to a container with a tight-fitting lid and store in the refrigerator for up to 2 weeks or freeze for up to 3 months.

AIP-FRIENDLY ITALIAN DRESSING MIX

This powdered dressing mix is super-convenient and versatile. You can use leftover prepared dressing as a marinade or drizzle for chicken, steak, asparagus, or zucchini, and the dry mix can double as a seasoning for rubs or marinades. Delicious and practical! Just make sure your Italian herb blend is AIP-safe: Read the ingredient list carefully and avoid red pepper flakes and seed-based herbs. As for oils, walnut oil is recommended for paleo, and avocado or extra-virgin olive oil for AIP.

● GLUTEN-FREE ● DAIRY-FREE ● PALEO ● AIP-FRIENDLY ● VEGAN

DIETARY LEVELS 1, 2, 3

SERVINGS About ½ scant cup (24 g) of dressing mix, which yields 7 batches of prepared dressing (⅔ cup [156 ml] per batch, or approximately 4½ cups [1.1 L] total).

PREP TIME 10 minutes

TOTAL TIME 10 minutes

FOR ITALIAN DRESSING MIX

2 tablespoons (36 g) plus 1 teaspoon fine sea salt

1 teaspoon freshly ground black pepper (omit for AIP)

1 tablespoon (7 g) onion powder

1 teaspoon garlic powder

2 tablespoons (5 g) Italian herb blend

1 teaspoon dried oregano

1 tablespoon (9 g) coconut sugar or maple sugar

FOR PREPARED DRESSING

1 tablespoon (6 g) Italian Dressing Mix

1 tablespoon (15 ml) water

2 tablespoons (30 ml) vinegar of choice (see note)

⅓ cup (79 ml) oil of choice, such as walnut (for paleo), or avocado or extra-virgin olive oil (for AIP)

To Make the Italian Dressing Mix

1. Combine all the ingredients in a spice grinder or small food processor and blend to a fine powder. Alternatively, mix the ingredients in a small bowl and stir well to combine without grinding. Pour the dry mix into a small jar with a tight-fitting lid and label it. The dry mix will keep in the pantry for up to 1 year.

To Make the Prepared Dressing

2. Combine the Italian Dressing Mix, water, and vinegar in a 2-cup (473 ml) glass measuring cup. Whisk vigorously with a fork to combine. Slowly drizzle in the oil in a steady stream, whisking constantly to emulsify. Alternately, combine all the ingredients in a jar with a tight-fitting lid and shake vigorously to combine.

For the best flavor, make the dressing at least 30 minutes in advance to allow the flavors to meld. Store the prepared dressing in the refrigerator for up to 2 weeks.

NOTE

My favorite vinegar to use in this dressing is white balsamic, followed by red wine vinegar and regular balsamic. White wine vinegar and apple cider vinegar are also good choices. All of these *can* be AIP-compliant, but be sure to read the labels carefully to avoid added sugars, colorings, flavorings, or noncompliant ingredients.

NIGELLA SEED VINAIGRETTE

This vinaigrette is delicate and versatile, and perfect drizzled over fresh, tender greens with no accoutrements besides, perhaps, toasted nuts and shredded carrot. It makes a small batch, so feel free to double it if you'd like extra dressing for the week. Nigella seeds, also known as black cumin and black caraway, have an aromatic, peppery onion flavor that lightly infuses this vinaigrette. They also contain thymoquinone, a powerful anti-inflammatory compound that may help reduce thyroid gland inflammation and lower thyroid antibodies.

● **GLUTEN-FREE**   ○ **DAIRY-FREE**   ● **PALEO**

DIETARY LEVELS 1, 2

SERVINGS 4

PREP TIME 10 minutes

TOTAL TIME 10 minutes

½ teaspoon nigella seeds

1 teaspoon Dijon mustard

1 teaspoon honey

1 tablespoon (15 ml) champagne vinegar or apple cider vinegar

¼ teaspoon fine sea salt

Pinch white pepper

½ cup (118 ml) walnut or avocado oil

Whisk together the nigella seeds, mustard, honey, vinegar, salt, and white pepper in a 2-cup (473 ml) glass measuring cup. Slowly drizzle in the oil, whisking vigorously with a fork to blend. Pro tip: Start by adding the oil very slowly, just a few drops at a time. After the vinegar mixture starts to absorb the oil and emulsify, you can drizzle in the oil a bit more rapidly. Store in the refrigerator for up to 2 weeks.

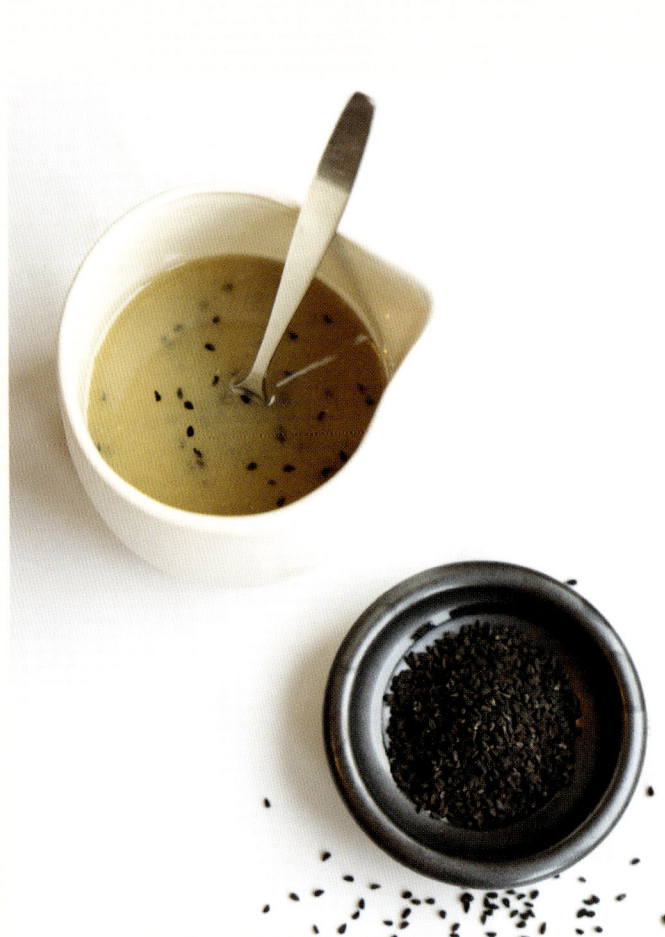

BRAZIL NUT "PARMESAN"

This surprisingly delicious alternative to traditional Parmesan packs a double-whammy of flavor and nutrients. Sprinkle it on your favorite pasta, roasted spaghetti squash, or salads for a healthy dose of thyroid-supportive selenium from Brazil nuts and B vitamins from the nutritional yeast.

● GLUTEN-FREE　● DAIRY-FREE　● PALEO　● VEGAN

DIETARY LEVELS 1, 2

SERVINGS 16
PREP TIME 5 minutes
TOTAL TIME 5 minutes

¾ cup (100 g) Brazil nuts

3 tablespoons (27 g) nutritional yeast

¾ teaspoon fine sea salt

¼ teaspoon garlic powder

¼ teaspoon onion powder

½ teaspoon Italian herb blend or herbs de Provence

Combine all the ingredients in a food processor and process just until the mixture resembles fine crumbs: Be careful not to overprocess into a paste. Store in an airtight container in the refrigerator for up to 3 weeks.

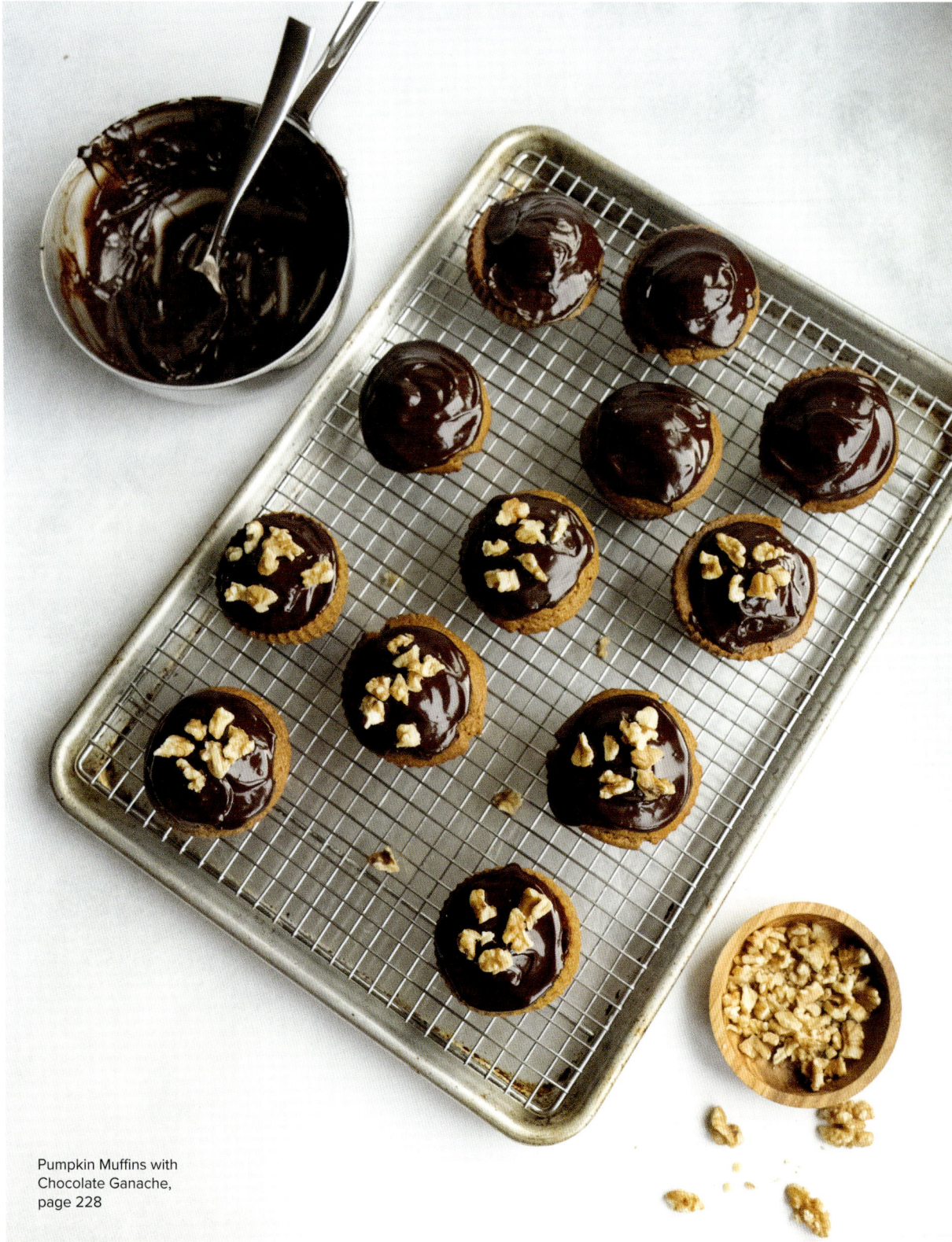

Pumpkin Muffins with
Chocolate Ganache,
page 228

15

Sweets and Sips

Thyroid-healthy eating doesn't have to mean saying goodbye to dessert: It means redefining it. Treats can do a whole lot more than taste good. They don't need to be packed with inflammatory white flour and sugar, and they definitely don't need to leave us feeling regretful or "naughty" after eating them. With a few smart tweaks and strategic additions, treats can fuel and support your body and still be a deliciously irresistible part of your thyroid-friendly menu.

   In this chapter, you'll find a collection of feel-good sweets and hydrating sips that strike a balance between indulgence and intention. Whether you're craving something cool and refreshing, rich and chocolatey, or fruity and fun, the options in the following pages will satisfy your sweet tooth without derailing your wellness goals. From protein-packed blondies to collagen-boosted bonbons and umbrella-worthy mocktails with functional benefits, these recipes are designed to spark joy—the kind that comes from sipping a frosty drink on a warm day, sharing a beautiful berry trifle with friends, and celebrating with treats that make you feel just as good afterward as they do in the moment.

PUMPKIN MUFFINS WITH CHOCOLATE GANACHE

These pumpkin muffins are moist, fluffy, and perfectly spiced, with just the right touch of subtle sweetness. They straddle the line between muffin and cupcake—balanced and not too sugary, but topped with a swirl of silky chocolate ganache that makes them feel extra special. A sprinkle of chopped walnuts or pecans adds the perfect bit of crunch. Chocolate lovers can fold a scoop of chocolate chips into the batter for a little extra decadence. Optional, but delightful.

● GLUTEN-FREE　　● DAIRY-FREE　　● PALEO　　● VEGAN

DIETARY LEVELS 1, 2

SERVINGS 12 muffins
PREP TIME 25 minutes
COOK TIME 20–25 minutes
TOTAL TIME 45–50 minutes + cooling time

FOR MUFFINS

1 cup (245 g) pumpkin puree
(not pumpkin pie filling)

½ cup (72 g) coconut sugar or maple sugar

2 tablespoons (40 g) pure maple syrup

¼ cup (56 g) full-fat coconut milk,
well-shaken

4 large eggs at room temperature

1 teaspoon pure vanilla extract

¼ cup (59 ml) melted unrefined coconut oil,
plus more for greasing

2 cups (192 g) superfine blanched almond flour

⅓ cup (38 g) tapioca flour

1 teaspoon baking soda

1½ teaspoons pumpkin pie spice

½ teaspoon cinnamon

¼ teaspoon fine sea salt

½ cup (88 g) dairy-free chocolate chips,
such as Hu Kitchen or Enjoy Life (optional)

FOR GANACHE FROSTING

⅓ cup (64 g) full-fat coconut milk,
well-shaken

⅔ cup (117 g) dairy-free chocolate chips

2 teaspoons pure maple syrup

Pinch fine sea salt

⅓ cup (40 g) chopped walnuts or toasted
pecans (optional)

To Make the Muffins

1. Preheat the oven to 350°F (175°C). Line a 12-cup muffin tin with paper or silicone cupcake liners. If using silicone liners, coat the insides with coconut oil to prevent sticking.

2. Combine the pumpkin puree, coconut or maple sugar, maple syrup, coconut milk, eggs, and vanilla extract in a large bowl and whisk until smooth. Stir in the coconut oil and whisk to combine.

3. Mix the flours, baking soda, spices, and salt in a separate bowl until well combined. Gradually whisk the dry ingredients into the wet until fully incorporated and no lumps remain. The mixture should have a cake batter consistency. Stir in the chocolate chips, if using.

4. Divide the batter evenly among the 12 prepared muffin cups, filling each almost but not quite full. Depending on the size of your muffin cups, you may have a little extra batter, especially if you add the chocolate chips. Fill the cups just below the rim to avoid overflow, and bake any remaining batter in a second batch.

5. Bake for 20 to 25 minutes or until a toothpick inserted in the center of a muffin comes out clean. Remove the muffins from the oven and let them cool in the pan for 10 minutes. Transfer to a wire rack to cool completely before frosting with chocolate ganache.

To Make the Ganache Frosting

6. Gently heat the coconut milk in a small saucepan over medium-low heat until it just begins to simmer—do not boil. Remove from the heat and add the chocolate chips. Let sit for 2 to 3 minutes to soften. Stir the mixture until smooth and glossy. Add the maple syrup and sea salt and stir to combine. The ganache should have a pudding-like consistency and be thick enough to spread. Dollop and spread the ganache while still warm and glossy atop the cooled muffins with the back of a spoon. Try to use up all the frosting: You won't regret it! Sprinkle with chopped toasted walnuts or pecans while the ganache is still soft, if desired.

The muffins will look and taste their best if kept at room temperature and enjoyed within 1 day, but leftovers may be refrigerated in an airtight container for up to 5 days.

CHERRY LIME GELATIN PARFAITS

This recipe transforms anti-inflammatory, gut-supportive ingredients into a delicious (and much healthier) rendition of a 1980s throwback dessert. Creamy coconut-lime whip adds a luxurious texture while balancing the fruitiness of the cherry gelatin. Tart cherry juice is packed with anthocyanins, powerful antioxidants that help reduce inflammation and support muscle recovery. Studies have shown that it can improve sleep quality by naturally boosting melatonin levels, making this a dessert that's as restorative as it is delicious!

● **GLUTEN-FREE**　　● **DAIRY-FREE**　　● **PALEO**　　● **AIP-FRIENDLY**

DIETARY LEVELS 1, 2, 3

SERVINGS 4

PREP TIME 30 minutes

INACTIVE TIME 4 hours

TOTAL TIME 4½ hours

FOR LIME CREAM

1 (14-ounce [392 g]) can full-fat coconut milk, shaken

2 teaspoons grass-fed gelatin

Pinch fine sea salt

¼ cup (59 ml) fresh lime juice (from about 2 limes)

½ teaspoon lime zest

2 tablespoons (40 g) honey or maple syrup, or to taste

FOR CHERRY GELATIN

2 cups (473 ml) 100 percent tart cherry juice

1 tablespoon (14 g) grass-fed gelatin

OPTIONAL GARNISHES

Lime wheels

Curls of lime zest

Pomegranate arils

Fresh cherries

Fresh mint leaves

To Make the Lime Cream

1. Pour the coconut milk into a small saucepan and sprinkle the gelatin over the top. Let sit for about 5 minutes to allow the gelatin to bloom, then place over medium heat and cook, stirring frequently, just until warmed through and the gelatin has dissolved. Do not boil.

2. Remove the saucepan from the heat and add the salt, lime juice, lime zest, and honey or maple syrup and stir to combine. Taste and adjust sweetness as desired. Pour the mixture into a medium mixing bowl (big enough to whip it in once chilled). Cover and refrigerate for at least 4 hours or until set.

To Make the Cherry Gelatin

3. Pour the tart cherry juice into a small saucepan and sprinkle gelatin over the top. Let sit for about 5 minutes to allow the gelatin to bloom. Place over medium heat and cook, stirring frequently, just until warmed through and the gelatin has dissolved. Do not boil. Remove the saucepan from the heat and divide the mixture evenly among 4 medium glasses. Refrigerate until set, at least 4 hours or overnight.

4. Assemble the parfaits. After the lime cream and cherry gelatin have set, beat the lime cream with an electric mixer on high speed until light and fluffy, about 2 to 3 minutes, stopping to scrape down the bowl. (It will start out chunky but will smooth out as it whips.) Spoon or pipe the whipped lime cream evenly over the cherry gelatin in each glass. Garnish as desired and enjoy! This dessert can be prepared up to 2 days in advance and will keep for up to 4 days in the refrigerator.

STRAWBERRY COLLAGEN BONBONS

You can't go wrong with the classic flavor combination of chocolate and strawberries. Dehydrated strawberries give these bonbons lots of pure fruit flavor without adding refined sugar or dairy, and they're also rich in vitamin C, which makes them the perfect partner for a dose of collagen, another key ingredient in these treats. Pairing collagen with a vitamin C–rich food like strawberries enhances its absorption and maximizes its benefits. And that's great news for Thyroid Thrivers, because collagen supports healthy skin, joints, and gut health, all of which can be impacted by thyroid disease.

● GLUTEN-FREE   ● DAIRY-FREE   ● PALEO

DIETARY LEVELS 1, 2

SERVINGS 12–15 bonbons
PREP TIME 30 minutes
INACTIVE TIME 30 minutes
TOTAL TIME 1 hour

1 cup (170 g) dehydrated strawberries

½ cup (109 g) coconut butter

½ cup (48 g) superfine almond flour

¼ cup (80 g) pure maple syrup

¼ cup (50 g) collagen powder

½ teaspoon lemon zest

1 teaspoon fresh lemon juice

⅛ teaspoon ground ginger

⅛ teaspoon cinnamon

1 teaspoon vanilla extract

Pinch fine sea salt

4 ounces (113 g) high-quality dairy-free dark chocolate (not chips), finely chopped

1. Place the dehydrated strawberries in a small food processor and blend to a fine powder. Add the remaining ingredients except the chocolate and blend to combine, stopping as needed to scrape down the sides of the bowl. The texture will be like cookie dough. Taste and adjust the mixture as desired.

2. You can either roll the mixture by hand into 1-inch (2.5 cm) balls or use a silicone mold to create shapes of your choice. Place in the freezer until firm, about 20 to 30 minutes.

3. Line a baking sheet with parchment paper.

4. Once the strawberry filling is firm, melt the chocolate. Place the chocolate in a small, microwaveable bowl. Microwave at 30-second intervals, stirring between each, just until chocolate is melted. Use 2 forks to dip each strawberry bonbon into the melted chocolate. Let the excess drip off, then place on the prepared baking sheet. Let sit until the chocolate has cooled and hardened. The bonbons can be refrigerated for up to 1 week or frozen for up to 3 months.

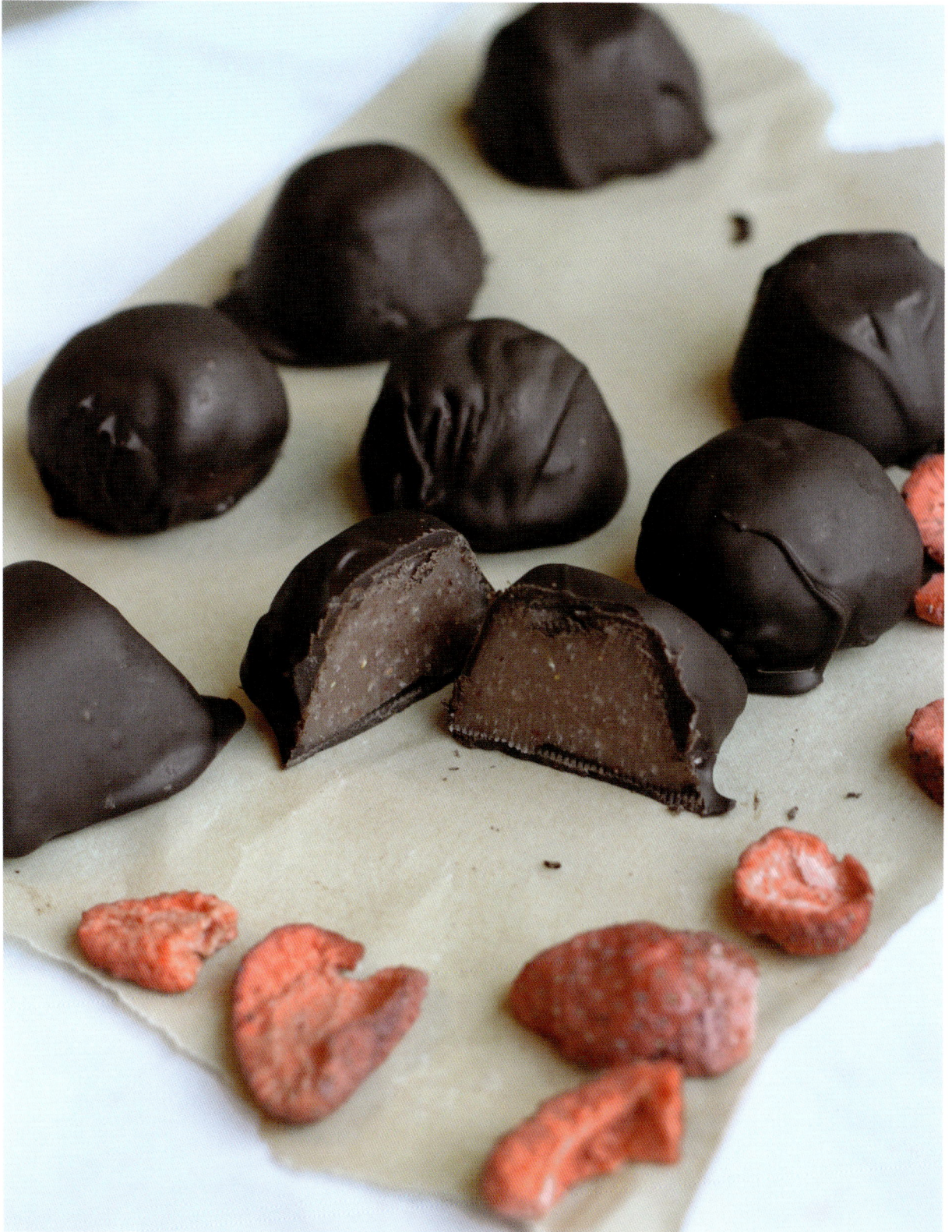

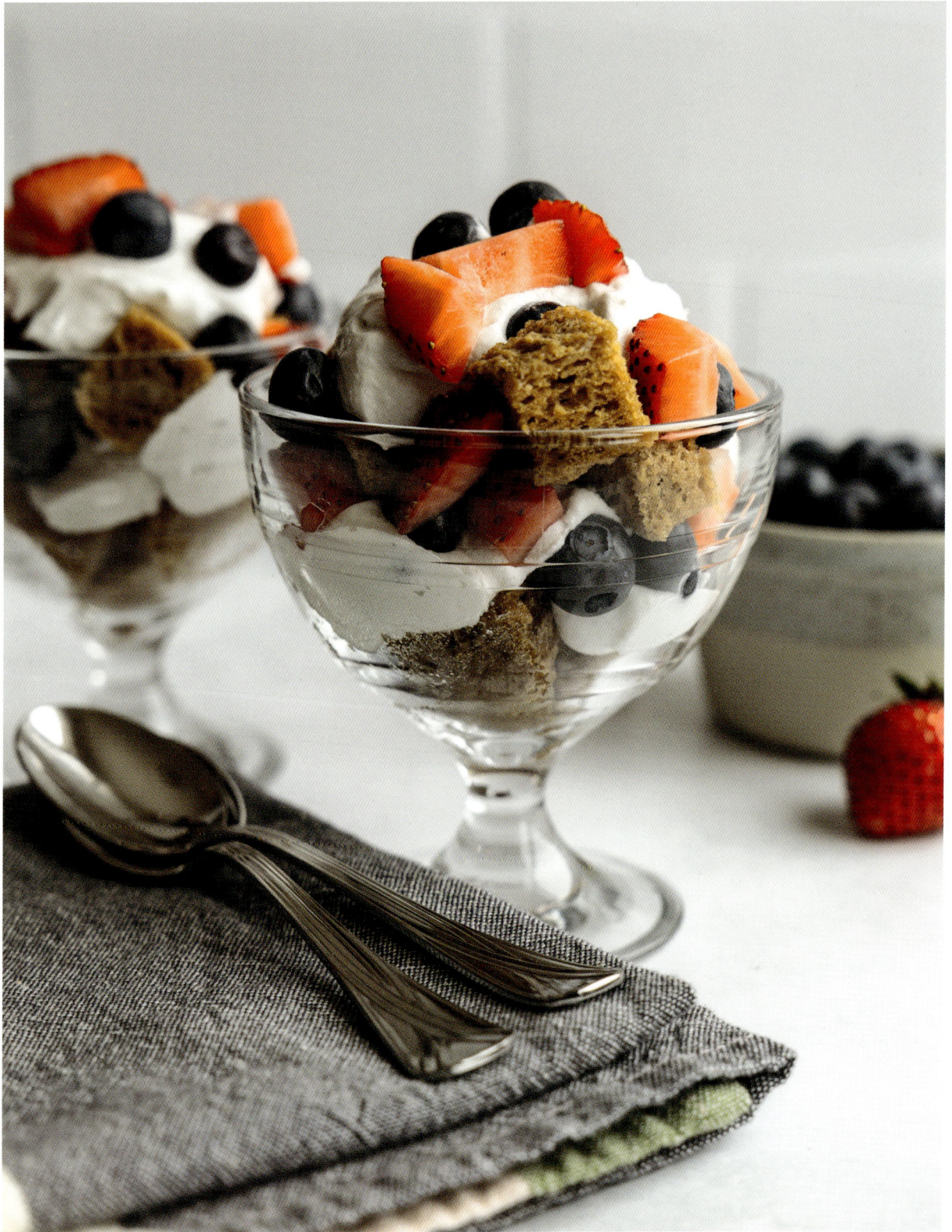

FRESH BERRY TRIFLE

Fluffy cubes of lemony almond cake, fresh berries, and cloudlike coconut cream combine to create this quick and easy dessert. For a convenient nonpaleo option, replace the homemade whipped coconut cream with a 9-ounce (270 g) tub of frozen dairy-free coconut whipped topping such as Cocowhip.

● **GLUTEN-FREE**   ● **DAIRY-FREE**   ● **PALEO**

DIETARY LEVELS 1, 2

SERVINGS 4
PREP TIME 30 minutes
COOK TIME 4 minutes
TOTAL TIME 34 minutes, plus cooling time

FOR CAKE

2 tablespoons (30 ml) melted unrefined coconut oil, plus more for greasing

2 eggs

1 tablespoon (15 ml) fresh lemon juice

½ teaspoon lemon zest

2 tablespoons (18 g) coconut sugar

1 teaspoon vanilla extract

¼ cup (24 g) plus 2 tablespoons (6 g) superfine almond flour

1 tablespoon (7 g) tapioca flour

½ teaspoon baking soda

¼ teaspoon fine sea salt

FOR PALEO-COMPLIANT WHIPPED COCONUT CREAM

1 (13.5-ounce [398 ml]) can heavy coconut cream, such as Let's Do Organic, chilled overnight

1 tablespoon (20 g) maple syrup

½ teaspoon vanilla extract

FOR ASSEMBLY

2 cups (290 g) fresh berries of choice

Fresh mint leaves (optional)

To Make the Cake

1. Grease a 7-inch (18 cm) round or 5 x 7-inch (12.7 x 18 cm) glass or ceramic microwave-safe baking dish with coconut oil.

2. Whisk the eggs vigorously in a small mixing bowl. Add the lemon juice, zest, coconut sugar, vanilla, and melted coconut oil. Combine the almond flour, tapioca flour, baking soda, and salt in a separate bowl and whisk well. Slowly add the dry ingredients to the wet, whisking until you have a smooth batter.

3. Pour the batter into the prepared baking dish. Microwave at 60 percent power for 3 to 4 minutes, checking for doneness by gently pressing the center. The cake will rise as it cooks, and it should spring back and feel dry to the touch. If it's still tacky, microwave in additional 30-second increments. Let the cake cool completely before cutting into small cubes for the trifle.

To Make the Paleo-Compliant Whipped Coconut Cream

4. Scoop the solid portion of the chilled coconut cream into a medium mixing bowl, reserving the liquid portion. Whip with a hand mixer fitted with the whisk attachment at high speed until fluffy. Add the maple syrup and vanilla extract and whip again to combine. Taste and adjust sweetness as desired. If the mixture is too thick, whip in 1 teaspoon of the reserved coconut liquid at a time until you reach the desired consistency. Skip this step if using store-bought whipped coconut cream.

To Assemble

5. Divide half of the cubed cake evenly between four 8- to 12-ounce (237–355 ml) glasses. Top with a generous dollop of whipped coconut cream and some of the berries. Repeat the layers, finishing with a final layer of berries. Top each serving with fresh mint (if using), and enjoy!

CHOCOLATE ALMOND PROTEIN BLONDIES

Who can turn down an ooey, gooey, chewy blondie? Luckily there's no reason to, because these are packed with nourishing ingredients and boast 10 grams of protein per serving, making them a perfect snack or post-workout treat.

● **GLUTEN-FREE**   ◐ **DAIRY-FREE**   ● **PALEO**

DIETARY LEVELS 1, 2

SERVINGS 12
PREP TIME 15 minutes
COOK TIME 30 minutes
TOTAL TIME 45 minutes, plus cooling time

¼ cup (54 g) unrefined coconut oil, melted, plus more for greasing

½ cup (128 g) almond butter

½ cup (161 g) maple syrup

2 eggs

2 teaspoons vanilla extract

1 teaspoon cinnamon

¼ teaspoon fine sea salt

½ cup (50 g) powdered collagen peptides

1 cup (96 g) almond flour

2 tablespoons (14 g) coconut flour

½ cup (88 g) + 2 tablespoons (22 g) paleo-compliant chocolate chips

Flaky sea salt for topping (optional)

1. Preheat the oven to 325°F (163°C). Grease an 8 x 8-inch (20 x 20 cm) square baking dish with coconut oil and line with parchment paper, leaving the parchment paper long to overhang the edges for easy removal.

2. Combine the wet ingredients in a medium bowl and stir until smooth and well mixed.

3. Combine the cinnamon, salt, collagen peptides, almond flour, and coconut flour in a separate bowl. Whisk until combined and no lumps remain. Add the dry ingredients to the wet and stir to combine. Stir ½ cup (88 g) of the chocolate chips into the mixture.

4. Pour the batter into the prepared baking dish and sprinkle with the remaining 2 tablespoons (22 g) of chocolate chips and flaky sea salt (if using). Bake in the center of the oven for 25 to 30 minutes or until the edges are golden brown and the center feels set to the touch.

5. Let cool completely before cutting into 12 squares. Store leftovers in an airtight container in the fridge for up to 1 week or freeze for up to 2 months.

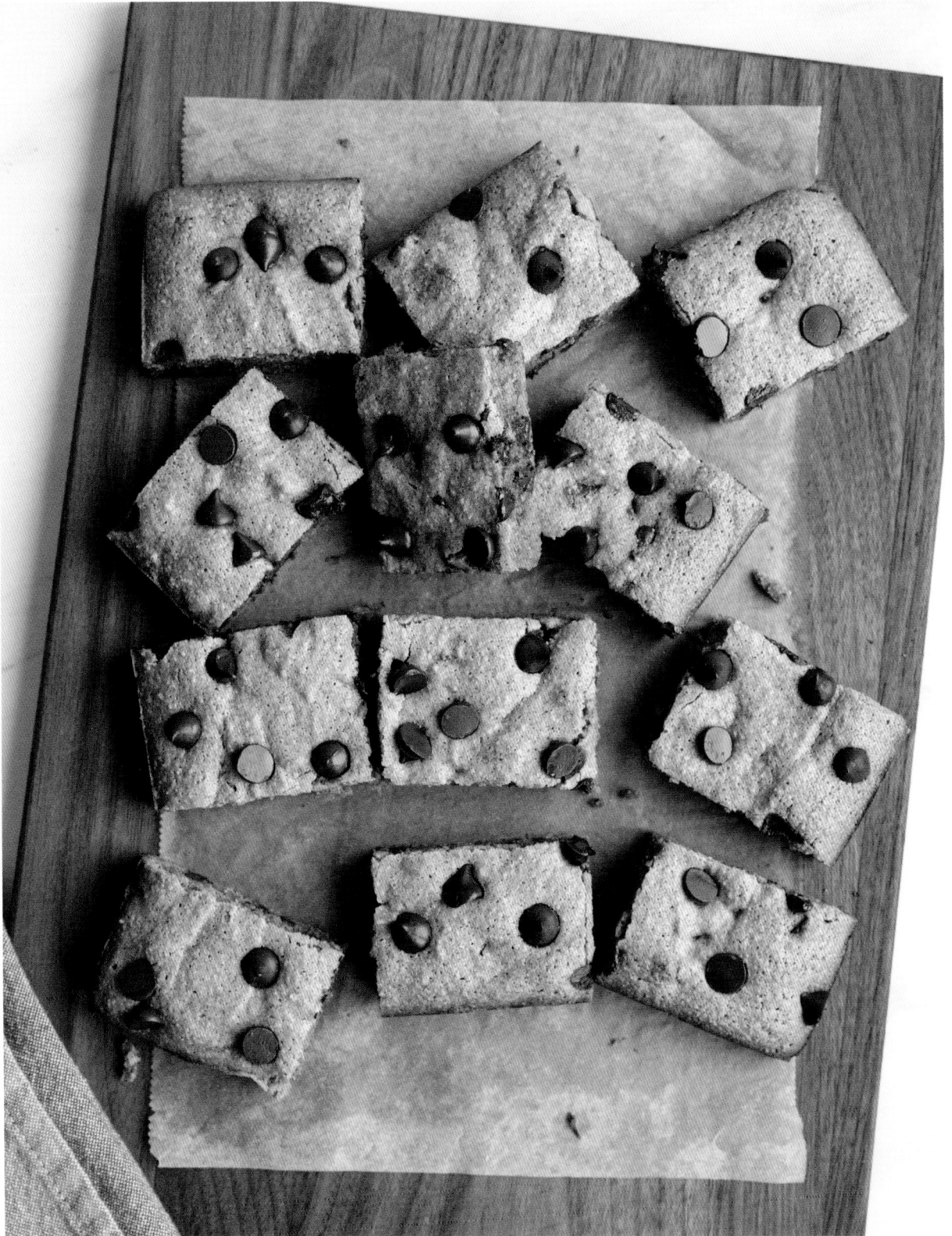

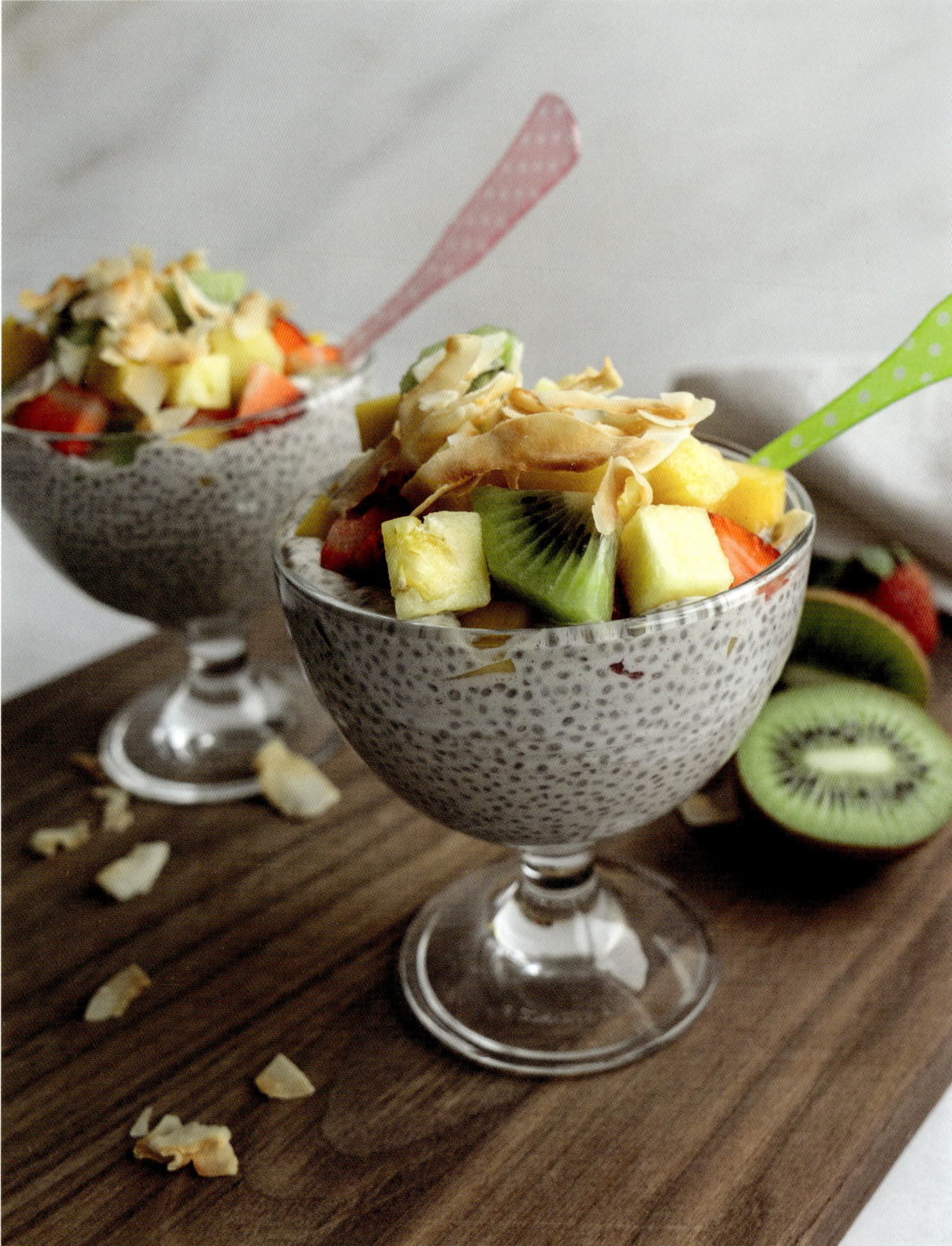

TROPICAL DELIGHT CHIA PUDDING

If you like piña coladas . . . then you'll love this chia pudding! Coconut milk is a dairy-free staple rich in medium-chain triglycerides (MCTs), which are renowned for their brain-, energy-, and weight loss–boosting benefits. It also happens to taste amazing, so here we're going to fully embrace its flavor and top it with an assortment of tropical fruit. Add a bit of crunch with some toasted wide-gauge coconut flakes and get ready to enjoy this mini-vacation in a bowl!

● **GLUTEN-FREE**   ● **DAIRY-FREE**   ● **PALEO**   ● **VEGAN**

DIETARY LEVELS 1, 2, 3

SERVINGS 3
PREP TIME 15 minutes
INACTIVE TIME 4 hours
TOTAL TIME 4 hours, 15 minutes

1 (14-ounce [392 g]) can full-fat coconut milk

2 tablespoons (40 g) maple syrup

¼ teaspoon ground cinnamon

¼ teaspoon ground cardamom

½ teaspoon vanilla extract

Pinch fine sea salt

⅓ cup (59 g) chia seeds

1½ cups (218–248 g) diced tropical fruit, such as pineapple, mango, bananas, kiwi, or papaya

2 tablespoons (10 g) wide coconut flakes, toasted (optional)

1. Whisk together the coconut milk, maple syrup, cinnamon, cardamom, vanilla, and salt in a medium mixing bowl until fully combined. Add the chia seeds and whisk vigorously to prevent clumping. Taste and adjust sweetness if desired.

2. Transfer the mixture to an airtight container and refrigerate for at least 4 hours, stirring halfway through to ensure even thickening.

3. Stir the pudding well, then scoop into serving bowls. Top with your favorite tropical fruits, garnish with toasted coconut flakes (if using), and enjoy!

ENERGIZING GREEN GODDESS SMOOTHIE

Feeling low, fatigued, or like you need a mini-cleanse? This energizing smoothie will fix you right up! Between the electrolyte-rich coconut water, the detoxifying cilantro and cucumber, the zippy ginger, the zingy lemon, and the subtle sweetness of pineapple and dates, this blend is the pick-me-up you're looking for. This recipe can easily be doubled so that you can have a grab-and-go snack at the ready for the next day. Want a protein boost? Add a scoop of your favorite protein powder (see page 247 for recommendations).

● **GLUTEN-FREE**   ● **DAIRY-FREE**   ● **PALEO**   ● **AIP-FRIENDLY**   ● **VEGAN**

DIETARY LEVELS 1, 2, 3

SERVINGS 1
PREP TIME 10 minutes
INACTIVE TIME 10 minutes
(for optional seed soaking)
TOTAL TIME 20 minutes

1 cup (237 ml) no-sugar-added coconut water

½ cup (85 g) frozen pineapple

½ cup (68 g) chopped cucumber

½ small avocado

⅓ cup (63 g) frozen spinach

¼ cup (4 g) fresh cilantro (optional)

Juice of ½ lemon

½-inch (1.3 cm) piece fresh ginger, peeled and sliced

1 pitted Medjool date, roughly chopped

½–1 tablespoon (5–11 g) chia seeds or ground flaxseeds (optional, omit for AIP)

Place all the ingredients except the seeds (if using) in a high-speed blender and blend until smooth. If using chia or flaxseeds, stir them into the smoothie after blending. Let sit for at least 10 minutes to allow the seeds to gel for easier digestion. Pour into a glass or to-go jar, sip, and enjoy your refreshing energy boost!

ANTI-INFLAMMATORY CHERRY ALMOND SMOOTHIE

Cherries and almonds are BFFs when it comes to flavor pairing. (The secret to great cherry pie? Almond extract!) This smoothie leverages that pairing for a rich, creamy, and anti-inflammatory blend. Why soak the almonds? It makes their nutrients more bioavailable and easier to digest and also softens them for a creamier smoothie.

● **GLUTEN-FREE**   ● **DAIRY-FREE**   ● **PALEO**   ● **VEGAN**

DIETARY LEVELS 1, 2

SERVINGS 2

PREP TIME 10 minutes, plus an overnight soak for the almonds

TOTAL TIME 10 minutes, plus overnight

2 cups (473 ml) filtered water

1 teaspoon fine sea salt

½ cup (73 g) raw almonds

2 cups (490 g) frozen cherries

¼ teaspoon almond extract

1 cup (237 ml) no-sugar-added, additive-free almond milk, coconut milk, or coconut water

1 banana

Protein powder of choice (optional, see page 247 for recommendations)

Up to 2 tablespoons (22 g) ground flaxseed or chia seeds (optional)

1. Combine filtered water with fine sea salt in a small mixing bowl, stirring to dissolve the salt. Rinse the almonds to remove any dust or debris, then add to the mixing bowl. Refrigerate for 8 to 12 hours or overnight.

2. Drain and rinse the almonds and add to a high-powered blender, along with the cherries; almond extract; almond milk, coconut milk, or coconut water; and banana. Blend on high speed for 1 to 2 minutes or until completely smooth. Stir in protein powder and ground flaxseed or chia seeds, if desired. If adding seeds, let the smoothie sit for 10 minutes before drinking to allow the seeds to gel, aiding digestion.

3. Pour into glasses and enjoy immediately. Leftovers can be stored in an airtight jar in the fridge for up to 24 hours.

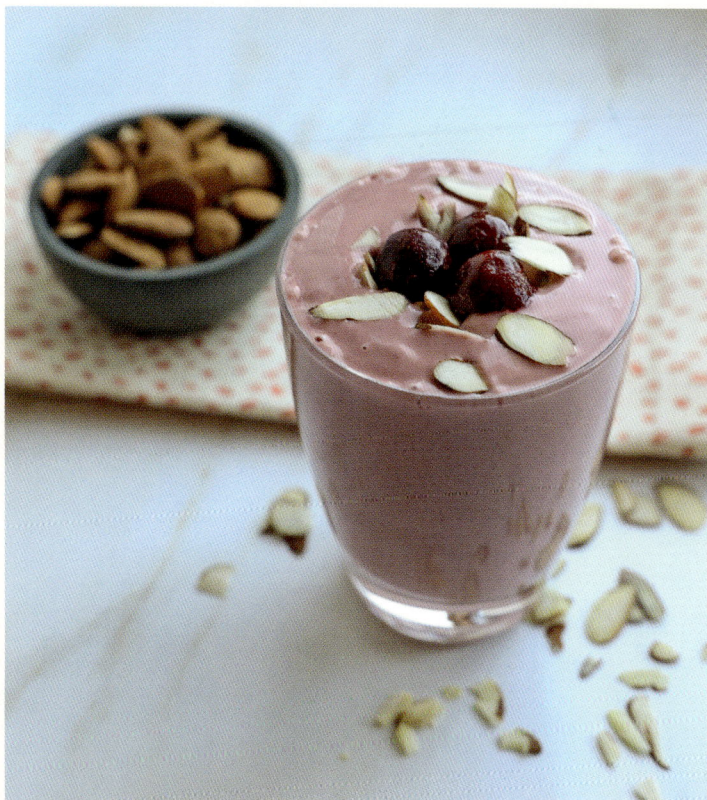

THYROID-FRIENDLY, SUGAR-SMART SMOOTHIES

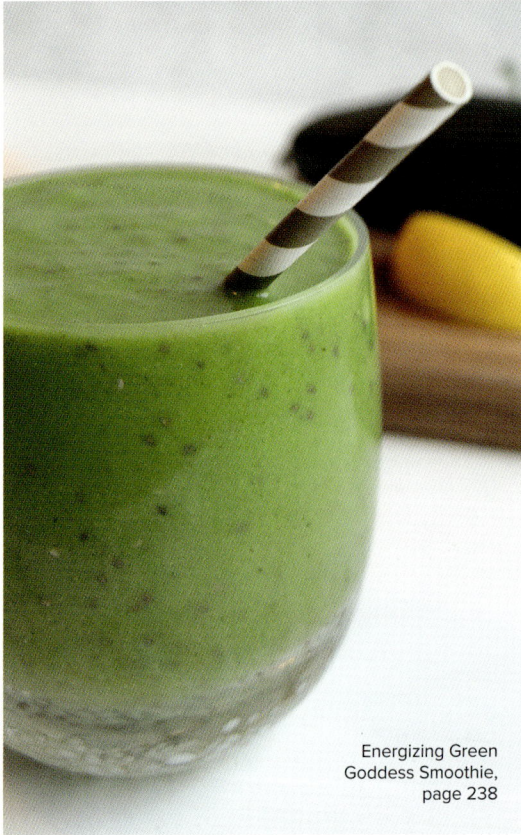

Energizing Green Goddess Smoothie, page 238

Smoothies have gotten a bad rep for being total sugar bombs, but they don't have to be! In fact, they can be a powerful way to support your body with a blast of phytonutrients, antioxidants, and the healthy carbs required for proper thyroid function. Balance is key, though, so here's how to craft and enjoy smoothies in a way that will keep you nourished and satisfied while avoiding the big blood sugar spikes and crashes that can zap your energy.

1. **Be Mindful of Sugar Content**

   - When possible, balance fruits with veggies, or use lower-sugar fruits like berries or kiwi.

   - Consider using green bananas instead of ripe ones for lower sugar and a higher dose of prebiotic (microbiome-supporting) fiber.

   - For liquid, choose water, unsweetened dairy-free milk (like coconut, almond, macadamia, and so on), or no-sugar-added coconut water instead of high-sugar fruit juices.

2. **Prioritize Protein**

   - Protein helps stabilize blood sugar, maintain lean muscle mass, and keeps you full. It also provides a counterweight to balance the healthy carbs in smoothies.

   - Add a scoop of your favorite thyroid-friendly protein powder to your smoothie (see page 247 for recommendations).

   - If you're not adding protein directly to your smoothie, serve the smoothie with a protein-rich side like Zesty Homemade Breakfast Sausage Patties (page 107) or a hard-boiled egg.

HIGH-SUGAR ADDITIONS	LOW-SUGAR ADDITIONS
Ripe bananas	Green bananas
Mango	Raspberries
Pears	Strawberries
Pomegranate	Blackberries
Cherries	Blueberries
Grapes	Kiwi
Figs	Cucumber
	Lemons
	Avocado

HIGH-FIBER SMOOTHIE INGREDIENTS

Avocado	10 g fiber/cup
Blackberries	8 g fiber/cup
Raspberries	8 g fiber/cup
Chia Seeds	6 g fiber/tablespoon
Blueberries	4 g fiber/cup
Banana	3 g fiber/medium banana
Strawberries	3 g fiber/cup
Flaxseed	2–3 g fiber/tablespoon

3. **Include Healthy Fats**

    • Fats slow digestion, balance blood sugar, keep you satisfied, and support hormone health.

    • Smoothie-friendly healthy fat options include avocado, nut and seed butters, canned coconut milk, chia seeds, or ground flaxseed.

    • It doesn't take much! Just a quarter of an avocado or a teaspoon or tablespoon of more concentrated fat sources per serving can be enough.

4. **Don't Forget the Fiber**

    • Consuming fiber is another way to keep blood sugar balanced while also supporting gut health, digestion, and satiety.

    • Smoothies often contain a good dose of fiber on their own, but they can be a great vehicle for supplemental sources of fiber like chia seeds, ground flaxseed, or psyllium husk. Remember to space high-fiber meals away from your thyroid medication for maximum absorption.

    • Plant-based protein powders are often high in fiber, so if you're using one, check the label to see how much fiber it contains.

5. **Be Smart About Goitrogens**

    • Goitrogenic foods such as cruciferous vegetables can impact iodine absorption and, therefore, thyroid function, but are safe in moderation.

    • Cooking or fermenting destroys or reduces goitrogenic compounds in most foods, so the rule of thumb is to enjoy goitrogenic foods cooked whenever possible.

    • An easy smoothie hack: Frozen vegetables are preblanched (cooked)! Save time and reduce your goitrogen consumption by using frozen rather than raw greens and cruciferous veggies (that is, kale, spinach, cauliflower) for smoothies.

NOTE: SMOOTHIES MAY NOT BE RIGHT FOR SOME PEOPLE

Thyroid patients are unfortunately more prone to gut health issues like intestinal permeability (that is, leaky gut), SIBO, and gut dysbiosis (an overgrowth of bad gut bacteria). Individuals who are coping with these issues might find the combination of increased fiber and raw (as opposed to cooked) fruits and vegetables difficult to digest and may experience bloating and discomfort as a result. If so, cooked alternatives like pureed soups may be better tolerated and easier to digest.

WATERMELON LIME CHIA FRESCA

Inspired by both agua fresca and chia fresca, this naturally hydrating beverage is the kind of thing you'll want to sip poolside: It's like a mini-vacay in a glass. Watermelon, coconut water, and sea salt provide natural electrolytes, while lime juice balances the sweetness with a citrusy burst of vitamin C. Chia seeds—which are surprisingly drinkable, thanks to their gel-like texture—lend plenty of fiber and a dose of omega-3s. You'll barely notice they're there, especially if you use a straw for stirring and sipping. In this watermelon-pink drink, they even resemble tiny watermelon seeds, which adds a fun visual touch. Prefer to skip them? Feel free: This drink is delicious either way.

● **GLUTEN-FREE**   ● **DAIRY-FREE**   ● **PALEO**   ● **VEGAN**

DIETARY LEVELS 1, 2

SERVINGS 4
(makes 4 cups [946 ml])

PREP TIME 10 minutes, plus 10 minutes for the chia seeds to soak

TOTAL TIME 20 minutes

3 cups (450 g) cubed watermelon, seedless or with seeds removed

1½ cups (355 ml) unsweetened, additive-free coconut water

Juice of 1½ limes, plus more as needed

1–2 teaspoons pure maple syrup, or to taste (optional)

¼ teaspoon fine sea salt

1 tablespoon (11 g) chia seeds

Ice, for serving

Lime wedges or wheels (optional)

1. Combine the watermelon, coconut water, lime juice, maple syrup (if using), and sea salt in a blender. Blend until smooth.

2. For a smoother texture, pour the mixture through a fine-mesh sieve, pressing gently with a silicone spatula to extract the juice. (Skip this step if you don't mind pulp!)

3. Stir in the chia seeds and let the mixture sit for at least 10 minutes to allow the chia seeds to gel, making them easier to digest. Taste and adjust the flavor with additional sweetener or lime juice if needed. Stir well before pouring over ice, and garnish with lime wedges or wheels, if desired. Store leftovers in a glass pitcher or jar and refrigerate for up to 3 days: Just shake or stir before serving!

GINGER APPLE SWITCHEL

Switchel just might be the original sports drink! Back in the eighteenth and nineteenth centuries it was often called "Haymaker's Punch" because it was enjoyed by farmers during the long, hot days of the hay harvest. They drank it to stay hydrated and replenish electrolyte minerals supplied by the vinegar, lemon juice, and honey or maple syrup. Today, switchel is a great way to get those same minerals and a palatable dose of blood sugar–balancing, gut-supportive, unfiltered apple cider vinegar. This version plays off those cidery notes with complementary spices and a touch of regular apple cider!

● **GLUTEN-FREE**   ● **DAIRY-FREE**   ● **PALEO**   ● **AIP-FRIENDLY**

DIETARY LEVELS 1, 2, 3

SERVINGS 5
(about 5 cups [1.2 L])

PREP TIME 5 minutes

COOK TIME 10 minutes

TOTAL TIME 15 minutes

4 cups (946 ml) filtered water, divided

2-inch (5 cm) piece fresh ginger root, thinly sliced

1 small cinnamon stick

1–2 tablespoons (20–40 g) honey, or to taste

1 cup (237 ml) apple cider or unsweetened apple juice

¼ cup (60 ml) unfiltered apple cider vinegar with the mother

1 tablespoon (15 ml) fresh lemon juice

1. Combine 1½ cups (355 ml) of the water with the ginger and cinnamon stick in a small saucepan. Bring to a boil, reduce the heat, cover, and simmer for about 10 minutes.

2. Remove from the heat and discard the ginger and cinnamon. Let cool slightly. While the liquid is still warm, stir in the honey until fully dissolved.

3. Combine the remaining 2½ cups (591 ml) of water, apple cider or juice, apple cider vinegar, and lemon juice in a pitcher and stir in the ginger-cinnamon infusion.

4. Refrigerate for at least 1 hour or overnight for a more well-balanced flavor, then pour over ice and enjoy!

CUCUMBER LIME INFUSION MOCKTAIL

Cucumber, lime, and ginger come together in this light and delicately flavored libation. Topped with chilled sparkling mineral water, it's crisp, hydrating, not too sweet, and perfect for warm weather!

● **GLUTEN-FREE**　　● **DAIRY-FREE**　　● **PALEO**　　● **AIP-FRIENDLY**

DIETARY LEVELS 1, 2, 3

SERVINGS About 6
PREP TIME 15 minutes
TOTAL TIME 15 minutes

1 medium cucumber, washed, unpeeled, and roughly chopped

1 cup (237 ml) no-sugar-added, additive-free coconut water

⅓ cup (79 ml) fresh lime juice (from 2–3 limes)

3-inch (7.6 cm) piece fresh ginger, peeled and sliced into coins

¼ cup (85 g) raw honey

Pinch fine sea salt

Ice cubes

32 ounces (4 cups [946 ml]) chilled, unflavored, additive-free sparkling mineral water, such as Sanpellegrino, Gerolsteiner, or Topo Chico

Freshly sliced lime or cucumber wheels (optional)

1. Combine the cucumber, coconut water, lime juice, ginger, honey, and sea salt in a blender. Blend on low to medium speed until *almost* but not fully pureed (this makes straining easier).

2. Place a fine-mesh strainer over a small mixing bowl. Pour the blended mixture through the strainer, pressing with a silicone spatula to extract as much liquid as possible.

3. Fill six 12-ounce (355 ml) glasses with ice. Pour about ⅓ cup (79 ml) of the strained mixture into each glass. Top each with about ⅔ cup (158 ml) sparkling water and stir to combine. Garnish with freshly sliced lime or cucumber wheels, if desired. The cucumber concentrate will keep refrigerated for up to 5 days when stored in an airtight jar: Add the sparkling water just before serving.

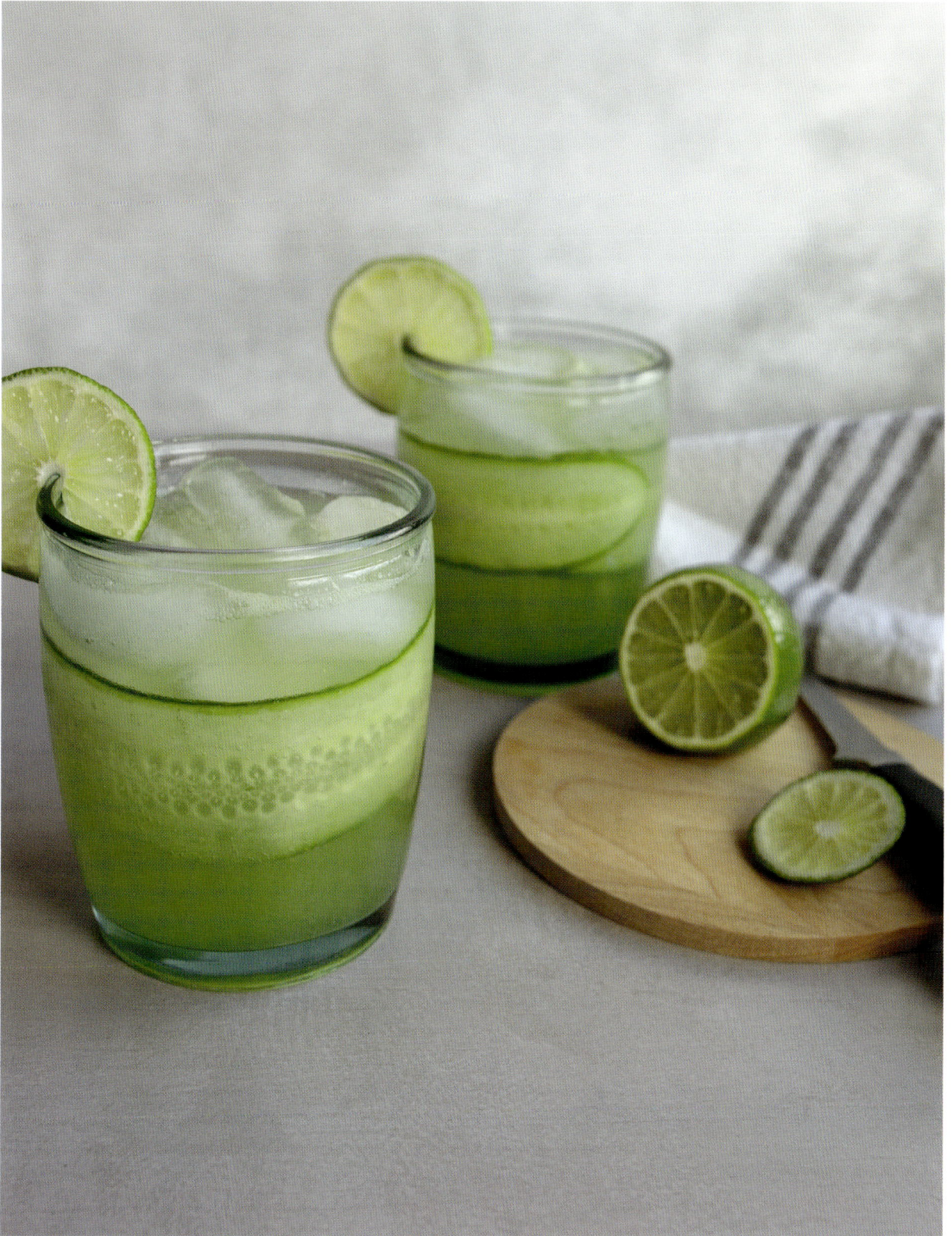

THYROID30
Support and Resources

YOU DID IT! You made it to the end of *The THYROID30 Cookbook.* Whether you're just getting started or already thriving, this chapter is your launchpad for turning inspiration into transformation. These hand-picked resources are designed to help you stay supported, inspired, and well-provisioned as you continue your THYROID30 journey.

Start Here: Your THYROID30 Support Hub

Visit the official resource page for cookbook readers: hypothyroidchef.com/cookbook

You'll find:

- Printable THYROID30 score sheets and digital trackers
- Bonus videos and tools to support your 30-day journey
- Details on how to join the Thrivers Club and participate in THYROID30 as part of a supportive community

JOIN US IN THE THRIVERS CLUB!

hypothyroidchef.com/membership

The Thrivers Club is where THYROID30 and the 8 Daily Rituals come to life! In our private membership community, you can:

- Participate in THYROID30 with a supportive group of fellow Thyroid Thrivers
- Access coaching, workshops, and meal plans
- Connect with others who get it
- Stay consistent and get ongoing support beyond THYROID30

Find-a-Thyroid-Doctor and At-Home Testing Resources

Sometimes the missing piece of the puzzle is a great practitioner or reliable labs. Here are trusted resources to help you take the next step:

- Functional Medicine Provider Directory, The Institute for Functional Medicine: ifm.org/find-a-practitioner
- Virtual Thyroid Care and Testing (United States only), Paloma Health: palomahealth.com
- At-Home Thyroid Testing (International), Let's Get Checked: letsgetchecked.com

Pantry Staples and Resources

These products are useful culinary tools for Thyroid Thrivers, and many of them can be used to prepare the recipes throughout this book.

- Bacon (uncured, sugar-free): Applegate Naturals, Pederson's Naturals, US Wellness Meats

- Bread (gluten-free): Canyon Bakehouse

- Bone broth: Bare Bones, Bonafide, Kettle & Fire

- Cacao powder or nibs: Nutiva

- Cereal (AIP): Lovebird

- Chia seeds: Nutiva

- Chocolate chips: Enjoy Life (dairy- and allergen-free), Hu Chocolate (paleo)

- Coconut aminos: Big Tree Farms

- Coconut cream: Let's Do Organic

- Coconut milk: Native Forest

- Coconut oil (organic, unrefined): Nutiva, Spectrum Culinary

- Coconut water (no sugar added): Harmless Harvest, Kirkland Organic No-Sugar-Added

- Coconut whipped topping (dairy-free): Cocowhip by So Delicious

- Collagen peptides: Great Lakes Wellness, Vital Proteins

- Crackers: Mary's Gone Crackers (gluten-free), Simple Mills (grain-free, paleo), Sweetpotato Awesome (AIP)

- Creamer (dairy-free, Paleo): Nut Pods

- Eggs (organic, pasture-raised): Vital Farms

- Fermented pickles and sauerkraut: Bubbies Fine Foods, Olive My Pickle, Wildbrine

- Ghee: 4th & Heart (grass-fed), Organic Valley (pasture-raised)

- Gluten-free all-purpose flour blends: Bob's Red Mill, King Arthur Measure for Measure, Thomas Keller's Cup4Cup

- Granola (grain-free): Autumn's Gold, Coconola

- Hot sauce (paleo): Tabasco (original), Chipotle Tabasco, Crystal, Frank's Red Hot

- Ice cream (dairy-free, check label to ensure gluten-free): Cosmic Bliss, So Delicious

- Mayonnaise: Follow Your Heart Soy-Free Vegenaise (egg-free, soy-free, vegan), Primal Kitchen or Sir Kensington's Avocado Oil Mayo (paleo)

- Meat sticks and snacks (grass-fed): Chomps, Epic Bison Bars, Paleo Valley

- Milk (dairy-free, paleo): Malk, Milkadamia, Three Trees

- Miso (organic, soy-free): Miso Master Chickpea Miso

- Nut butters: Artisana, MaraNatha, NuttZo

- Nutritional yeast: Lewis Labs (certified gluten-free)

- Oils: Spectrum Culinary

- Pasta (gluten- and/or grain-free): Jovial

- Pizza crust: Capello's Almond Flour Crust (paleo), Caulipower (gluten-free)

- Plantain chips: Artisan Tropic, Barnana

- Prosciutto di Parma: Products with this protected "di Parma" designation of origin (PDO) have no ingredients other than pork and sea salt.

- Protein powder: Be Well by Kelly, EarthChimp (plant-based), Equip: Prime (grass-fed beef-based)

- Pumpkin seeds: Go Raw (sprouted)

- Salami (uncured, sugar-free): Applegate Naturals

- Salt: Maldon Sea Salt Flakes (finishing salt), Selina Naturally Celtic Sea Salt (fine ground, for general use)

- Sambal oelek (paleo): Sky Valley

- Snack bars: Lara Bars (gluten-free), Rx Bars (paleo)

- Sriracha (Paleo): Yellowbird

- Sunflower seeds: Go Raw (sprouted)

- Tahini (organic): Artisana, Seed + Mill, Woodstock

- Tea and coffee alternatives: Pique, Sip Herbals

- Tortillas and tortilla chips (grain-free): Siete Foods

- Water filter: The Epic Water Filters Pure Filter removes thyroid-disrupting chemicals like chlorine and fluoride without stripping essential minerals. Rated #1 by the Environmental Working Group.

BIBLIOGRAPHY

Abbott, Robert D., Adam Sadowski, and Angela G. Alt. "Efficacy of the Autoimmune Protocol Diet as Part of a Multi-disciplinary, Supported Lifestyle Intervention for Hashimoto's Thyroiditis." *Cureus,* April 27, 2019. https://doi.org/10.7759/cureus.4556.

American Thyroid Association. "General Information/Press Room | American Thyroid Association," February 12, 2024. www.thyroid.org/media-main/press-room.

Bolk, Nanne, Wilmar M. Wiersinga, Henk F. Fliers, Peter J. Tijssen, and A. Anton M. Prummel. "Effects of Evening vs Morning Levothyroxine Intake: A Randomized Double-Blind Crossover Trial." *Archives of Internal Medicine* 170, no. 22 (2010): 1996–2003. https://jamanetwork.com/journals/jamainternalmedicine/fullarticle/776486.

Capriello, Silvia, Ilaria Stramazzo, Maria Flavia Bagaglini, Nunzia Brusca, Camilla Virili, and Marco Centanni. "The Relationship Between Thyroid Disorders and Vitamin A: A Narrative Minireview." *Frontiers in Endocrinology* 13 (October 11, 2022). https://doi.org/10.3389/fendo.2022.968215.

Cleveland Clinic. "SIBO (Small Intestinal Bacterial Overgrowth)," March 19, 2025. https://my.clevelandclinic.org/health/diseases/21820-small-intestinal-bacterial-overgrowth-sibo.

Galanty, Agnieszka, Marta Grudzińska, Wojciech Paździora, Piotr Służały, and Paweł Paśko. "Do Brassica Vegetables Affect Thyroid Function?—A Comprehensive Systematic Review." *International Journal of Molecular Sciences* 25, no. 7 (April 3, 2024): 3988. https://doi.org/10.3390/ijms25073988.

Hussein, Suha Majeed Mohammed, and Rasha Mohammed AbdElmageed. "The Relationship Between Type 2 Diabetes Mellitus and Related Thyroid Diseases." *Cureus,* December 25, 2021. https://doi.org/10.7759/cureus.20697.

Knezevic, Jovana, Christina Starchl, Adelina Tmava Berisha, and Karin Amrein. "Thyroid-Gut-Axis: How Does the Microbiota Influence Thyroid Function?" *Nutrients* 12, no. 6 (June 12, 2020): 1769. https://doi.org/10.3390/nu12061769.

Krysiak, Robert, Witold Szkróbka, and Bogusław Okopień. "The Effect of Gluten-Free Diet on Thyroid Autoimmunity in Drug-Naïve Women with Hashimoto's Thyroiditis: A Pilot Study." *Experimental and Clinical Endocrinology and Diabetes* 127, no. 7 (July 2019): 417–422. https://pubmed.ncbi.nlm.nih.gov/30060266/

Lai, Ying-Wen, and Shih-Ming Huang. "Tea Consumption Affects the Absorption of Levothyroxine." *Frontiers in Endocrinology* 13 (September 12, 2022). https://doi.org/10.3389/fendo.2022.943775.

Osowiecka, Karolina, and Joanna Myszkowska-Ryciak. "The Influence of Nutritional Intervention in the Treatment of Hashimoto's Thyroiditis—A Systematic Review." *Nutrients* 15, no. 4 (February 20, 2023): 1041. https://doi.org/10.3390/nu15041041.

Romano, Renata Marino, Jeane Maria De Oliveira, Viviane Matoso De Oliveira, Isabela Medeiros De Oliveira, Yohandra Reyes Torres, Paula Bargi-Souza, Anderson Joel Martino Andrade, and Marco Aurelio Romano. "Could Glyphosate and Glyphosate-Based Herbicides Be Associated with Increased Thyroid Diseases Worldwide?" *Frontiers in Endocrinology* 12 (March 19, 2021). https://doi.org/10.3389/fendo.2021.627167.

Sachmechi, Issac, Amna Khalid, Saba Iqbal Awan, Zohra R. Malik, and Mohaddeseh Sharifzadeh. "Autoimmune Thyroiditis with Hypothyroidism Induced by Sugar Substitutes." *Cureus,* September 7, 2018. https://doi.org/10.7759/cureus.3268.

Wang Xia, Yingying Ouyang, Jun Liu, Minmin Zhu, Gang Zhao, Wei Bao, Frank B. Hu. "Fruit and Vegetable Consumption and Mortality from All Causes, Cardiovascular Disease, and Cancer: Systematic Review and Dose-Response Meta-analysis of Prospective Cohort Studies." *BMJ* 349, (July 29, 2014): g4490. https://doi.org/10.1136/bmj.g4490.

ACKNOWLEDGMENTS

First and foremost, to James and Noah, for loving me no matter what I eat or how I feel, and for all the taste-testing, grocery runs, dish-doing, and emotional support. Your patience and encouragement carried me through every step of this journey.

To my mom, Barbara Mahar Lincoln, for believing in this dream since I was tall enough to turn on the stove, and for showing me how to lead with the heart. And to my siblings, Kim, Carrie, Michael, and Dan. You inspire me daily with your incredible hearts and gifts. Finally, to my dad, I wish I could have cooked even one meal for you, but I feel you in the kitchen with me every day.

To Jill Alexander, Heather Godin, Megan Buckley, and the Fair Winds team. Thank you for your guidance, vision, and belief in this project.

To Mary Shomon, whose pioneering advocacy has helped so many of us find the answers we need to thrive. I'm lucky to call you friend and mentor.

To Dr. Christine White Deeble, your rare gifts as a healer changed my life. Without you, none of this would've happened.

To Cindy Bryson, your gifts of support, insight, and intuition have helped me grow into and understand my own gifts.

To my Thrivers Club community, for endless inspiration, love, and encouragement. We thrive best when we thrive together.

To everyone who's supported my work, thank you for the likes, comments, reviews, and for buying this book. Even if we've never met, I feel our connection.

To the Alley Chats, for your collective strength and courage, and for never making me feel like an outsider for having dietary restrictions. To Krissy, for decades of laughs, pep talks, and reminding me to chase big dreams even when it's scary. And to all the friends and fellow cooks who added color and flavor to this journey.

To my fellow thyroid advocates, Angela Brown, Alison Marras, Kate Jay, Rachel Hill, Danna Bowman, Annabel Bateman, and too many others to name—thank you for your support and for being on this shared mission.

To Dr. Sandra Scheinbaum and the Functional Medicine Coaching Academy, for validating and elevating my work and teaching me why it matters.

To all the experts whose work contributed to this guide: Dr. Izabella Wentz, Dr. Antonio C. Bianco, Dr. Alan Christianson, Dr. Jeffrey Bland, Dr. Mark Hyman, Dr. Amy Myers, Dr. Eric Balcavage, Dr. Kelly Halderman, Dr. Emily Kiberd, Dr. Becky Campbell, Dr. Jacob Teitelbaum, Dr. Joni Labbe, Kiran Krishnan, Mickey Trescott, Nadia Ahrens, LICSW, Debra Atkinson, Lara Adler, and The Institute for Functional Medicine.

We've come so far as a community in empowering better health, and I'm grateful to those who have lit the way. When we heal ourselves, we help heal the world.

ABOUT THE AUTHOR

GINNY MAHAR, FMCHC, is a Le Cordon Bleu–trained chef, functional medicine certified health coach, and creator of Hypothyroid Chef, a popular online hub for thyroid-friendly recipes and lifestyle support. Diagnosed with hypothyroidism in 2011 (and later, Hashimoto's), Ginny turned her personal health challenges into a mission to empower others with the tools, recipes, and strategies that helped her restore her health and start living fully again.

With more than two decades of experience as a chef, food writer, and cooking instructor, Ginny brings a flavor-first approach to healing that has resonated with thousands of Thyroid Thrivers worldwide. In 2017, she launched THYROID30, a thirty-day whole-life wellness program designed to help people with thyroid conditions create sustainable, nourishing habits. The program has been endorsed by leading experts including Dr. Mark Hyman and Dr. Terry Wahls.

In addition to her functional medicine training, Ginny is certified in culinary medicine through the Harvard CHEF Coaching program, combining her professional culinary expertise with evidence-based nutrition and behavior change science.

She hosts the *Thyroid-Healthy Bites* podcast and the *Hypothyroid Chef Show* on YouTube, where she shares simple, delicious recipes and real-world strategies for thriving with thyroid issues. Ginny also leads the Thrivers Club, a supportive coaching community where members participate in monthly wellness challenges—including her signature THYROID30 reset.

Ginny lives in western Montana with her husband and son, where she enjoys growing her own food, spending time outdoors, and savoring life one thyroid-friendly bite at a time.

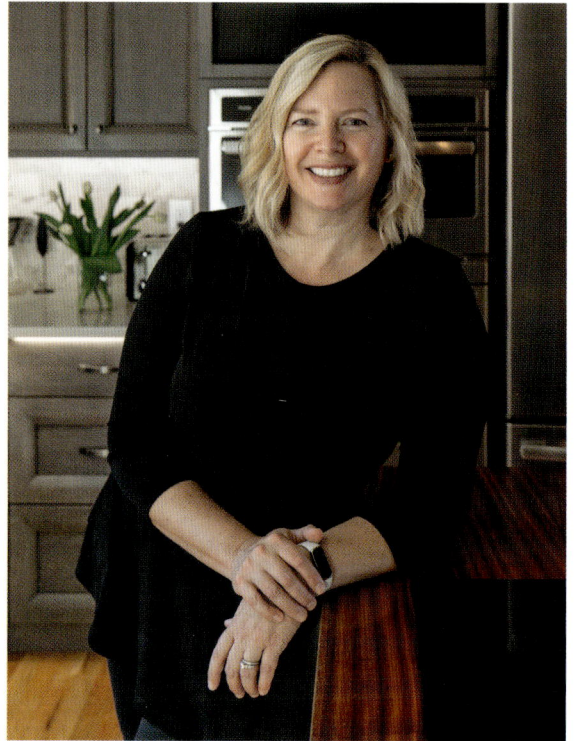

Learn more about Ginny at hypothyroidchef.com.

Scan the QR code or visit hypothyroidchef.com/cookbook for free resources, video demos, and a special invite to the Thrivers Club.

INDEX